STUDY GUIDE
Robert R. Smith

ESSENTIALS *of*
ANATOMY & PHYSIOLOGY

MARTINI
◆
BARTHOLOMEW

PRENTICE HALL Upper Saddle River, NJ 07458

Production Editor: *James Buckley*
Special Projects Manager: *Barbara A. Murray*
Acquisitions Editor: *David Brake*
Supplement Editor: *Laura Edwards*
Production Coordinator: *Benjamin Smith*
Supplement Cover Manager: *Paul Gourhan*

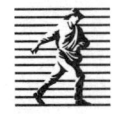

© 1997 by **PRENTICE-HALL, INC.**
Simon & Schuster/A Viacom Company
Upper Saddle River, NJ 07458

All rights reserved. No part of this book may be
reproduced, in any form or by any means,
without permission in writing from the publisher.

Printed in the United States of America

10 9 8 7 6 5 4 3 2 1

ISBN 0-13-359936-1

Prentice-Hall International (UK) Limited, *London*
Prentice-Hall of Australia Pty. Limited, *Sydney*
Prentice-Hall Canada, Inc., *Toronto*
Prentice-Hall Hispanoamericana, S.A., *Mexico*
Prentice-Hall of India Private Limited, *New Delhi*
Prentice-Hall of Japan, Inc., *Tokyo*
Simon & Schuster Asia Pte. Ltd., *Singapore*
Editora Prentice-Hall do Brasil, Ltda., *Rio de Janeiro*

Contents

	Preface	v
	Introduction	vii
1	An Introduction to Anatomy and Physiology	1
2	The Chemical Level of Organization	17
3	Cellular Structure and Function	32
4	The Tissue Level of Organization	46
5	The Integumentary System	62
6	The Skeletal Structure	74
7	The Muscular System	100
8	Neural Tissue and the Central Nervous System	124
9	The Peripheral Nervous System and Integrated Functions	146
10	Sensory Function	162

11	The Endocrine System	**176**
12	Blood	**190**
13	The Heart	**203**
14	Blood Vessels and Circulation	**213**
15	The Lymphatic System and Immunity	**229**
16	The Respiratory System	**242**
17	The Digestive System	**256**
18	Nutrition and Metabolism	**269**
19	The Urinary System	**279**
20	The Reproductive System	**295**
21	Development and Inheritance	**310**
	Answer Key	**323**

Preface

It is my expressed hope that students using the *Study Guide* in conjunction with *Essentials of Anatomy and Physiology*, by Frederic Martini and Edwin Bartholomew, will find it an invaluable reinforcement of difficult concepts presented during the duration of their course.

The sequence of topics within the Study Guide parallels that of the text and also incorporates the Three-Level Learning System that students encounter in the text's end of chapter material. This system will be familiar to those of you conversant with Bloom's Taxonomy. It provides a means for students to accurately gauge their level of comprehension of topics. The Level 1 questions are keyed directly to chapter objectives and offer a review of facts and terms. The Level 2 exercises encourage students to synthesize concepts, and Level 3 questions promote critical thinking. Each level contains appropriate question types including matching, multiple choice, completion, essay, labeling and concept mapping.

In addition, an introductory chapter has been been included that provides important tips on helping students study. This chapter, I hope, will provide students with guidelines for absorbing information on the various topics within the broader field of Anatomy and Physiology.

I would like to acknowledge the students and colleagues who have had an impact on this work. Particular thanks go to my editors, David Brake and Laura Edwards. Finally and most importantly, I thank my my wife, Peggy, for her continuing support of a very time intensive project.

Of course, any errors or omissions found by the reader are attributable to the author, rather than to the reviewers. Readers with comments, suggestions, relevant reprints, or corrections should contact me at the address below.

R. R. Smith
c/o Prentice Hall
1208 E. Broadway
Suite 200
Tempe, AZ 85282

Format and Features

The Three Level Review System utilized in the *Essentials of Anatomy and Physiology* text and all of its supplements affords each student a logical framework for the progressive development of skill as he or she advances through material of increasing levels of complexity. The three-tiered organization is designed to help students (1) learn basic facts, ideas, and principles; (2) increase their capacity for abstraction and concept integration; and (3) think critically in applying what they have learned to specific situations.

Level 1, a review of Chapter Objectives, consists of exercises that test the student's mastery of vocabulary and recall of information through objective-based multiple choice, completion, matching, and illustration labeling questions.

Level 2 focuses on Concept Synthesis, a process that actively involves the student in combining, integrating, and relating the basic facts and concepts mastered in Level 1. In addition to multiple choice, completion, and short answer/essay questions, this level incorporates a feature that is unique to this study guide: the development and completion of concept maps. The examples provided give students a framework of information that encourages them to complete the map. Once completed, these maps help the user to understand relationships between ideas and to differentiate related concepts. In addition, they have been designed to serve as models that will encourage students to develop new maps of their own.

Another feature of Level 2 is the use of Body Treks with Robo, the micro-robot. The organ systems of the human body are examined by combining fantasy with actual techniques that are currently being used experimentally to study anatomical features and monitor physiological activity. The treks are written to demonstrate the interrelationship of concepts in a unique and dynamic way.

Level 3 activities promote Critical Thinking and Application skills through the use of life experiences, plausible clinical situations, and common diagnostic problems. These techniques draw on the students' analytical and organizational powers, enabling them to develop associations and relationships that ultimately may benefit their decision-making ability in clinical situations and everyday life experiences.

An answer key for each section has been provided at the end of the study guide.

INTRODUCTION

Learning to Apply Yourself: How to Study Anatomy & Physiology

STUDY HINTS

by Jeffrey L. Smith
Delgado Community College

Studying any subject, especially one as complex as human anatomy and physiology, is not a hit-or-miss proposition. There are systematic habits and skills that can be developed to increase the efficiency of the studying process. Some of these are the following:

- Make sure that you choose a suitable place for study. A comfortable desk or chair with good, over-the-shoulder lighting is ideal. A flat surface is useful to have—a desk or table top of comfortable height will do nicely. There should not be a lot of distractions in your study area. Loud talking, televisions, and blaring radios distract from the learning process.
- Establish a regular schedule of study. You should set aside 30 to 60 minutes each day for study. This is far better than trying to study for three hours at a stretch on one or two days of the week.
- Start each study session by quickly reviewing the previously covered material. The key to mastery is repetition. A quick review within 24 hours of having studied new material will greatly reinforce what was learned. A very easy way to do this is to read through the study outline that is provided at the end of each chapter of your textbook.
- Develop a systematic approach to studying. Science is a systematic way of looking at the world, and your approach to learning science should also be systematic. The approach detailed below is one that has proven very useful to a large number of students. References to specific features of *Essentials of Anatomy and Physiology* have been included to help you get the most out of your text.

If you are studying this material as part of a formal college course, then you will in all probability be attending formal lectures. Always read the chapter once before attending lecture. You will find that the lecture is much more meaningful to you if you have already read the material at least once. Here are some guidelines to follow when studying each chapter:

1. Begin each chapter by reading the chapter objectives. These will tell you what the author considers to be the most important points.
2. Read the chapter in the textbook.
   - As you read, pay particular attention to the terminology. One of the things that makes anatomy and physiology difficult for the new student is the extensive vocabulary. You will be introduced to more new terms in this course than are found in the typical foreign language course. They must be mastered, and you should begin immediately.
   - Pay attention to the illustrations and tables. A large amount of information is contained in these, and to bypass them eliminates about fifty percent of the information in the textbook.
   - When you come to the Concept Check Questions at key locations in each chapter, take a few minutes to answer the questions. They are designed to serve as intellectual "speed bumps"—they will tell you whether you have been reading too fast or not paying enough attention to what you have been reading. Some test chiefly memory, others require a bit of thought, but if you have been concentrating on what you have read you should be able to answer all of them quickly and easily. If you find that you are stumped, you probably need to reread the preceding material. (You can check your answers in Appendix I of the text.)
   - Where recall of material covered in previous chapters is important for understanding new material, cross references have been provided. Blue "chain links" icons are used to call attention to these references, and to remind you that very few things about the human body can be studied in isolation. Whenever you see the links icon, stop for a moment to make sure you remember the material that is referred to. If not, go back and refresh your memory.
   - Topics in the *Applications Manual* are referenced in the text at the point where the material is most relevant. The title of the discussion follows the AM button logo. Your instructor may assign some of these, and you may wish to read others to shed additional light on the text material, or because you are interested in the topic.
3. After you have completed reading the text, be sure to read the Summary Outline at the chapter's end. This Summary Outline is a summary of the major topics and vocabulary included in the chapter. It constitutes an excellent review, and is one of the most useful features of your notebook.
4. Answer the end-of-chapter questions carefully. The Level 1 questions test your recall of specific pieces of information. The Level 2 questions call for more extended answers; they require an understanding of concepts and the ability to synthesize ideas. Level 3 questions help you to develop your critical thinking skills and allow you to apply your knowledge to actual clinical situations.

This *Study Guide* contains many additional questions and exercises to help you master the material of this course. The most important idea to remember is: "Do not become discouraged." To the beginning student the mysterious polysyllabic terms encountered in human anatomy and physiology can be intimidating. Keep in mind that with a systematic approach to study and sufficient time, anyone can master the subject. The secret is to stay with it. As you proceed through the subject you will find that mastery of previous material makes the new material much easier, and eventually you will develop a "critical mass" of information that will permit you to move forward with confidence. The rewards of success are worth the time and energy. Besides all the practical application, there is a great deal of satisfaction in understanding how your body is constructed and how it functions.

The sections that follow provide more detailed discussions of techniques you may find useful for reading your text, taking notes in lecture, and studying.

Reading a Textbook

How do you read a textbook? Simple. You sit at a desk or in a comfortable chair and read it, right? Probably not. Do you do any of the following things when reading a textbook?

1. Hope for many large pictures and graphs because they take up space that could be used for words?
2. Continually flip several pages ahead to see how close you are to the end of the chapter?
3. Stare at a page for several minutes before discovering that your mind was somewhere else?
4. Look back at the previous page and discover that you read it but don't remember any of it?

These are pretty good indicators of someone whose mind is drifting elsewhere. Authors write novels expecting you to read them in comfortable chairs. They're filled with drama, romance, suspense, and intrigue that keeps you turning pages to find out what happens next. If a novel doesn't hold your attention, you simply stop reading it. Textbooks have facts and concepts. Because a course textbook is rarely an exciting page turner, you must develop techniques to keep your attention centered on your task.

Most students prefer not to read a chapter before the professor covers the material in class. To be honest, it is probably easier to read the chapter after having heard about it first in lecture. However, it is much more efficient to listen to the lecture having already covered the material in the book. If you get bogged down in the reading, you can always go back, slow down, or take a break. If you get lost in lecture, there is no going back. Always read the chapter before the professor lectures about it. You are eventually going to read it several times; why not read it once a few days earlier? It will make your lecture material much easier to understand.

The SQ3R Study Formula

The five-step **SQ3R** formula (**S**urvey, **Q**uestion, **R**ead, **R**ecite, **R**eview) may, at first, appear too time consuming. Try it, keeping in mind that you'll be using your study time much more efficiently. You won't have to reread the chapter as many times, and you will save time in the future.

Here are the five steps to SQ3R:

Survey

This consists of previewing the material before you begin to study it. In the first few minutes before beginning to read the chapter, do the following steps:

1. Read the title of the chapter.
2. Read the chapter outline (usually at the end of the chapter) if one is present.
3. Read the introduction or first few paragraphs at the beginning of the chapter. This gives you a general overview of what the chapter is about.
4. Thumb through the entire chapter, page by page:
   - Read the headings of sections. Some of these should be familiar. Don't worry if some headings seem foreign to you.
   - Read the first sentence of each paragraph.
   - Glance over the pictures, tables, and diagrams. Again, if they don't make sense now, don't worry about it.
   - Read the summary or concluding paragraph at the end of the chapter.

That's it. In about 10 minutes, you have become much more familiar with the chapter. Just as if you'd seen a preview of a movie or a television show, you now know something about the chapter. You have some idea of how long the chapter is, how easy or difficult it might be, and how you might want to break it up into smaller pieces. You can double your comprehension later by first getting a vague familiarity with the information to be studied.

Question

It is much easier to study material if you are doing it with the intention of answering questions. If you have an idea of what questions you are trying to answer, the material in the chapter will have more meaning. Read over the Chapter Objectives, the Concept Check Questions, and the study questions at the back of the chapter. If you have some idea of what to be looking for, the important points will be more likely to stand out when you reach them during your reading.

Read

It is easier to master material that is in smaller pieces. Twenty years ago, many textbooks consisted of 20 chapters over 80 pages each. Today, most textbooks have more chapters with fewer pages each. If the material you have reviewed in steps 1 and 2 (Survey and Questions) appeared difficult, break up the chapter further into even smaller pieces before you start reading. For example, if it is a difficult or unfamiliar 20-page chapter, try to break it into four or five smaller subsections of four to five pages each.

Read the chapter or section with the idea of finding the answers to those questions and objectives you saw earlier. You will get much more out of your reading now that you have an idea of what you are looking for.

Don't simply *read* the chapter or section. You *must* use strategies for keeping your attention focused on the material. This is particularly important if you aren't feeling alert. Specifically, try one or more of the following:

- *Outline the material.* Any time you write about something (versus simply reading it), you are much more likely to retain it. This takes longer than underlining, but is much more effective. To outline, you must actively think about what you are reading.
- *Make flash cards.* This doesn't take as much time as outlining, and it forces you to think about potential questions.
- *Write answers to the Chapter Objective or Study Questions.* Try to use your own wording. Why not just run through the answers in your head? (1) You may not realize that you can't answer the question until you try, and (2) you are much more likely to remember something that you have written.

Should you underline or highlight important sentences or phrases? This requires the least effort and is probably better than just reading alone. However, students who highlight their books often make the following errors:

- Highlighting unimportant material. Many students have little idea of what to highlight.
- Highlighting familiar material while skipping unfamiliar material. There is a tendency to assume something that you already know must be more important. However, focusing on the familiar material means you aren't learning anything new.
- Highlighting with the idea of "I will study this later." Reading the chapter again later leads to more highlighting until most of the pages are yellow, pink, and blue. This makes the chapter even harder to read, and has wasted much time.

Do not try to answer questions by simply thumbing through the book's index and searching for answers. At best, this will result in piecemeal memorization of words and phrases without understanding their meaning or significance. Taking this unfortunate shortcut is very common because it gives students the mistaken impression that they are making progress in learning the material.

Once you have completed a section, don't immediately go on to the next section. Give the material a few minutes to settle in. The idea here is to master smaller pieces of the textbook without skipping over challenging material.

Recite

Although this literally means audibly saying the answers to questions (quietly to yourself or to another person), you might get the same benefit by writing the answers down on paper. Go through the learning objectives and try to answer the questions. Review your flash cards and try to recite answers to them aloud or on paper. Don't simply think of the answer; say it or write it. Studies have shown that retention of material is much greater if you say or write the answers to questions rather than simply reading them. If you can't say it or write it, you probably don't know it. Many students claim that they "go blank" on exams. It is likely that they would have "gone blank" during this step as well. It would be a very good idea to answer the Chapter Objectives in writing during reciting. There is a Latin proverb that applies here: "qui scribit bis legit," or "he who writes reads twice." For centuries, scholars have recognized that writing out something is very effective when trying to learn a subject thoroughly.

Review

The brain is very proficient at forgetting one-time events. You are most likely to retain information in long-term memory if you refresh your memory at regular intervals. Take several minutes for a break, and then review what you have just covered. Read what you underlined, review your outlines, or quiz yourself with the flash cards. You often get brief breaks between other activities (work, school, home, or on the bus). Use this time to review the study questions or learning objectives and the answers you have written for them.

Mastering any new learning technique takes time, practice, and refinement, but is worth the effort in the future. Don't give up on the SQ3R formula without really trying it in earnest for a few weeks. On the first few tries, you will be thinking about both the technique and the material in the book. Once you get accustomed to the technique, you will be able to devote all of your attention to the reading.

The secret to successful learning is keeping your mind actively involved in the material while avoiding distractions. It is difficult to keep your mind from wandering when reading a textbook. SQ3R gives you a specific purpose for your studying. It may seem like a lot of effort, but the time you invest in studying will be much more efficient. Thus, in the future you will have more time for other activities, and you will be less frustrated.

The SOAR Study Formula

Like SQ3R, the **SOAR** formula (**S**urvey, **O**rganize, **A**nticipate, **R**ecite, **R**eview) is a logical stepwise method for studying textbooks. Remember: reading is not studying. It is possible to sit and read something and not retain any of it. The SQ3R and SOAR formulas are techniques for studying a textbook, and should help anyone retain more of what they are studying. SOAR may be even better than SQ3R for students of Anatomy and Physiology. The following is a summary of the four steps of SOAR.

Survey

Like SQ3R, SOAR begins with a general survey of the chapter. The survey steps are the same:

1. Read the title of the chapter.
2. Read the chapter outline.
3. Read the introduction or first few paragraphs at the beginning of the chapter.
4. Thumb through the entire chapter, page by page.
   - Read the headings of sections.
   - Read the first sentence of each paragraph.
   - Glance over the pictures, tables, and diagrams.
   - Read the summary at the end of the chapter.

Organize

Well-organized information is much easier to remember. There are several different ways to organized the information in the chapter as you read it. You should try each until you find a particular method that works best for you.

1. Read the chapter and outline it or make concept maps of the information. When possible, avoid making long lists: always try to limit lists to about five subjects by subdividing into categories.
2. Read the chapter and take notes, either in a spiral-bound notebook or on note cards.

Again, underlining and highlighting "important" material may seem more effective than it really is. Unless you are certain that this method works well for you, don't use highlighters.

Anticipate

The word anticipate here refers to successfully predicting what an instructor might ask on an exam. In effect, you place yourself in the role of a teacher. If your instructor provides learning objectives, this step is simple; he or she will ask questions that test your understanding of those objectives. Students who consistently make high grades on exams can often look at paragraphs in a text and say, "That looks like something my instructor would ask." Students who cannot imagine what an instructor would ask must resort to trying learn everything. Soon, they get frustrated and quit. The student who can spot major ideas and differentiate them from examples (supporting information) has much less material to remember. The chapter objectives should help you with the task of anticipating questions.

Merely anticipating the questions is half the task. You must prove to yourself that you can correctly answer the questions. Making flash cards on 3"x5" or 5"x8" index cards is an excellent technique for review or study of unfamiliar terminology. Do not simply use other people's cards; you don't learn how to anticipate questions on your own. If you are having trouble, talk to your instructor.

Recite and Review

Instead of Recite and Review, many students make the mistake of trying to Read and Reread as their study strategy. It is probably a better idea to go through the chapter with the idea that it will be the last time you look at the material. If you have correctly followed the previous steps, you should have some written materials such as notes, outlines, or flash cards that you can study. You cannot learn effectively by simply reading alone.

- **Recite.** To recite literally refers to saying what you have learned aloud. As silly as this sounds, if you recite what you have learned aloud, you are much more likely to remember it later. You can either say it to yourself, to a study partner, or anyone who is willing to listen. The important thing is that you can repeat the information, quietly, aloud, or on paper, without reading it.
- **Review.** The more you review something (that is, the more times you must think about it), the more likely it will stay in your memory. Your brain is particularly adept at forgetting even interesting information if you don't reinforce that information through repetition. To move information from short-term memory to long-term memory, you need to refresh the circuits in your brain by reviewing previously studied material at reasonable intervals. Look over what you have highlighted or underlined, read your chapter outlines, review your flash cards and set aside those that you have really mastered. Always give yourself enough lead time to allow for review of material at a comfortable pace. Study ahead of time, some every day, and you should be able to spend the evening before an exam reciting and reviewing only.

An outstanding form of review is to place yourself in the role of teacher. The reason is well expressed by the Latin saying, "qui docet discit"—"he who teaches, learns." If you have a study partner in the class, review the material on a regular basis, and place yourselves in the role of teacher rather than student. Make a commitment to know it well enough to explain it to someone who doesn't know it. If you can do this, you will have no difficulty on an exam. Too many students try only to learn it well enough to fake it on a multiple-choice test.

The two methods for reading a textbook just described should help you focus your attention on the material and should make the time you spend reading much more efficient. Try the method that seems to fit your learning style and personality the best, and feel free to alter some steps as you see fit.

Effective Note-Taking

Lecture notes are frequently your best source of information when studying for exams. When an instructor covers material in lecture, you should assume that it must be more important than material that he or she omitted. Nevertheless, effective note-taking is a neglected skill. Each semester, many dejected students go to their instructor's office for help. Although they often claim to have taken usually voluminous lecture notes, those notes often amount to pages of disjointed words and diagrams copied verbatim from the chalkboard. Many professors refuse to use the chalkboard at all; students who daydream in those classes often have no lecture notes at all. Taking poor notes may be a worse curse than having no textbook.

Why is effective note-taking such a neglected learning strategy? There are several reasons:

- *Poor Listening Skills.* People tend to listen (not just hear, but really devote their attention) to someone speaking for periods of about thirty seconds, followed by variable periods of inattention. Many students become alert only when the professor writes something on the chalkboard. After they mindlessly copy the few words into their notebooks, their attention wanders off until the professor uses the chalkboard again.
- *Selective Note-Taking.* There is a tendency to write down what you want to hear or expect to hear; for example, material that you already knew before taking the class. This may also pose a problem when these students underline or highlight their books, because they underline or highlight the material they already know and ignore unfamiliar material, when it would make more sense to write down only the unfamiliar material.
- *Laziness.* If writing complete lecture notes seems like too much effort, then maybe you aren't setting high enough goals for yourself. When you are actively taking good lecture notes, a 50-minute class period seems like 20 minutes. When you are daydreaming and staring at the clock, it seems like hours.

How can you improve your note-taking skills? That depends on your current note-taking skills. If you are a slow writer, you should go straight to a department store and buy a portable tape recorder now. You may not need it later, but it is always better to have a taped lecture as insurance if you get bogged down or lost in lecture.

Even with the lecture taped, you need to develop effective note-taking skills. Keep the following in mind:

- You *cannot* listen to every word that your instructor says. If you attempt to write down every word, you will succeed only in writing down the first five words of several hundred sentences.
- You *cannot* listen to your instructor and paraphrase the lecture into complete sentences. To do so, you would have to hear the complete sentence, think about it, paraphrase it, and then begin to write it. While doing that, you are missing the next two sentences.

To take effective notes, you are going to have to come to class prepared. This means familiarizing yourself with the lecture topic before your professor covers it in lecture. For some inexplicable reason, many students obstinately resist this suggestion. However, the same students invariably read the chapter a day or two after the professor covers that material in class. Thus, they are spending the same amount of time reading the chapter. They are simply doing it one or two days too late to be most effective.

Although no two people take notes the same way, the following suggestions might improve your note-taking skills:

1. Use large notebooks (8½"x11" instead of smaller, stenographer-type notebooks).
2. Leave a generous left-hand margin to allow insertion of material, pictures, and diagrams. Use lined paper with a 3" left margin. If you cannot find this at an office supply store, try to find lined paper with no margin, and remember to leave yourself about 3" at the left.
3. Use a ballpoint or rollerball pen. If you make a mistake, just draw line through it; you may discover later that you needed that information after all. Erasing takes time, and is irreversible.
4. Learn to outline. You cannot possibly write down everything your professor says, and it takes time to think and paraphrase the lecture. The only way to take complete notes is to write brief phrases and try to organize them logically. An outline is ideal for this.
5. Make important material stand out. Place an asterisk (*) next to important material, or underline it, or circle it. If you don't understand something during the lecture, make a note of it. It may help to write **l.i.u.** (=**l**ook **i**t **u**p) in the left-hand margin when something is unclear during lecture.
6. Don't write in longhand. Although you may be accustomed to writing in attractive longhand, it takes much longer to make curved lines, particularly on capitalized letters. Write just as fast as you can while still leaving something that is readable to you. Forget penmanship. Your finished product may be half writing and half printing, but as long as it is legible, that's fine.
7. Develop your own shorthand and abbreviations. There are many words and figures of speech that are common to many college courses. Whenever you can, use abbreviations for these phrases or words. (Think how much time you will save, for example, by just writing "hom" or "h," instead of "homeostasis" each time the term comes up in lecture.)
8. Write as fast as necessary to ensure understandable notes. Write as much as you can during the period. Don't simply write what the professor puts on the chalkboard. It is easy to eliminate less important material later. When you are taking notes, you don't know what is going to be important and what isn't. Write down everything you can while you have the chance.
9. Rewrite your notes soon after class. No kidding! Rewriting your notes takes little effort, and it is a wonderful form of mental reinforcement. Even if you are extremely conscientious in taking notes, there are going to be some points (typically examples of concepts) that you didn't have time to write during class. It is an excellent practice to spend some time rewriting your notes, preferably soon after the class. This will allow you to arrange the information logically, write more legibly, and add points that you remember from the lecture but didn't have time to write. Students who tape the lectures have the added advantage of being able to rewrite their notes while listening to the lecture a second time. This may seem like too much trouble, but it is very effective. Rewriting notes doesn't take much time, the completed product is easier to study, and you can do it even if you are tired.

Is all this really worth it? There are estimates that, for each day you spend in completing a college degree, you will earn an additional $1,000 during your lifetime. If you don't complete the degree, you can throw that all away; a partial college degree is worth the same as no degree.

Many "A" students are following the suggestions above, and don't seem a bit overtaxed by the process. You are competing with them for slots in nursing school, graduate school, and the job market. If they are doing so much work, then why are *you* the one who is always feeling stressed out? Working efficiently is not stressful. Wasting your time with study habits that don't work is extremely stressful. None of the time you are putting in is working, and your poor grades make it appear that you aren't doing anything.

There is a Latin phrase, "quae nocent docent," which means "things that hurt teach!" One good thing about mistakes is that we can *learn* from them. If your current study habits are not working, change them!

Cramming

Cramming is the term used to describe a long period of intensive studying just before an exam. Some books on "Making It in College" applaud the practice as the best way to get high grades with the least effort. They may be right, and if high grades with least work are all you are after, it might be right for you. Who would benefit from cramming?

- Students who are taking classes whose content is irrelevant to their future endeavors
- Students whose grade-point averages are so low that they must take "fluff" courses to raise it

Unfortunately, this doesn't describe most students who cram. Instead those who cram are usually:

- Students who procrastinate
- Students with little ability to manage time
- Students with little motivation or direction in their college studies
- Students who fear that they won't be able to remember information longer than one day
- Students who like to feel that they are "beating the system."

A few college study manuals advocate cramming with the following warning: Cramming is most useful if you are not learning new information during the cram session. But reviewing familiar material the night before an exam is not what most people call "cramming." People generally think of cramming as studying the bulk of the material for the first time the day, evening, or morning before an exam. As such, it is only useful as a last ditch effort to salvage an exam grade without resorting to cheating. You may get the grade you wanted, but you are unlikely to retain much of the material for long. In short, it is better than not studying at all. The fact that you must resort to it should alert you to your lack of effective time management.

The best way to study the night before an exam is to be so well prepared that you don't have to do anything but quiz yourself and organize your thoughts. The priority you should have the night before the exam is getting 7 to 8 hours sleep. The only organ in your body that benefits from regular sleep is your brain. Staying up all night before an exam deprives your cerebrum of needed rest; it is the only organ that is going to get you through the exam successfully. Don't compromise your brain by overtaxing it the 24 hours prior to an exam.

Learning the Language of Anatomy and Physiology

by Martha Newsome
Tomball College

Medical books bristle with difficult-looking terminology such as rhinorrhagia and osteomyelitis. Why are the words so difficult to understand? Is a doctor who writes "rhinorrhagia" on the chart just trying to be more impressive than one who records "a bloody nose?"

Not at all. Medical personnel learn and use a special language, not to make communication harder but to make it easier. The terms of this language offer two great advantages over words in common usage:

- *Precision*: Unlike many everyday words, the technical terms used by doctors, nurses, and researchers have very exact and specific meanings.
- *Universality*: A technical term will mean the same thing to a doctor in Lima as it does to one in Beijing.

Medical technicians, doctors, and nurses record and discuss patient information utilizing such terminology. The statement, "The patient broke his arm," is much too general for medical records. There are three large bones (and numerous smaller ones) in the upper and lower limb; the identity of the precise bone involved is obviously important both to the patient and to all those entrusted with his or her care.

Although a technical vocabulary is essential to facilitate diagnosis and treatment, learning all these terms isn't easy. The length and unfamiliarity of the words are likely to be barriers for the beginning student. Your anatomy and physiology text introduces dozens of new terms in the first chapter alone. Regional terms such as cephalic, brachial, gluteal, popliteal and others may seem impossible to learn.

What, then, is the best approach to such a daunting task?

1. **Relax! Realize that not all information will be retained the first time you are exposed to it.**

    Learning comes with time, experience, and repetition. If you are on a career pathway in the allied health professions, subsequent courses will reinforce the terminology introduced in this text. Every student who has gone on to become a successful nurse, doctor, technician, or therapist has overcome this challenge. Commitment is the key!

2. **Divide and Conquer!**

    Morphemes are the smallest parts of words that still have meaning. A study of morphemes in medical terminology is very useful to the anatomy and physiology student. For instance, an analysis of the word automobile will uncover two roots, auto and mobile. Determining the meaning of each of the roots is a great help in understanding the complete term. Auto is from a Greek word for "self" and mobile from a Latin word for "moving." The combined word is defined as a vehicle that moves by some sort of self-propulsion. When a term with one or more familiar roots is encountered in later reading, you can recall the meaning of the roots to deduce the definition of the term. This technique of relating one word to another is called word "association." As an example, try determining the meaning of the word autobiography in this way. (*Bio* means "life" and *graphy* is defined as "writing or record.")

    This type of exercise is of considerable benefit to the student learning the "foreign language" of anatomy and physiology. Try a medical term like *osteomyelitis* with the same approach. First, if possible, divide the term in question into separate parts to discern the meaning of each component. For example, osteomyelitis could be dissected into the following:

osteo-
-myel-
-itis

When noting these component parts of the word, try word association to help deduce the definition:
- You may be familiar with such terms as osteoporosis or osteoarthritis, common disorders affecting the bones. Indeed, the word root *osteo* means "bone."
- The term *myel* is derived from *myelon*, meaning bone marrow. This is a less familiar term. You will probably need to focus your studies on word arts such as these that are not as easy to recognize.
- Most people recognize appendicitis as an inflammation or infection of the appendix. Many names of diseases contain the suffix *itis* connected to the term for the organ or tissue that is inflamed or infected. The term *itis*, therefore, means "inflammation or infection of."

The definition of *osteomyelitis* is thus "an inflammation of the bone and bone marrow."

Most of the word roots used in medicine are derived from Greek or Latin. Many of them occur again and again in various forms and combinations. When you master the most common ones, difficult words become easier to understand. A medical dictionary is a very helpful reference book for finding the meanings of word roots. Some of the more common prefixes, suffixes, and combining forms derived from foreign word roots are given in Table A-1.

A more complete list of word roots, prefixes, suffixes, and combining forms can be found on the end papers of the main text, *Essentials of Anatomy & Physiology*.

3. **Repetition and association are the keys to learning word roots, and thereafter medical terminology.**
   - Make a flash card for each unfamiliar term and its definition. Study these cards during a wait at the bank or the dentist's office.
   - Create a visual association by drawing a picture next to the written word root. For example, a picture of a simple cell could be drawn next to the term *cyto-*.
   - Associate a word with another memorable word or phrase. Often a silly one is best: For example, you may tell yourself that you'll break your arm if you forget the term *brachial*. You'll be surprised how well this can work. And once the term brachial is learned, you'll also know the location of such anatomical entities as the brachial artery and vein, the brachialis muscle, and the brachial nerve plexus.
   - Categorize terms to facilitate learning. Terms describing color, for example, such as *erythros* (red), *leuko* or *alba* (white), *cyan* (blue), and *melan* (black), can be associated together.
   - Practice spelling terms to reinforce your visualization of the roots and combining forms they contain.
   - Use the text or a medical dictionary to determine the proper pronunciation of words and practice vocalizing them. Words such as pharynx, carotid, and many others are frequently mispronounced.
   - Some students will not ask questions in class for fear of mispronouncing a term. Overcome this anxiety and use the terminology as often as possible in the classroom. It is better to make the mistake in the classroom than in the clinic.
   - Read the clinical discussions in this manual to develop a greater awareness of the role of word roots in the naming of various diseases.

TABLE A-1 AN INTRODUCTION TO WORD CONSTRUCTION

Word Root	Definition	Example	Example Definition
a-	without	anucleate	without a nucleus
bi-	two	bilateral	involving both sides of the body
-cyte	cell	osteocyte	bone cell
epi-	on	epicardium	layer of connective tissue on the heart
ex-	out; away from	exocytosis	movement out of the cell
hem-	blood	hemorrhage	bleeding
hyper-	above; excessive	hypertrophy	increase in the size of cell, such as muscle cell
hypo-	below; under	hypothyroidism	underproduction of thyroid hormone
gen-/genesis	producing; forming	osteogenesis	bone formation
intra-	within	intracellular	inside of the cell
inter-	between	intermolecular	between molecules
-lysis	breakdown	hemolysis	destruction or rupture of the red blood cell
macro-	large	macrocyte	cell that is larger than normal
micro-	small	microscopic	pertains to something so small it must be viewed with a microscope
peri-	around	periodontal disease	disorder of the gums surrounding the teeth
sub-	under; below	sublingual gland	salivary gland that opens under the tongue
trans-	across; through	transport	movement across or through

CHAPTER 1

An Introduction to Anatomy and Physiology

■ Overview

Are you interested in knowing something about your body? Have you ever wondered what makes your heart beat or why and how muscles contract to produce movement? If you are curious to understand the what, why, and how of the human body, then the study of anatomy and physiology is essential for you. The term anatomy is derived from a Greek word which means to cut up, or anatomize (dissect) representative animals or human cadavers which serve as the basis for understanding the structure of the human body. Physiology is the science that attempts to explain the physical and chemical processes occurring in the body. Anatomy and Physiology provide the foundation for personal health and clinical applications.

Chapter 1 is an introduction to anatomy and physiology citing some of the basic functions of living organisms, defining various specialties of anatomy and physiology, identifying levels of organization in living things, explaining homeostasis and regulation, and introducing some basic anatomical terminology. The information in this chapter will provide the framework for a better understanding of anatomy and physiology, and includes basic concepts and principles necessary to get you started on a successful and worthwhile trek through the human body.

☐ LEVEL 1   REVIEW OF CHAPTER OBJECTIVES

1. Describe the basic functions of living organisms.
2. Define anatomy and physiology and describe the various specialties of each discipline.
3. Identify the major levels of organization in living organisms from the simplest to the most complex.
4. Identify the organ systems of the human body, their functions, and the major components of each system.
5. Explain the significance of homeostasis.
6. Describe how positive and negative feedack are involved in homeostatic regulation.
7. Use anatomical terms to describe body sections, body regions, and relative positions.
8. Identify the major body cavities and their subdivisions.

Chapter 1 An Introduction to Anatomy and Physiology

[L1] Multiple Choice:

Place the letter corresponding to the correct answer in the space provided.

OBJ. 1 ____ 1. Creating subsequent generations of similar organisms describes the basic function of:

    a. development
    b. reproduction
    c. assimilation
    d. growth

OBJ. 1 ____ 2. All of the basic functions in living things necessitate a common need for:

    a. excretion
    b. circulation
    c. energy
    d. growth

OBJ. 1 ____ 3. All of the following selections include functions in living organisms except:

    a. oxygen, carbon dioxide
    b. growth, reproduction
    c. response, adaptability
    d. absorption, movement

OBJ. 2 ____ 4. Anatomy is the study of ___ and physiology is the study of ___.

    a. function, structure
    b. animals, plants
    c. cells, microorganisms
    d. structure, function

OBJ. 2 ____ 5. Systemic anatomy considers the structure of major ___, while surface anatomy refers to the study of ___.

    a. anatomical landmarks, organ systems
    b. organ systems, superficial markings
    c. superficial markings, macroscopic anatomy
    d. external features, anatomical landmarks

OBJ. 2 ____ 6. The specialized study which analyzes the structure of individual cells is:

    a. histology
    b. microbiology
    c. cytology
    d. pathology

OBJ. 3 ____ 7. The smallest living units in the body are the:

    a. elements
    b. sub-atomic particles
    c. cells
    d. molecules

Level -1-

[OBJ. 3] ___ 8. The level of organization that reflects the interactions between organ systems is the:

    a. cellular level
    b. tissue level
    c. molecular level
    d. organism

[OBJ. 4] ___ 9. The two regulatory systems in the human body include:

    a. nervous and endocrine
    b. digestive and reproductive
    c. muscular and skeletal
    d. cardiovascular and lymphatic

[OBJ. 5] ___ 10. Homeostasis refers to:

    a. body parts in proper relative size and form
    b. treating diseases with small doses of drugs
    c. interbreeding in groups of the same species
    d. stabilizing internal conditions in physiological systems

[OBJ. 6] ___ 11. When a variation outside of normal limits triggers an automatic response that corrects the situation, the mechanism is called:

    a. positive feedback
    b. crisis management
    c. negative feedback
    d. homeostasis

[OBJ. 6] ___ 12. When the initial stimulus produces a response that exaggerates the stimulus, the mechanism is called:

    a. autoregulation
    b. negative feedback
    c. extrinsic regulation
    d. positive feedback

[OBJ. 7] ___ 13. When a person is lying down face up in the anatomical position, the individual is said to be:

    a. prone
    b. rostral
    c. supine
    d. proximal

[OBJ. 7] ___ 14. Moving from the wrist toward the elbow is an example of moving in a _____ direction.

    a. proximal
    b. distal
    c. medial
    d. lateral

4 Chapter 1 An Introduction to Anatomy and Physiology

OBJ. 7 ___ 15. RLQ is an abbreviation as a reference to designate a specific:
   a. section of the vertebral column
   b. area of athe cranial vault
   c. region of the pelvic girdle
   d. abdominopelvic quadrant

OBJ. 7 ___ 16. A sagittal section results in the separation of:
   a. anterior and posterior portions of the body
   b. superior and inferior portions of the body
   c. dorsal and ventral portions of the body
   d. right and left portions of the body

OBJ. 7 ___ 17. The process of choosing one sectional plane and making a series of sections at small intervals is called:
   a. parasagittal sectioning
   b. resonance imaging
   c. serial reconstruction
   d. sectional planing

OBJ. 8 ___ 18. The subdivisions of the dorsal body cavity include:
   a. the thoracic and abdominal cavities
   b. the abdominal and pelvic cavities
   c. the pericardial and pleural cavities
   d. the cranial and spinal cavities

OBJ. 8 ___ 19. The subdivisions of the ventral body cavity include:
   a. the pleural and pericardial cavities
   b. the thoracic and abdominopelvic cavities
   c. the pelvic and abdominal cavities
   d. the cranial and spinal cavities

OBJ. 8 ___ 20. The heart and lungs are located in the _____ cavity.
   a. pericardial
   b. thoracic
   c. pleural
   d. abdominal

OBJ. 8 ___ 21. The ventral body cavity is divided by a flat muscular sheet called the:
   a. mediastinum
   b. pericardium
   c. diaphragm
   d. peritoneum

OBJ. 8 ___ 22. Checking for tumors or other tissue abnormalities is best accomplished by the use of:
   a. computerized tomography
   b. X-ray
   c. ultrasound
   d. magnetic resonance imaging

Level -1-

Level 1 Review of Chapter Objectives 5

[L1] Completion:

Using the terms below, complete the following statements.

digestion	transverse	responsiveness	urinary
endocrine	liver	integumentary	positive feedback
organs	histologist	pericardial	medial
regulation	excretion	physiology	peritoneal
tissues	mediastinum	distal	molecules
digestive			

OBJ. 1 23. Moving your hand away from a hot stove is an example of a basic function called _____.

OBJ. 1 24. In order for food to be utilized by cells in the human body, it must first be broken down by the process of _____.

OBJ. 1 25. Harmful waste products are discharged into the environment by the process of _____.

OBJ. 2 26. A person who specializes in the study of tissue is called a _____.

OBJ. 2 27. The study of the functions of the living cell is called cell _____.

OBJ. 2 28. In complex organisms such as the human being cells unite to form _____.

OBJ. 3 29. At the chemical level of organization, atoms interact to form _____.

OBJ. 3 30. The cardiovascular system is made up of structural units called _____.

OBJ. 4 31. The kidneys, bladder, and ureters are organs which belong to the _____ system.

OBJ. 4 32. The esophagus, large intestine, and stomach are organs which belong to the _____ system.

OBJ. 4 33. The organ system to which the skin belongs is the _____ system.

OBJ. 5 34. The term that refers to the adjustments in physiological systems that are responsible for the preservation of homeostasis is homeostatic _____.

OBJ. 6 35. A response that is important in accelerating processes that must proceed to completion rapidly is _____.

OBJ. 6 36. The two systems usually controlled by negative feedback mechanisms are the nervous and _____ system.

OBJ. 7 37. Tenderness in the right upper quadrant (RUQ) might indicate problems with the _____.

OBJ. 7 38. A term that means "close to the long axis of the body" is _____.

OBJ. 7 39. A term that means "away from an attached base" is _____.

OBJ. 7 40. A plane that is perpendicular to the long axis of the body is a _____ section.

OBJ. 8 41. The subdivision of the thoracic cavity which houses the heart is the _____ cavity.

OBJ. 8 42. The large central mass of connective tissue that surrounds the pericardial cavity and separates the two pleural cavities is the _____.

OBJ. 8 43. The Abdominopelvic cavity is also known as the _____ cavity.

6 Chapter 1 An Introduction to Anatomy and Physiology

[L1] Matching:

Match the terms in column "B" with the terms in column "A." Use letters for answers in the spaces provided.

	COLUMN "A"	COLUMN "B"
OBJ. 1	___ 44. Excretion	A. Disease
OBJ. 1	___ 45. Respiration	B. Steady state
OBJ. 2	___ 46. Gross anatomy	C. Oxygen
OBJ. 2	___ 47. Pathology	D. Endocrine
OBJ. 3	___ 48. Internal cell structures	E. Waste
OBJ. 4	___ 49. Heart	F. Stimulus
OBJ. 4	___ 50. Pituitary	G. Skull
OBJ. 5	___ 51. Homeostasis	H. Macroscopic
OBJ. 6	___ 52. Receptor	I. Cardiovascular
OBJ. 7	___ 53. Cranial	J. Organelles
OBJ. 7	___ 54. Prone	K. Abdominopelvic
OBJ. 8	___ 55. Peritoneal	L. Face up

[L1] Drawing/Illustration Labeling:

Identify each numbered structure by labeling the following figures:

OBJ. 7   **FIGURE 1.1** Planes of the Body

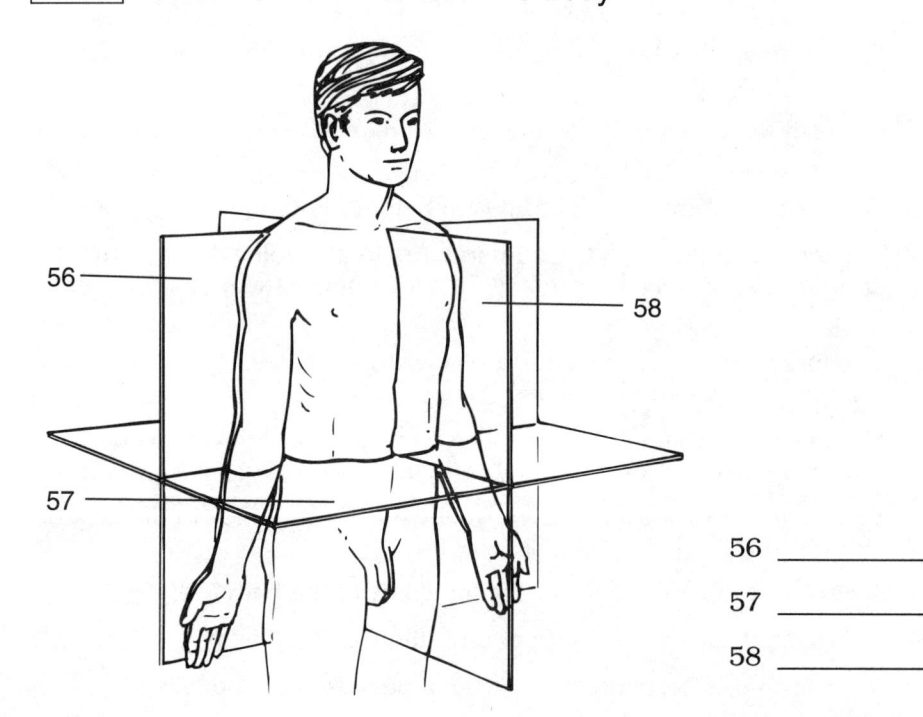

56 _____

57 _____

58 _____

Level 1 Review of Chapter Objectives 7

OBJ. 7   **FIGURE 1.2**   Human Body Orientation & Direction

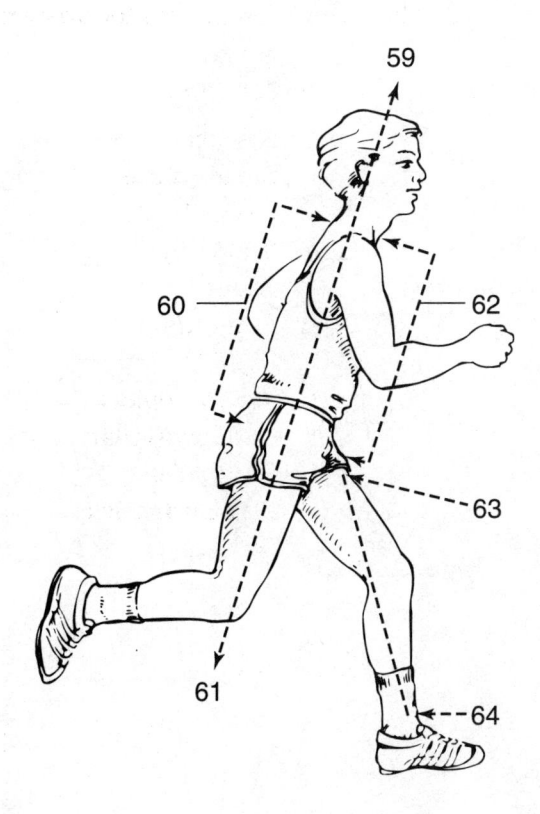

59 _____
60 _____
61 _____
62 _____
63 _____
64 _____

8 Chapter 1 An Introduction to Anatomy and Physiology

OBJ. 7 **FIGURE 1.3** Regional Body References

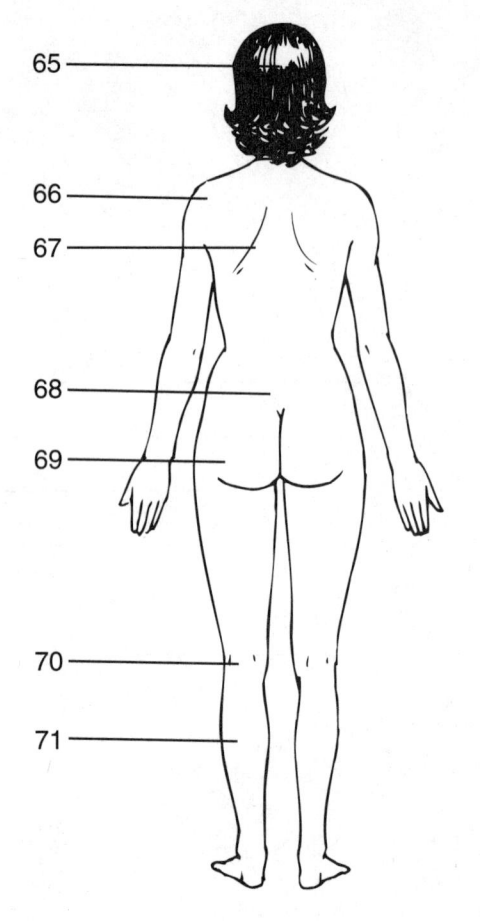

Posterior view
(dorsal)

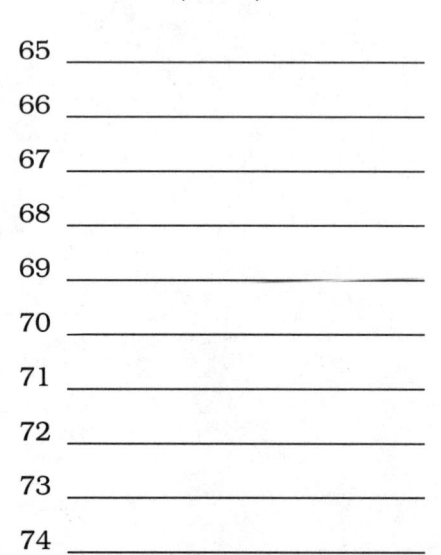

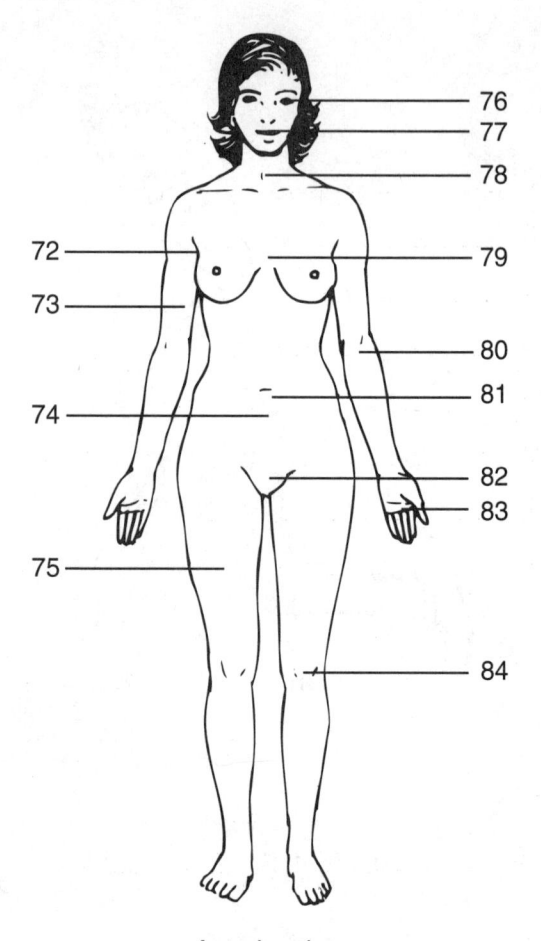

Anterior view
(ventral)

65 _____
66 _____
67 _____
68 _____
69 _____
70 _____
71 _____
72 _____
73 _____
74 _____

75 _____
76 _____
77 _____
78 _____
79 _____
80 _____
81 _____
82 _____
83 _____
84 _____

Level 1

Level 1   Review of Chapter Objectives   9

OBJ. 8   **FIGURE 1.4**   Body Cavities – Sagittal View

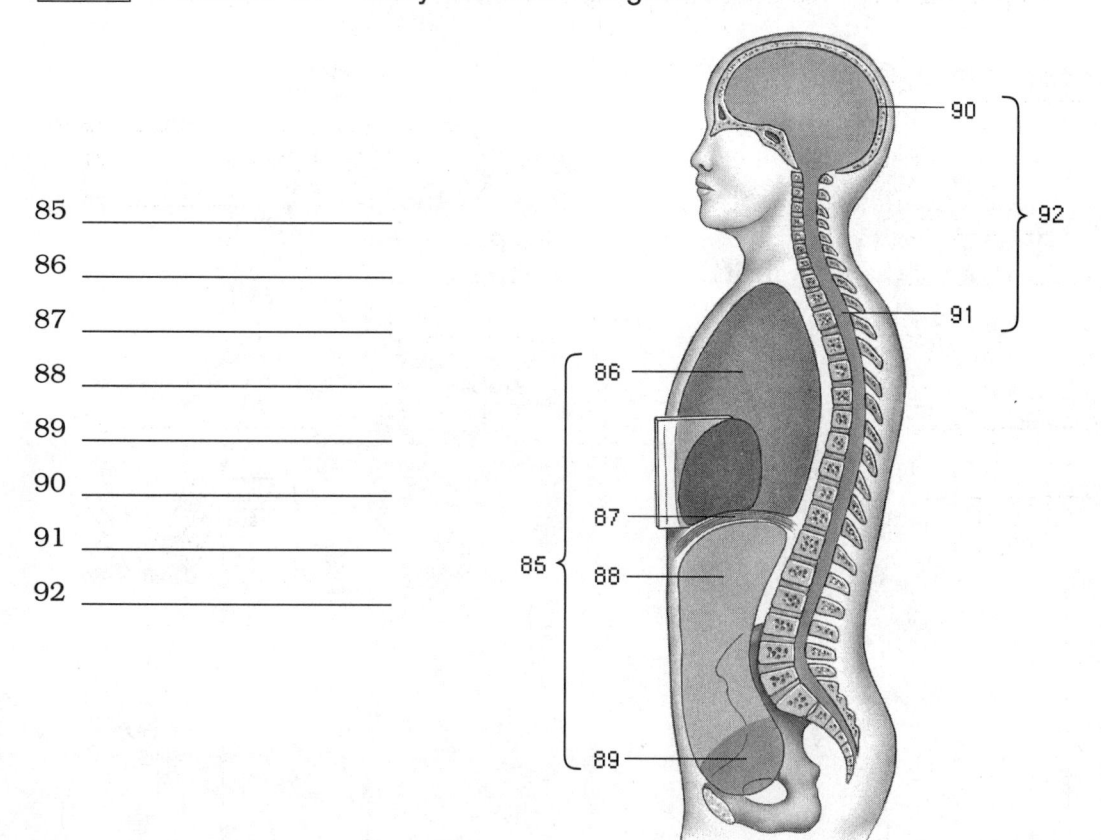

85 _____
86 _____
87 _____
88 _____
89 _____
90 _____
91 _____
92 _____

OBJ. 8   **FIGURE 1.5**   Body Cavities – Anterior View

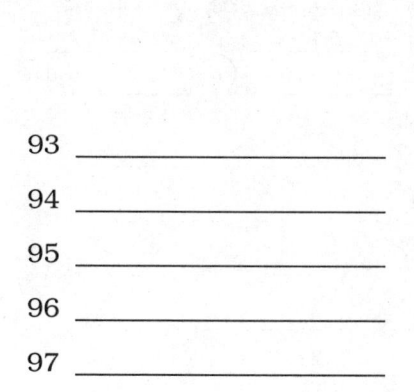

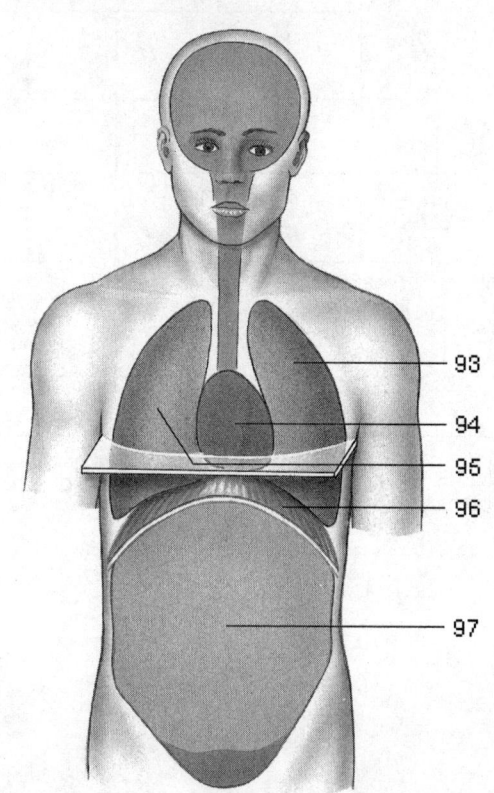

93 _____
94 _____
95 _____
96 _____
97 _____

When you have successfully completed the exercises in L1 proceed to L2.

Level -1-

Chapter 1 An Introduction to Anatomy and Physiology

☐ LEVEL 2 CONCEPT SYNTHESIS

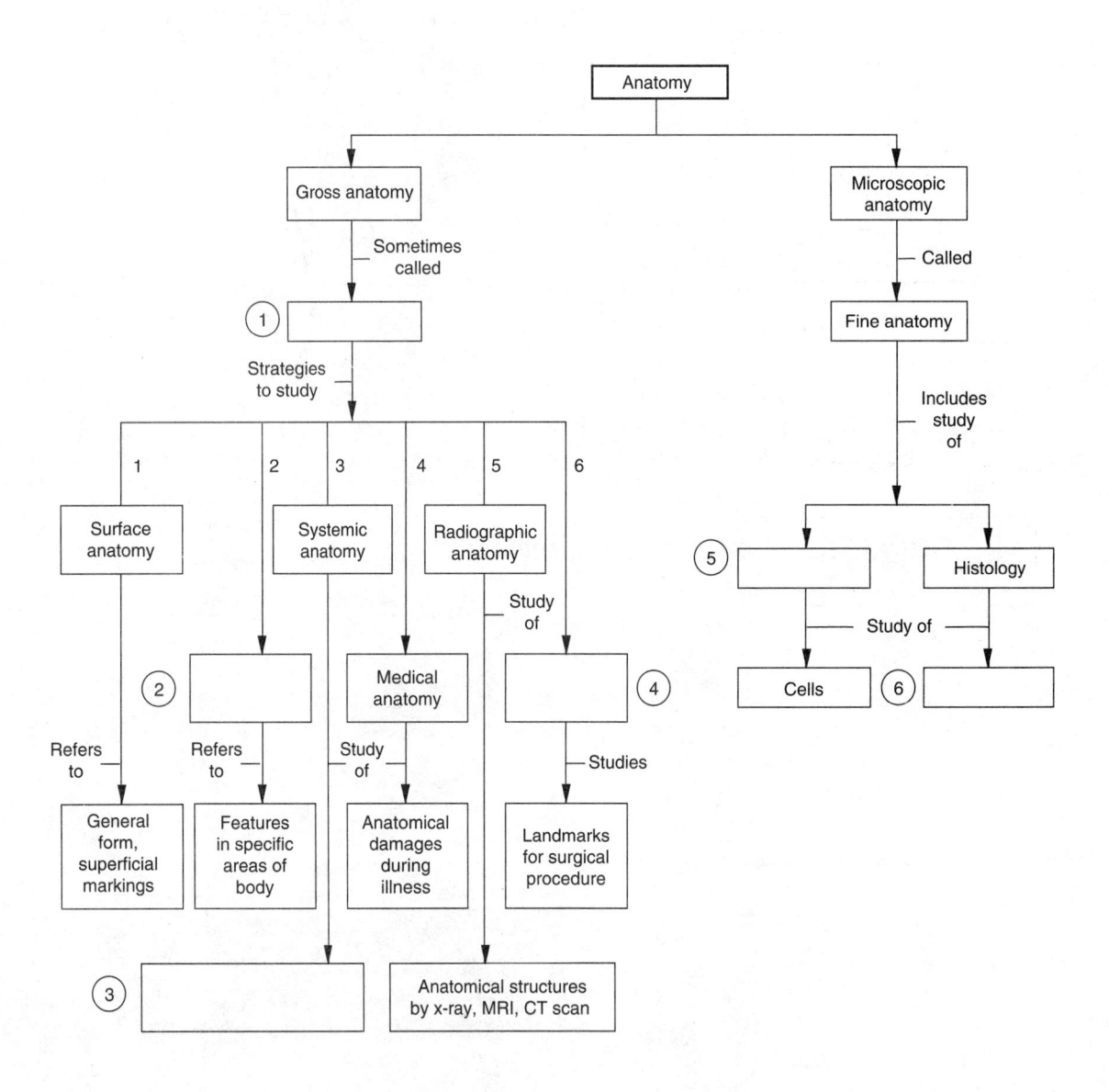

Concept Map I:

Using the following terms, fill in the numbered, blank spaces to complete the concept map. Follow the numbers which comply with the organization of the map.

- Surgical Anatomy
- Cytology Tissues
- Structure of Organ Systems
- Regional Anatomy
- Macroscopic Anatomy
- Tissues

Level 2   Concept Synthesis   11

Concept Map II:

Using the following terms, fill in the numbered, blank spaces to complete the concept map. Follow the numbers which comply with the organization of the concept map.

- Pelvic Cavity
- Heart
- Spinal Cord
- Abdominopelvic Cavity
- Cranial Cavity
- Two Pleural Cavities

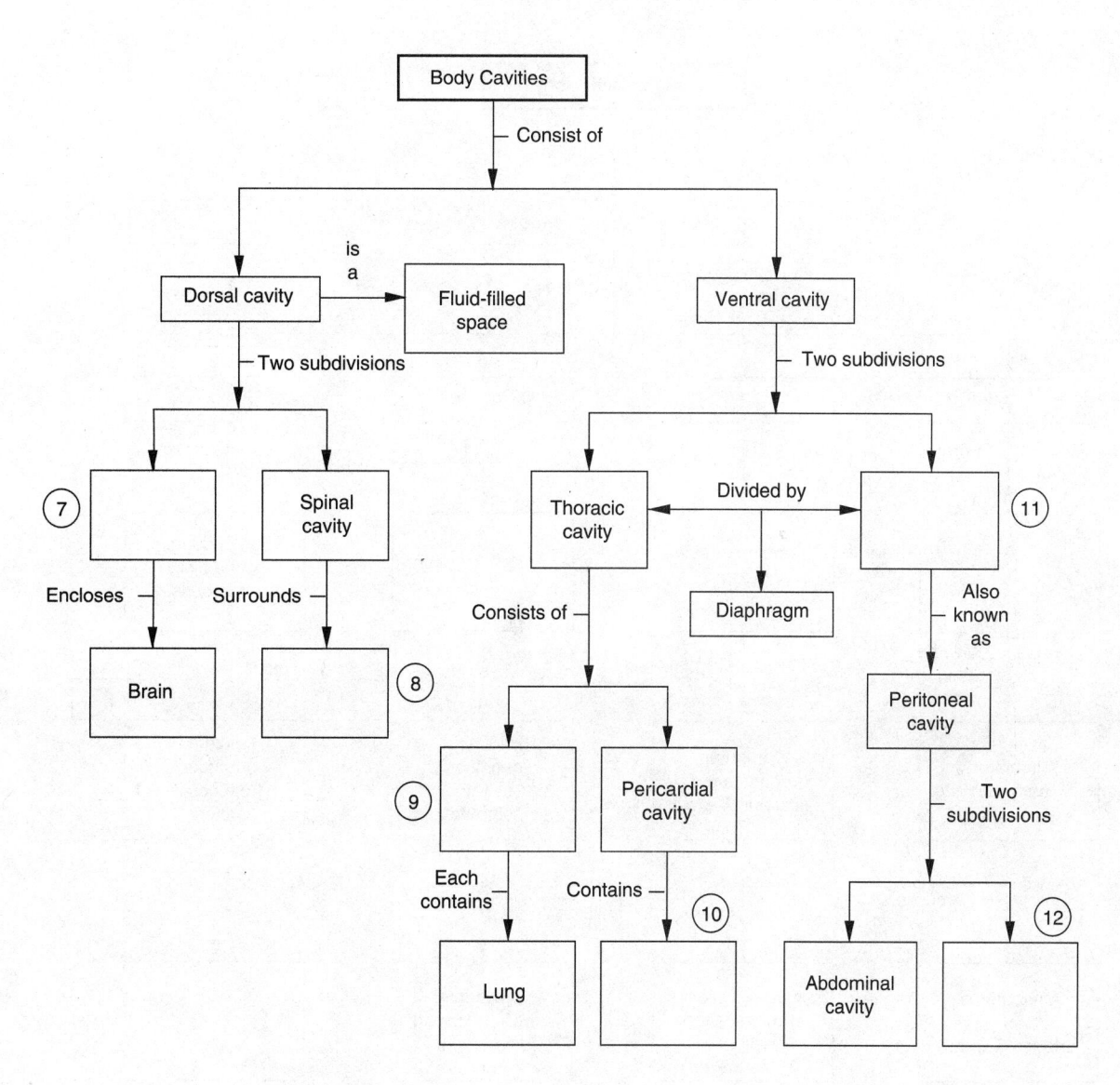

Chapter 1 An Introduction to Anatomy and Physiology

Concept Map III:

Using the following terms, fill in the numbered blank spaces to complete the concept map. Follow the numbers which comply with the organization of the concept map.

- High-energy Radiation
- CT Scans
- Echogram
- Radio Waves
- Radiologist

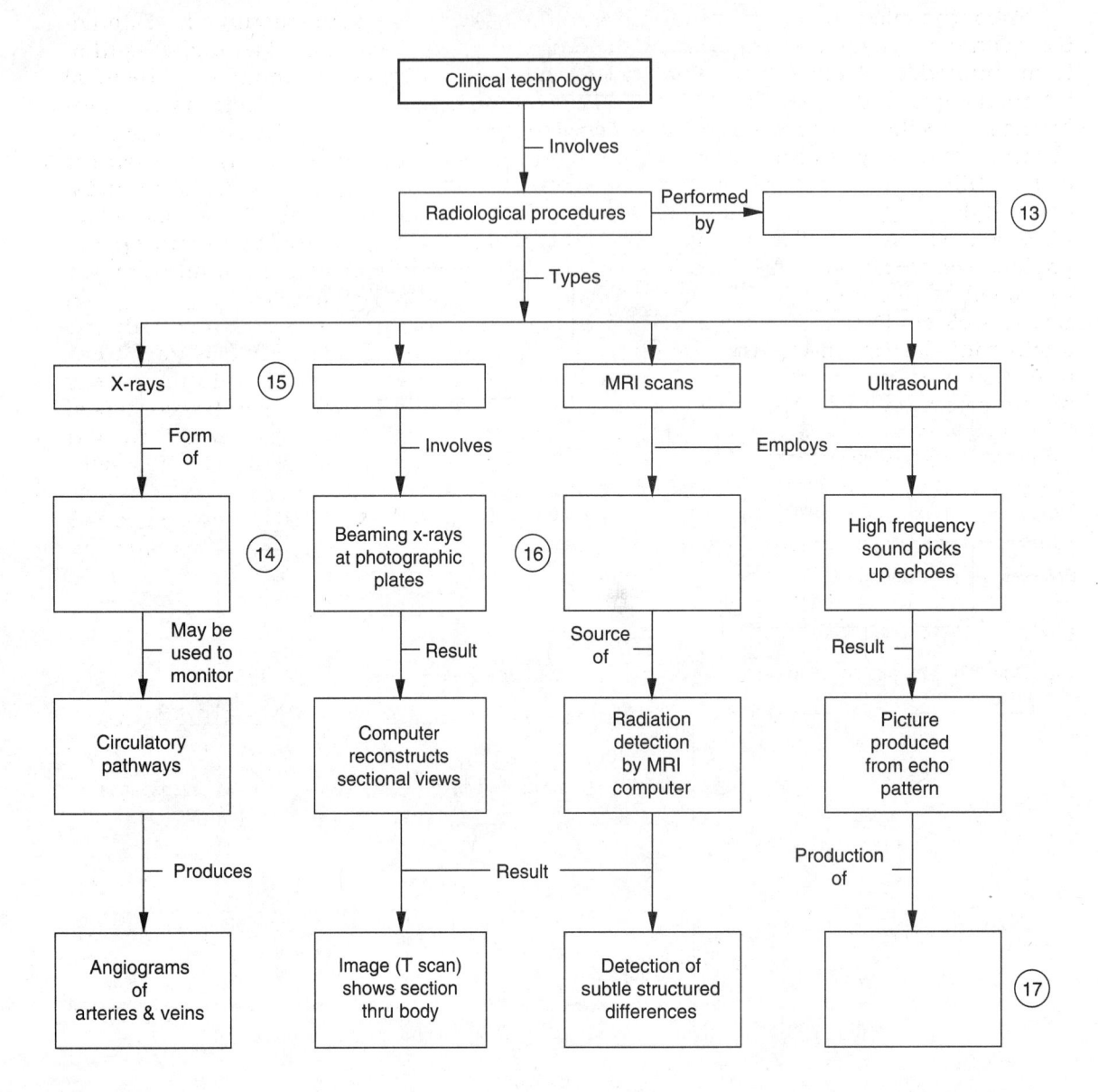

```
                    Clinical technology
                           │
                         Involves
                           ▼
    Radiological procedures ──Performed by──▶ [ 13 ]
                           │
                         Types
          ┌────────────┬──┴──────────┬────────────┐
          ▼            ▼             ▼            ▼
        X-rays       [ 15 ]      MRI scans     Ultrasound
          │            │             │             │
        Form of     Involves       Employs         │
          ▼            ▼             ▼             ▼
       [ 14 ]    Beaming x-rays  [ 16 ]      High frequency
                 at photographic              sound picks
                 plates                       up echoes
          │            │             │             │
       May be        Result       Source of     Result
       used to         │             │             │
       monitor         ▼             ▼             ▼
          ▼        Computer      Radiation      Picture
      Circulatory  reconstructs  detection      produced
      pathways     sectional     by MRI         from echo
                   views         computer       pattern
          │            │             │             │
       Produces      Result        Result     Production of
          ▼            ▼             ▼             ▼
      Angiograms   Image (T scan)  Detection of  [ 17 ]
      of arteries  shows section   subtle structured
      & veins      thru body       differences
```

Level 2

Body Trek:

Using the terms below, fill in the blanks to complete the trek through the levels of organization in the human body.

Tissues   Organelles   Cells   Organism
Atoms   Systems   Molecules Organs

Robo, the micro-robot, is introduced into the body by way of the mouth where immediate contact is made with the lining of the oral cavity, which consists of a mucous epithelium. Immediate feedback to Mission Control gives information about the chemical interactions taking place. Robo discloses that protons, neutrons, and electrons are combining in specific numbers and arrangements to form (18) _____. These units use the electrons to form chemical bonds which hold the units together to make larger structures called (19) _____. These structures, in turn, unite to form still larger structures, called (20) _____, which are organized to form specific functions. These last structures float within a liquid substance called protoplasm, and are enclosed by a double phospholipid cell membrane. Robo senses many of these membrane-enclosed units. They are the smallest functional and structural units of life and are called (21) _____. As Robo's trek continues it is quite evident that these structural units combine with one another into larger collections called (22) _____. Four kinds are detected as Robo treks into other areas of the body. Epithelium is rather plentiful in the mouth, while other areas of the body include the presence of muscle, nerve, and connective tissue types. Combinations of these four tisssue types form more organized and complex structural and functional units called (23) _____, which, when combined with other functionally-similar units, form the next higher level of organization called body (24) _____. The complex, complete, living being is referred to as an (25) _____. With the completion of Robo's investigation, Mission Control programs a convenient exit by way of the mouth, and preparations will be made for the next body trek.

[L2] Multiple Choice:

Place the letter corresponding to the correct answer in the space provided.

_____ 26. Beginning with cells and proceeding through increasing levels of complexity, the correct sequence is:

   a. cells, tissues, organs, system
   b. cells, organs, tissues, system
   c. cells, system, tissues, organs
   d. system, organs, tissues, cells

_____ 27. Damage at the cellular, tissue, or organ level often affects the entire system. This supports the view that:

   a. each level is totally independent of the others
   b. each level has its own specific function
   c. each level is totally dependent on the other
   d. the lower levels depend on the higher levels

_____ 28. Anatomical position refers to a person standing erect, feet facing forward and:

   a. arms hanging to sides with palms of hands facing anteriorly and the thumbs located medially
   b. arms in a raised position with palms of hands facing forward and the thumbs to the outside
   c. arms hanging to sides with palms of hands facing forward and the thumbs to the outside
   d. arms in a raised position with palms of hands facing dorsally and the thumbs to the outside

14 Chapter 1 An Introduction to Anatomy and Physiology

_____ 29. If an observer is facing someone in front of him, the left side is to the observer's:
   a. left
   b. right
   c. dorsal side
   d. proximal side

_____ 30. Resistance to X-ray penetration is called radiodensity. From the following selections, choose the one that correctly shows the order of increasing radiodensity of materials in the human body.
   a. air, liver, fat, blood, bone, muscle
   b. air, fat, liver, blood, muscle, bone
   c. air, fat, blood, liver, muscle, bone
   d. air, liver, blood, fat, muscle, bone

_____ 31. In a homeostatic system, the mechanism which triggers an automatic response that corrects the situation is:
   a. the presence of a receptor area and an effector area
   b. an exaggeration of the stimulus
   c. temporary repair to the damaged area
   d. a variation outside of normal limits

_____ 32. If the temperature of the body climbs above 99 degrees F, negative feedback is triggered by:
   a. increased heat conservation by restricted blood flow to the skin
   b. the individual experiences shivering
   c. activation of the positive feedback mechanism
   d. an increased heat loss through enhanced blood flow to the skin and sweating

[L2] Completion:

Using the terms below, complete the following statements.

appendicitis	adaptability	stethoscope
nervous	sternum	knee
elbow		

33. Activities of the nervous and endocrine systems to control or adjust the activities of many different systems simultaneously is _____.
34. The system which performs crisis management by directing rapid, short-term, and very specific responses is the _____ system.
35. The popliteal artery refers to the area of the body in the region of the _____.
36. Tenderness in the right lower quadrant of the abdomen may indicate _____.
37. Moving proximally from the wrist brings you to the _____.
38. Auscultation is a technique that employs the use of a _____.
39. If a surgeon makes a midsagittal incision in the inferior region of the thorax, the incision would be made through the _____.

Level 2   Concept Synthesis

[L2]   Short Essay Answer:

Briefly answer the following questions in the spaces provided below.

40. Despite obvious differences, all living things perform the same basic functions. List five (5) functions that are active processes in living organisms.

41. Show your understanding of the levels of organization in a complex living thing by using arrows and listing in correct sequence from the simplest level to the most complex level.

42. What is the major difference between negative feedback and positive feedback?

43. What are the two (2) essential functions of body cavities in the human body?

When you have successfully completed the exercises in L2 proceed to L3.

LEVEL 3 CRITICAL THINKING/APPLICATION

Using principles and concepts learned in Introduction to Anatomy and Physiology, answer the following questions. Write your answers on a separate sheet of paper.

1. Unlike the abdominal viscera, the thoracic viscera is separated into two compartments by an area called the mediastinum. What is the clinical importance of this compartmental arrangement?

2. The events of childbirth are associated with the process of positive feedback. Describe the events which confirm this statement.

3. A radioactive tracer is introduced into the heart to trace a possible blockage in the blood vessels in or around the uterus. Give the sequence of body cavities that would be included as the tracer travels in the blood from the heart through the aorta to the blood vessels of the uterus.

4. What is the purpose of the large barium "milk shake" given to a patient before being X-rayed for a stomach ailment?

CHAPTER 2

The Chemical Level of Organization

■ Overview

Technology within the last 40 to 50 years has allowed humans to "see and understand" the unseen within the human body. Today, instead of an "organ system view" of the body, we are able to look through the eyes of scientists using sophisticated technological tools and see the "ultramicro world" within ourselves. Our technology has permitted us to progress from the "macro-view" to the "micro-view" and to understand that the human body is made up of atoms, and that the interactions of these atoms control the physiological processes within the body.

The study of anatomy and physiology begins at the most fundamental level of organization, namely individual atoms and molecules. The concepts in Chapter 2 provide a framework for understanding how simple components combine to make up the more complex forms that comprise the human body. Information is provided that shows how the chemical processes need to continue throughout life in an orderly and timely sequence if homeostasis is to be maintained.

The student activities in this chapter stress many of the important principles that make up the science of chemistry, both inorganic and organic. The tests are set up to measure your knowledge of chemical principles and to evaluate your ability to apply these principles to the structure and functions of organ systems within the human body.

☐ LEVEL 1   REVIEW OF CHAPTER OBJECTIVES

1. Describe an atom and an element.
2. Describe the different ways in which atoms combine to form molecules and compounds.
3. Use chemical notation to symbolize chemical reactions.
4. Distinguish among the major types of chemical reactions that are important for studying physiology.
5. Describe the role of enzymes in metabolism.
6. Distinguish between organic and inorganic compounds.
7. Explain how the chemical properties of water make life possible.
8. Describe the pH scale and the role of buffers in body fluids.
9. Describe the physiological roles of inorganic compounds.
10. Discuss the structure and function of carbohydrates, lipids, proteins, nucleic acids, and high-energy compounds.

Chapter 2 The Chemical Level of Organization

[L1] Multiple Choice:

Place the letter corresponding to the correct answer in the space provided.

OBJ. 1 ____ 1. The smallest chemical units of matter of which no chemical change can alter their identity are:
- a. electrons
- b. mesons
- c. protons
- d. atoms

OBJ. 1 ____ 2. The protons in an atom are found:
- a. outside the nucleus only
- b. in the nucleus and in energy shell
- c. in the nucleus only
- d. in energy shells only

OBJ. 2 ____ 3. The unequal sharing of electrons in a molecule of water is an example of:
- a. an ionic bond
- b. a polar covalent bond
- c. a double covalent bond
- d. a triple covalent bond

OBJ. 2 ____ 4. The formation of cations and anions illustrates the attraction between:
- a. ionic bonds
- b. polar covalent bonds
- c. nonpolar covalent bonds
- d. double covalent bonds

OBJ. 3 ____ 5. The symbol 2H means:
- a. one molecule of hydrogen
- b. two molecules of hydrogen
- c. two atoms of hydrogen
- d. a, b, and c are correct

OBJ. 4 ____ 6. From the following choices, select the one which diagrams a typical decomposition reaction:
- a. A + B → AB
- b. AB + CD → AD + CB
- c. AB → A + B
- d. C + D → CD

OBJ. 4 ____ 7. A + B → AB is an example of a(n) _____ reaction.
- a. reversible
- b. synthesis
- c. decomposition
- d. a, b, and c are correct

Level 1   Review of Chapter Objectives   19

OBJ. 5 ___ 8. Organic catalysts made by a living cell to promote a specific reaction are called:
   a. nucleic acids
   b. buffers
   c. enzymes
   d. metabolites

OBJ. 6 ___ 9. The major difference between inorganic and organic compounds is that inorganic compounds are usually:
   a. small molecules held together partially or completely by ionic bonds
   b. made up of carbon, hydrogen, and oxygen
   c. large molecules which are soluble in water
   d. a and c are correct

OBJ. 6 ___ 10. The four major classes of organic compounds are:
   a. water, acids, bases, and salts
   b. carbohydrates, fats, proteins, and water
   c. nucleic acids, salts, bases, and water
   d. carbohydrates, lipids, proteins, and nucleic acids

OBJ. 7 ___ 11. The ability of water to maintain a relatively constant temperature and then prevent rapid changes in body temperature is due to its:
   a. solvent capacities
   b. molecular structure
   c. boiling and freezing point
   d. capacity to absorb and distribute heat

OBJ. 8 ___ 12. To maintain homeostasis in the human body, the normal pH range of the blood must remain at:
   a. 6.80 to 7.20
   b. 7.35 to 7.45
   c. 7.0
   d. 6.80 to 7.80

OBJ. 9 ___ 13. A solute that dissociates to release hydrogen ions and causes a decrease in pH is:
   a. a base
   b. a salt
   c. an acid
   d. water

OBJ. 9 ___ 14. A solute that removes hydrogen ions from a solution is:
   a. an acid
   b. a base
   c. a salt
   d. a buffer

20 Chapter 2 The Chemical Level of Organization

OBJ. 10 ____ 15. A carbohydrate molecule is made up of:
    a. carbon, hydrogen, oxygen
    b. carbon, oxygen, nitrogen, hydrogen, phosphorus
    c. carbon, hydrogen, oxygen, phosphorus
    d. carbon, hydrogen, nitrogen

OBJ. 10 ____ 16. Carbohydrates are most important to the body in that they serve as primary sources of:
    a. tissue growth and repair
    b. metabolites
    c. energy
    d. digestible forms of food

OBJ. 10 ____ 17. The building blocks of proteins consist of chains of small molecules which are called:
    a. peptide bonds
    b. amino acids
    c. R groups
    d. amino groups

OBJ. 10 ____ 18. Special proteins that are involved in metabolic regulation are called:
    a. transport proteins
    b. contractile proteins
    c. structural proteins
    d. enzymes

OBJ. 10 ____ 19. The three basic components of a single nucleotide of a nucleic acid are:
    a. a sugar
    b. a phosphate group
    c. a nitogen base
    d. a, b and c are correct

OBJ. 10 ____ 20. The most important high-energy compound found in the human body is:
    a. DNA
    b. RNA
    c. ATP
    d. b and c are correct

[L1] Completion:

Using the terms below, complete the following statements.

glucose	inorganic	solute	atomic weight
Na_2SO_4	protons	endergonic	buffers
decomposition	solvent	salt	exergonic
ionic bond	organic	catalysts	covalent bonds
acid	dehydration synthesis		

Level -1-

OBJ. 1   21. The atomic number of an atom is determined by the number of _____.

Level 1   Review of Chapter Objectives   21

OBJ. 1   22. The total number of protons and neutrons in the nucleus of an atom is the _____.

OBJ. 2   23. Atoms that complete their outer electron shells by sharing electrons with other atoms result in the formation of a(n) _____.

OBJ. 2   24. When one atom loses an electron and another accepts that electron, the result is the formation of a(n) _____.

OBJ. 3   25. The chemical notation that would indicate sodium sulfate would be _____.

OBJ. 4   26. A reaction that breaks a molecule into smaller fragments is called _____.

OBJ. 4   27. Reactions that release energy are said to be _____ and reactions that absorb heat are called _____ reactions.

OBJ. 5   28. Compounds that accelerate chemical reactions without themselves being permanently changed are called _____.

OBJ. 6   29. Compounds that contain the elements carbon and hydrogen and usually oxygen are _____.

OBJ. 6   30. Acids, bases and salts are examples of _____ compounds.

OBJ. 7   31. The fluid medium of a solution is called the _____ and the dissolved substance is called the _____.

OBJ. 8   32. A solution with a pH of 4.0 is _____.

OBJ. 8   33. Compounds in body fluids that maintain pH within normal limits are called _____.

OBJ. 9   34. The interaction of an acid and a base in which the hydrogen ions of the acid are replaced by the positive ions of the base results in the formation of a(n) _____.

OBJ. 10   35. The most important metabolic "fuel" in the body is _____.

OBJ. 10   36. The linking together of chemical units by the removal of water to create a more complex molecule is called _____.

[L1]   Matching:

Match the terms in column "B" with the terms in column "A." Use letters for answers in the spaces provided.

	COLUMN "A"	COLUMN "B"
OBJ. 1 ____ 37.	Electron	A. Two products; two reactants
OBJ. 2 ____ 38.	Inert gases	B. Hydroxyl group
OBJ. 2 ____ 39.	Polar covalent bond	C. Produces ions
OBJ. 3 ____ 40.	NaCl	D. Inorganic acid
OBJ. 4 ____ 41.	Exchange reaction	E. Bicarbonate ion
OBJ. 5 ____ 42.	Enzyme	F. Unequal sharing of electrons
OBJ. 6 ____ 43.	HCl	G. Catalyst
OBJ. 6 ____ 44.	NaOH	H. Sodium hydroxide
OBJ. 7 ____ 45.	Dissociation	I. Negative electrical charge
OBJ. 8 ____ 46.	O-	J. Uracil
OBJ. 8 ____ 47.	H+	K. Thymine
OBJ. 9 ____ 48.	HCO3-	L. Sodium Chloride
OBJ. 10 ____ 49.	DNA nitrogen base	M. Hydrogen ion
OBJ. 10 ____ 50.	RNA nitrogen base	N. Stable

22 Chapter 2 The Chemical Level of Organization

[L1] Drawing/Illustration Labeling:

Identify each numbered structure by labeling the following figures:

OBJ. 2   **FIGURE 2.1**   Identification of Types of Bonds

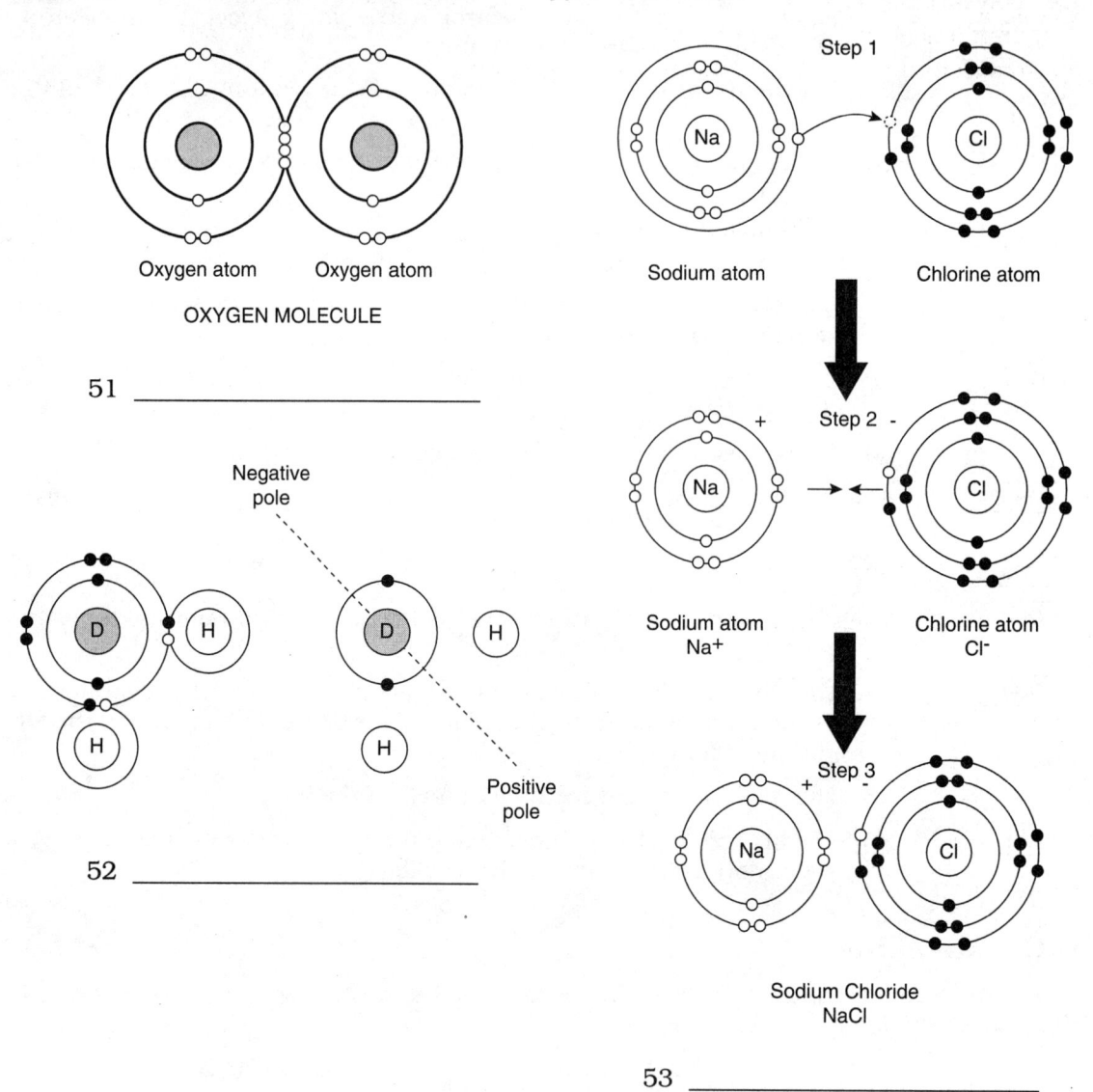

Oxygen atom   Oxygen atom
OXYGEN MOLECULE

51 _____

Negative pole

Positive pole

52 _____

Step 1
Sodium atom   Chlorine atom

Step 2
Sodium atom   Chlorine atom
Na+   Cl-

Step 3
Sodium Chloride
NaCl

53 _____

Level
-1-

Level 1 Review of Chapter Objectives 23

OBJ. 10 **FIGURE 2.2** Identification of Organic Molecules

(Select from the following terms to identify each molecule.)

polysaccharide   cholesterol   monosaccharide
amino acid   DNA   polyunsaturated fatty acid
disaccharide   saturated fatty acid

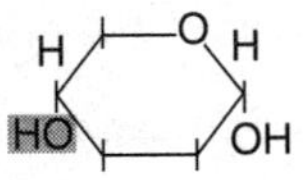

54 _____

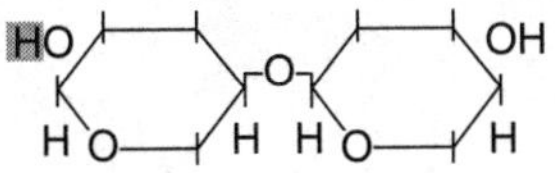

55 _____

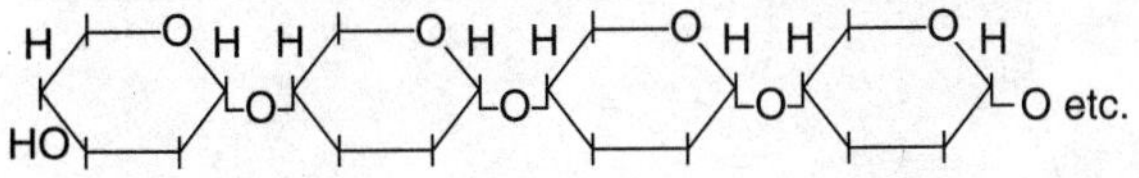

56 _____

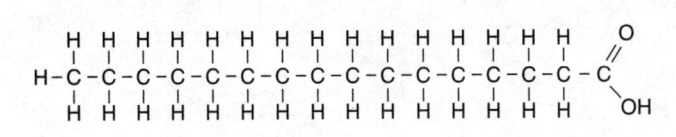

57 _____

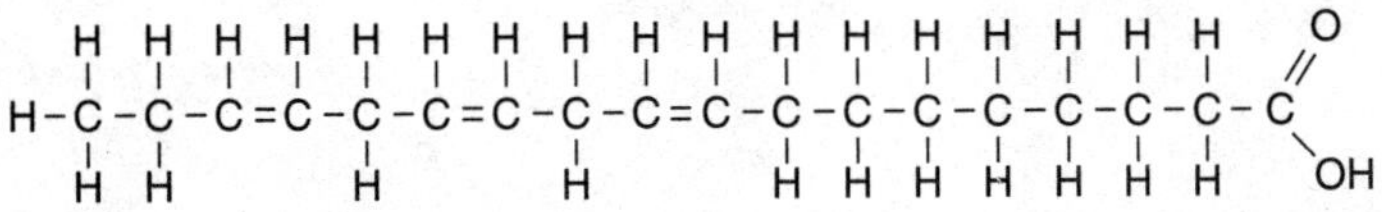

58 _____

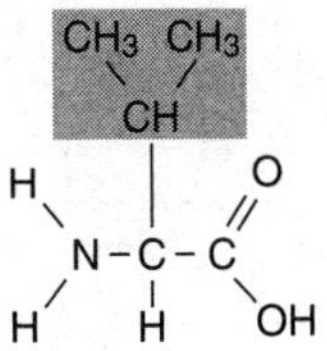

59 _____

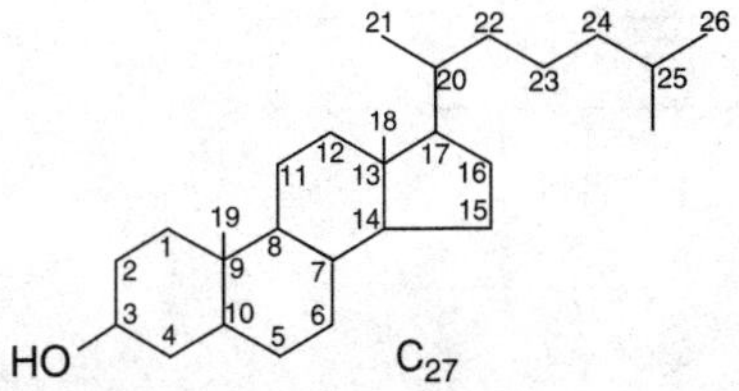

60 _____

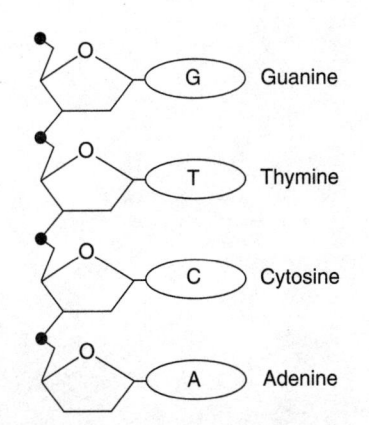

61 _____

When you have successfully completed the exercises in L1 proceed to L2.

LEVEL 2 CONCEPT SYNTHESIS

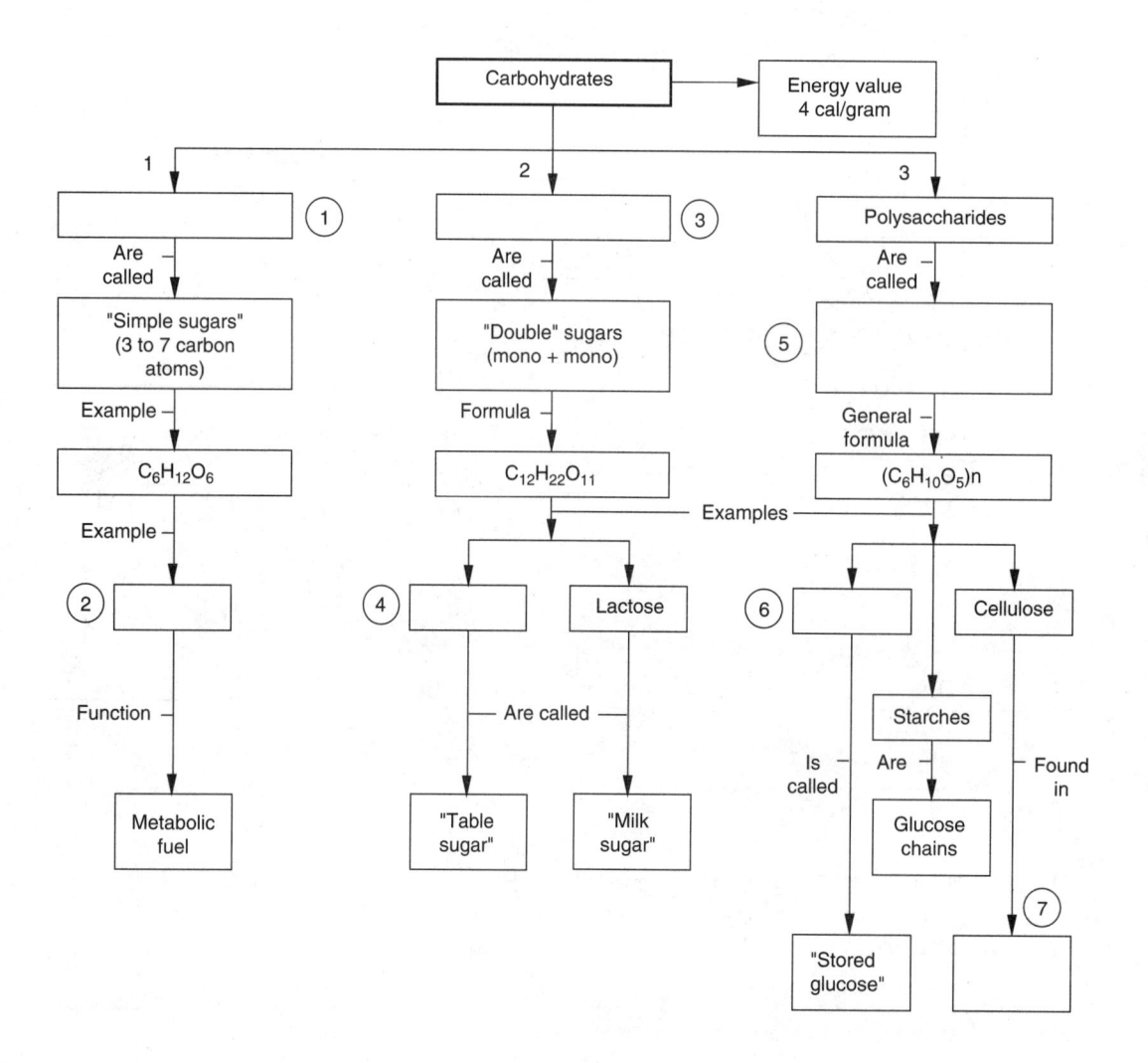

Concept Map I:

Using the following terms, fill in the numbered, blank spaces to complete the concept map. Follow the numbers to comply with the organization of the map.

- Monosaccharides
- Glucose
- Plants
- Sucrose
- Glycogen
- Disaccharides
- Complex carbohydrates

```
                        Carbohydrates ──► Energy value
                              │             4 cal/gram
             ┌────────────────┼────────────────┐
             1                2                3
             ▼                ▼                ▼
         ┌───────┐ ①      ┌───────┐ ③     Polysaccharides
         │       │         │       │
         Are               Are              Are
         called            called           called
           ▼                 ▼                ▼
      "Simple sugars"   "Double" sugars   ┌───────┐ ⑤
      (3 to 7 carbon    (mono + mono)     │       │
         atoms)
           │                 │              │
        Example           Formula         General
           ▼                 ▼             formula
         C₆H₁₂O₆          C₁₂H₂₂O₁₁          ▼
                                          (C₆H₁₀O₅)n
        Example ─┐      ──── Examples ────
                 ▼      ▼         ▼        ▼        ▼
               ② ┌──┐  ④┌──┐  Lactose   ⑥ ┌──┐  Cellulose
                 │  │   │  │                │  │
              Function  └─Are called─┘      │        │
                 ▼       ▼         ▼       Is       Found
              Metabolic "Table"  "Milk"   called     in
                fuel    sugar"   sugar"    │  Are ─ Starches
                                           ▼   ▼      │
                                        "Stored  ⑦   Glucose
                                        glucose"     chains
```

Answers: $C_6H_{12}O_6$, $C_{12}H_{22}O_{11}$, $(C_6H_{10}O_5)n$

Level 2 Concept Synthesis

Concept Map II:

Using the following terms, fill in the numbered, blank spaces to complete the concept map. Follow the numbers to comply with the organization of the map.

- Saturated
- Glyceride
- Di-
- Phospholipid
- Glycerol + fatty acids
- Steroids

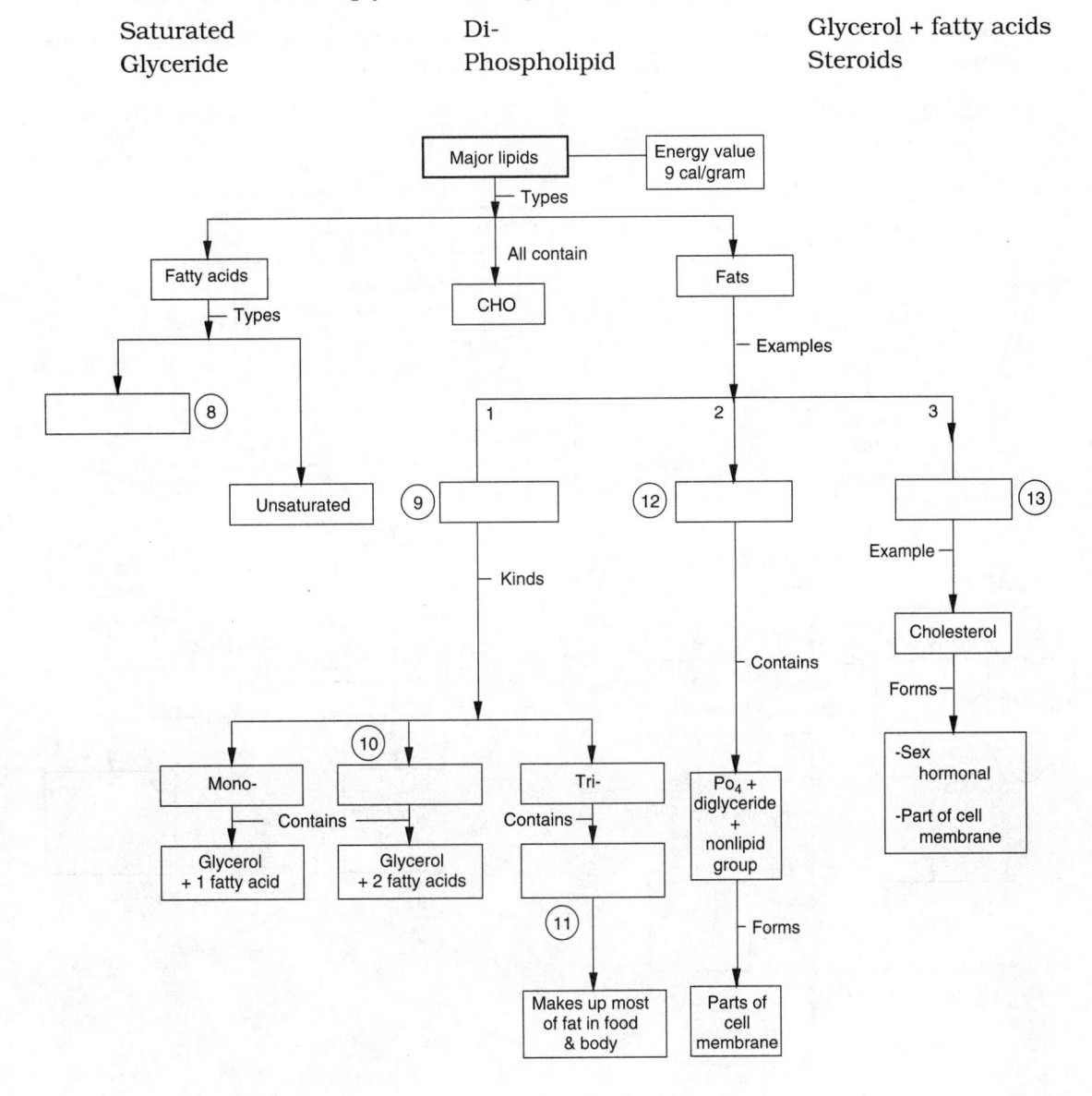

Chapter 2 The Chemical Level of Organization

Concept Map III:

Using the following terms, fill in the numbered, blank spaces to complete the concept map. Follow the numbers to comply with the organization of the concept map.

- Variable group
- -COOH
- Globular proteins
- Enzymes
- Keratin
- Amino acids
- Amino group

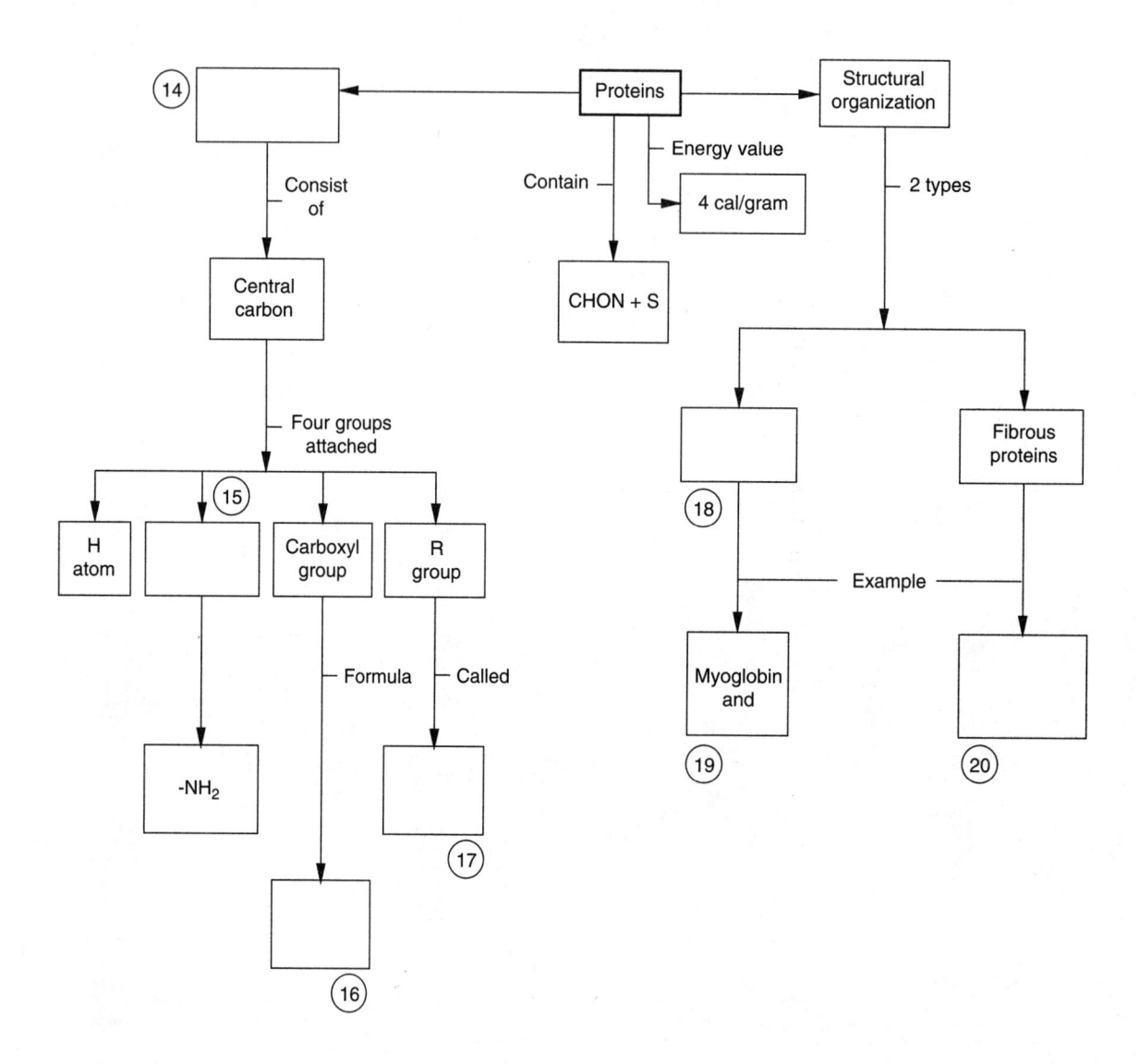

14. Amino acids
15. Amino group
16. -COOH
17. Variable group
18. Globular proteins
19. Enzymes
20. Keratin

Level 2   Concept Synthesis   27

Concept Map IV:

Using the following terms, fill in the numbered, blank spaces to complete the concept map. Follow the numbers to comply with the organization of the concept map.

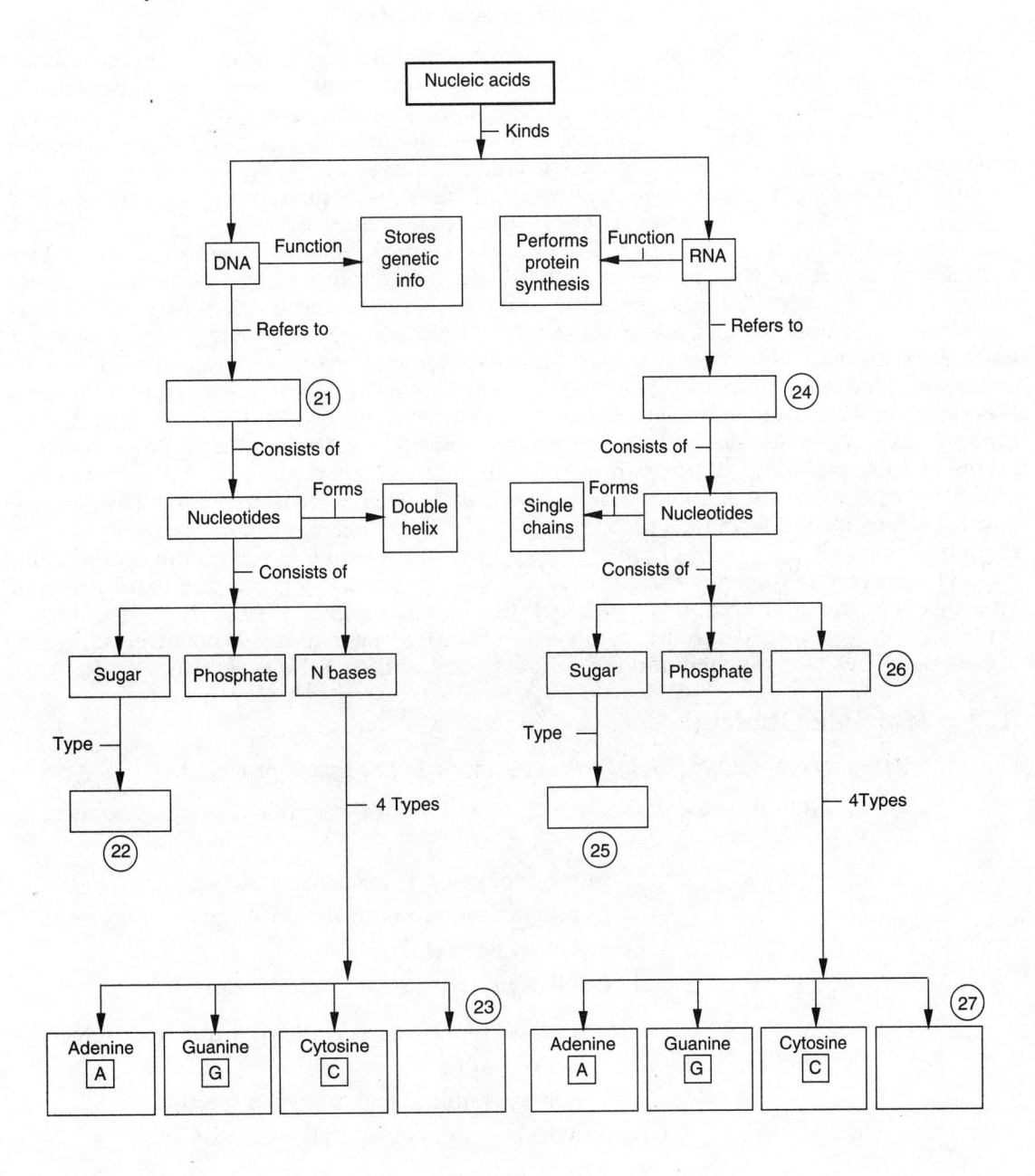

- Ribonucleic acid
- Uracil
- Deoxyribose
- Deoxyribonucleic acid
- Thymine
- N bases
- Ribose

28 Chapter 2 The Chemical Level of Organization

Body Trek:

Using the terms below, fill in the blanks to complete the trek through the chemical organization in the body.

Neutrons	Negatively	Isotope
Protons	Electrons	Molecule
Oxygen gas	Shells	Polar covalent
Nucleus	Double covalent bond	

Robo's task to monitor chemical activity begins with a trek outside the body. The robotic "engineers" have decided to place Robo in a cyclotron, an aparatus used in atomic research. Once inside the cyclotron, Robo's sensors immediately detect an environment that has negative particles called (28)_____, which are whirling around in cloud-like formations called (29) _____. The particles are travelling at a high rate of speed and appear to be circling stationary particles in a central region. This dense central region is called the (30) _____, and contains positively charged particles called (31) _____. With the exception of hydrogen in its natural state, all the central regions "observed" also contain particles which are neutral and are called (32) _____. Robo's electronic systems appear to be overloading and there is difficulty monitoring all the electrical acivity in the surrounding environment. Feedback to Mission Control reads, "Oops! There goes an atom that looks almost exactly like hydrogen, but it has two (2) neutrons rather than one." The substance is called deuterium and is chemically identified as a(n) (33) _____ of hydrogen. It is commonly used as a radioactive tracer in research laboratories. Robo next signals the presence of oxygen atoms. In the atmosphere these atoms are constantly in "search" of atoms of their own kind. When two of the atoms of oxygen come into contact with one another there is a chemical interaction between them with each atom equally sharing two pairs of electrons and forming a(n) (34) _____. This chemical union results in the formation of one (35) _____ of (36) _____. When a single oxygen atoms comes into contact with two hydrogen atoms a(n) (37) _____ bond is formed due to an unequal sharing of electrons. The result is a molecule in which the region around the oxygen atoms is (38) _____ charged and the region around the hydrogen atoms is positively charged. Robo's body trek is completed and the robot is retrieved from the cyclotron.

[L2] Multiple Choice:

Place the letter corresponding to the correct answer in the space provided.

_____ 39. Whether or not an atom will react with another atom will be determined primarily by the:

      a. number of protons present in the atom
      b. number of electrons in the outermost energy shell
      c. atomic weight of the atom
      d. number of neutrons and protons in the atom

_____ 40. The symbol 2H$_2$O means that two identical molecules of water are each composed of:

      a. 4 hydrogen atoms and 2 oxygen atoms
      b. 2 hydrogen atoms and 2 oxygen atoms
      c. 4 hydrogen atoms and 1 oxygen atom
      d. 2 hydrogen atoms and 1 oxygen atom

_____ 41. Lipid deposits are important as energy reserves because:

      a. they appear as fat deposits on the body
      b. they are readily broken down to release energy
      c. the energy released from lipids is metabolized quickly
      d. lipids provide twice as much energy as carbohydrates

Level 2 Concept Synthesis 29

_____ 42. Proteins differ from carbohydrates in that they:
    a. are not energy nutrients
    b. do not contain carbon, hydrogen, and oxygen
    c. always contain nitrogen
    d. are inorganic compounds

_____ 43. If an atom has an atomic number of 92 and its atomic weight is 238, how many protons does the atom have?
    a. 238
    b. 92
    c. 146
    d. 54

_____ 44. The atomic structure of hydrogen looks like which of the following?

a. (1 p+, 1 n) 1e⁻
b. (1 n) 2e⁻
c. (1 p+, 1 n) 2e⁻
d. (1 p+) 1e⁻

_____ 45. Which of the following selections represents the pH of the weakest acid?
    a. 8.0
    b. 2.0
    c. 3.2
    d. 6.7

_____ 46. The type of bond that has the most important effects on the properties of water and the shapes of complex molecules is the:
    a. hydrogen bond
    b. ionic bond
    c. covalent bond
    d. polar covalent bond

[L2] Completion:

Using the terms below, complete the following statements.

    peptide bond   hydrolysis   ionic bonds
    inorganic compounds   dehydration synthesis   alkaline

47. Electrical attraction between opposite charges produces a strong _____.
48. Small molecules held together partially or completely by ionic bonds are _____.
49. If the pH is above 7 with hydroxyl ions in the majority, the solution is _____.
50. The process that breaks a complex molecule into smaller fragments by the addition of a water molecule(s) is _____.
51. Glycogen, a branched polysaccharide composed of interconnected glucose molecules, is formed by the process of _____.
52. The attachment of a carboxylic acid group of one amino acid to the amino group of another forms a connection called a(n) _____.

30 Chapter 2 The Chemical Level of Organization

[L2] Short Essay:

Briefly answer the following questions in the spaces provided below.

53. Suppose an atom has 8 protons, 8 neutrons and 8 electrons. Construct a diagram of the atom and identify the subatomic particles by placing them in their proper locations.

54. In a water (H_2O) molelecule the unequal sharing of electrons creates a polar covalent bond. Why?

55. List the characteristics of water that make life possible.

56. List the four major classes of organic compounds found in the human body and give an example of each.

57. Using the four kinds of nucleotides that make up a DNA molecule, construct a model that will show the correct arrangement of the components which make up each nucleotide.

Level =2= **When you have succesfully completed the exercises in L2 proceed to L3.**

☐ LEVEL 3 CRITICAL THINKING/APPLICATION

Using principles and concepts learned in Chapter 2, answer the following questions. Write your answers on a separate sheet of paper.

1. Why might "baking soda" be used to relieve excessive stomach acid?
2. Using the glucose molecule ($C_6H_{12}O_6$), demonstrate your understanding of dehydration synthesis by writing an equation to show the formation of a molecule of sucrose ($C_{12}H_{22}O_6$).
3. Even though the recommended dietary intake for carbohydrates is 55-60 percent of the daily caloric intake, why do the carbohydrates account for less than 3 percent of our total body weight?
4. You are interested in losing weight so you decide to eliminate your intake of fats completely. You opt for a fat substitute such as Olestra, which contains compounds that cannot be used by the body. Why might this decision be detrimental to you?

CHAPTER 3

The Cellular Level of Organization: Cell Structure

■ Overview

Cells are highly organized basic units of structure and function in all living things. In the human body all cells originate from a single fertilized egg and additional cells are produced by the division of the preexisting cells. These cells become specialized in a process called differentiation, forming tissues and organs that perform specific functions. The "roots" of the study of anatomy and physiology are established by understanding the basic concepts of cell biology. This chapter provides basic principles related to the structure of cell organelles and the vital physiological functions that each organelle performs.

The following exercises relating to cell biology will reinforce your ability to learn the subject matter and to synthesize and apply the information in meaningful and beneficial ways.

☐ LEVEL 1   REVIEW OF CHAPTER OBJECTIVES

1. Discuss the basic concepts of the cell theory.
2. List the functions of the cell membrane and the structural features that enable it to perform those functions.
3. Describe the transport mechanisms that cells use to transport substances across the cell membrane.
4. Describe the organelles of a typical cell and indicate their specific functions.
5. Explain the functions of the cell nucleus.
6. Summarize the process of protein synthesis.
7. Describe the process of mitosis and explain its significance.
8. Define differentiation and explain its importance.

Level 1 Review of Chapter Objectives

[L1] Multiple Choice:

Place the letter corresponding to the correct answer in the space provided.

OBJ. 1 ____ 1. Which of the following is a part of the cell theory?
- a. Each cell maintains homeostasis.
- b. Cells are the smallest functioning units of life.
- c. New cells are produced by the division of preexisting cells.
- d. a, b, and c are correct

OBJ. 2 ____ 2. The outer boundary of the intracelluar material is called the:
- a. cytosol
- b. extracellular fluid
- c. cell membrane
- d. cytoplasm

OBJ. 2 ____ 3. The major components of the cell membrane are:
- a. carbohydrates, fats, proteins, water
- b. carbohydrates, lipids, ions, vitamins
- c. amino acids, fatty acids, carbohydrates, cholesterol
- d. phospholipids, proteins, cholesterol

OBJ. 2 ____ 4. Most of the communication between the interior and exterior of the cell occurs by way of:
- a. the phospholipid bilayer
- b. anchor proteins
- c. protein channels
- d. receptor proteins

OBJ. 3 ____ 5. The mechanism by which glucose can enter the cytoplasm without expending ATP energy is via:
- a. a carrier protein
- b. an anchor protein
- c. cilia
- d. recognition protein

OBJ. 3 ____ 6. All transport through the cell membrane can be classified as either:
- a. active or passive
- b. diffusion or osmosis
- c. pinocytosis or phagocytosis
- d. a and b are correct

OBJ. 4 ____ 7. The primary components of the cytoskeleton, which gives the cell strength and rigidity and anchors the position of major organelles are:
- a. microvilli
- b. microtubules
- c. microfilaments
- d. thick filaments

34 Chapter 3 The Cellular Level of Organization: Cell Structure

OBJ. 4 ____ 8. Approximately 95 percent of the energy needed to keep a cell alive is generated by the activity of the:
   a. mitochondria
   b. ribosomes
   c. nucleus
   d. microtubules

OBJ. 4 ____ 9. Nucleoli are nuclear organelles that:
   a. contain the chromosomes
   b. are responsible for producing DNA
   c. control nuclear operations
   d. synthesize the components of ribosomes

OBJ. 4 ____ 10. The three major functions of the endoplasmic reticulum (ER) are:
   a. hydrolysis, diffusion, osmosis
   b. detoxification, packaging, modification
   c. synthesis, storage, transport
   d. pinocytosis, phagocytosis, storage

OBJ. 4 ____ 11. The functions of the Golgi apparatus include:
   a. synthesis, storage, alteration, packaging
   b. isolation, protection, sensitivity, organization
   c. strength, movement, control, secretion
   d. neutralization, absorption, assimilation, secretion

OBJ. 5 ____ 12. Ribosomal proteins and RNA are produced primarily in the:
   a. nucleus
   b. nucleolus
   c. cytoplasm
   d. mitochondria

OBJ. 5 ____ 13. A sequence of three nitrogen bases can specify the identity of:
   a. a specific gene
   b. a single DNA molecule
   c. a single amino acid
   d. a specific peptide chain

OBJ. 7 ____ 14. The process where RNA polymerase uses the genetic information to assemble a strand of mRNA is:
   a. translation
   b. transcription
   c. initiation
   d. elongation

OBJ. 7 ____ 15. If the DNA triplet is TAG, the corresponding codon on the mRNA strand will be:
   a. AUC
   b. AGC
   c. ATC
   d. ACT

Level -1-

Level 1 Review of Chapter Objectives 35

OBJ. 7 ___ 16. The four stages of mitosis in correct sequence are:

  a. prophase, anaphase, metaphase, telophase
  b. prophase, metaphase, telophase, anaphase
  c. prophase, metaphase, anaphase, telophase
  d. prophase, anaphase, telophase, metaphase

OBJ. 8 ___ 17. The process of differentiation resulting in the appearance of characteristic cell specialization involves:

  a. irreversible alteration in protein structure
  b. the presence of an oncogene
  c. gene activation or repression
  d. the process of fertilization

[L1] Completion:

Using the terms below, complete the following statements:

gene	translation	nuclear pores	interphase
cytoskeleton	anaphase	ribosomes	phospholipid layer
nucleus	differentiation	cell theory	endocytosis

OBJ. 1 18. "Cells are the fundamental building blocks of life" is one concept in the _____.

OBJ. 2 19. Structurally, the cell membrane is called a(n) _____.

OBJ. 3 20. Intracellular membrane proteins are bound to a network of supporting filaments called the _____.

OBJ. 3 21. The packaging of extracellular materials in a vesicle at the cell surface for importation into the cell is called _____.

OBJ. 4 22. The cell organelles responsible for the synthesis of proteins using information provided by nuclear DNA are _____.

OBJ. 5 23. Chemical communication between the nucleus and cytosol occurs through the _____.

OBJ. 5 24. The organelle that determines the structural and functional characteristics of the cell is the _____.

OBJ. 6 25. Triplet codes needed to produce a specific peptide chain comprise the makeup of a(n) _____.

OBJ. 6 26. The construction of a functional polypeptide using the information provided by an mRNA strand is called _____.

OBJ. 7 27. Somatic cells spend the majority of their functional lives in a state known as _____.

OBJ. 7 28. The phase of mitosis in which the chromatid pairs separate and the daughter chromosomes move toward opposite end of the cells is _____.

OBJ. 8 29. The specialization process that causes a cell's functional abilities to become more restricted is called _____.

Chapter 3 The Cellular Level of Organization: Cell Structure

[L1] Matching:

Match the terms in column "B" with the terms in column "A." Use letters for answers in the spaces provided.

COLUMN "A"   COLUMN "B"

OBJ.	#	Column A		Column B
OBJ. 2	30.	Receptor proteins	A.	Protein "factories"
OBJ. 3	31.	Identifier proteins	B.	Carrier-mediated
OBJ. 3	32.	Active transport	C.	High concentration in cytosol
OBJ. 3	33.	Sodium ions	D.	DNA nitrogen base
OBJ. 3	34.	Potassium ions	E.	Chromosomes
OBJ. 4	35.	Ribosomes	F.	Nuclear division
OBJ. 4	36.	Golgi apparatus	G.	Major histocompatibility complex
OBJ. 5	37.	Nucleus	H.	RNA nitrogen base
OBJ. 5	38.	DNA strands	I.	Cell control center
OBJ. 6	39.	Thymine	J.	Cell specialization
OBJ. 6	40.	Uracil	K.	High concentration in extracellular fluid
OBJ. 7	41.	Mitosis	L.	Membrane turnover
OBJ. 8	42.	Differentiation	M.	Binds hormones

Level -1-

Level 1   Review of Chapter Objectives   37

[L1] Drawing/Illustration Labeling:

Identify each numbered structure by labeling the following figures:

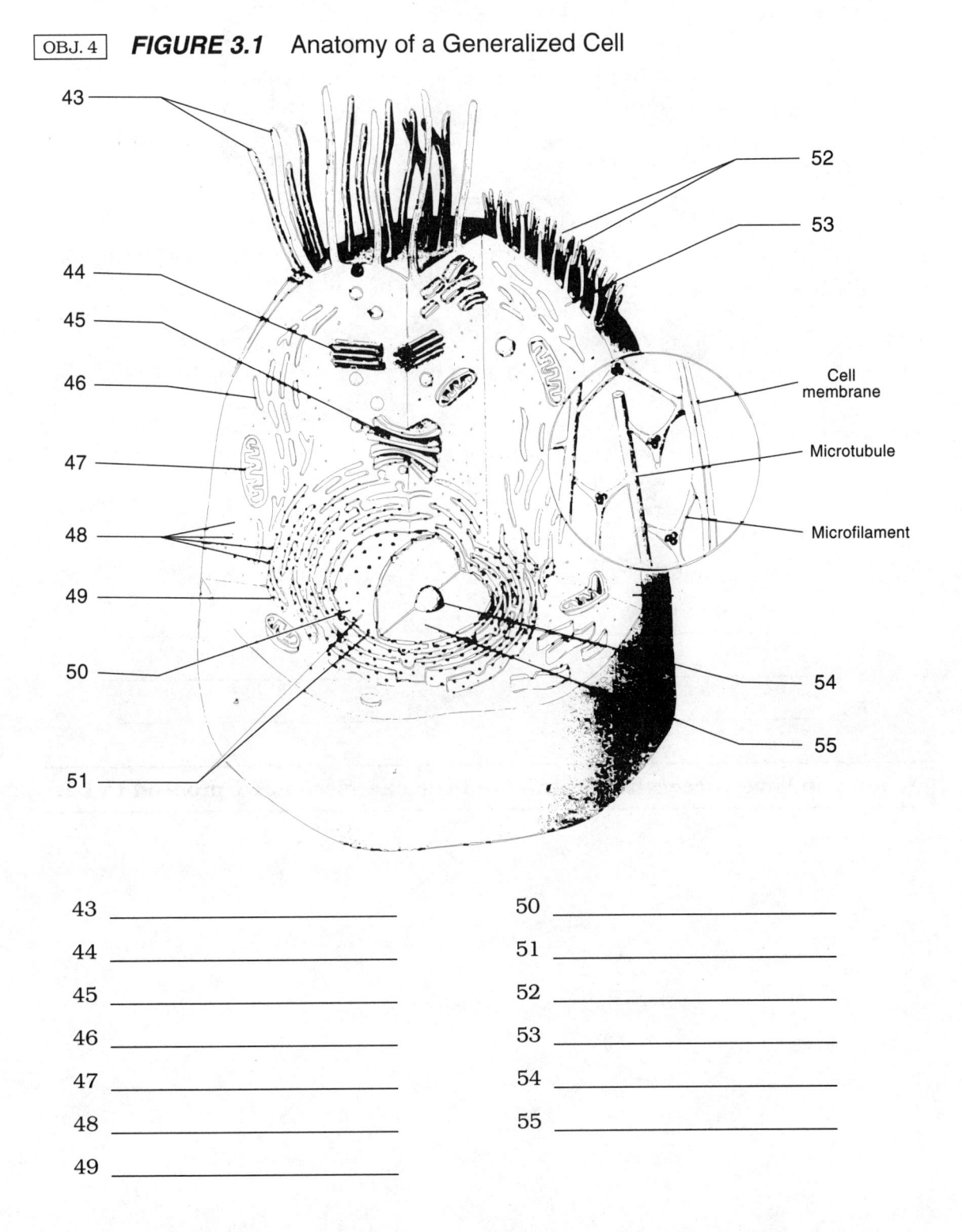

OBJ. 4   **FIGURE 3.1**   Anatomy of a Generalized Cell

43 _____	50 _____
44 _____	51 _____
45 _____	52 _____
46 _____	53 _____
47 _____	54 _____
48 _____	55 _____
49 _____	

38 Chapter 3   The Cellular Level of Organization: Cell Structure

OBJ. 10 **FIGURE 3.2**   The Stages of Mitosis

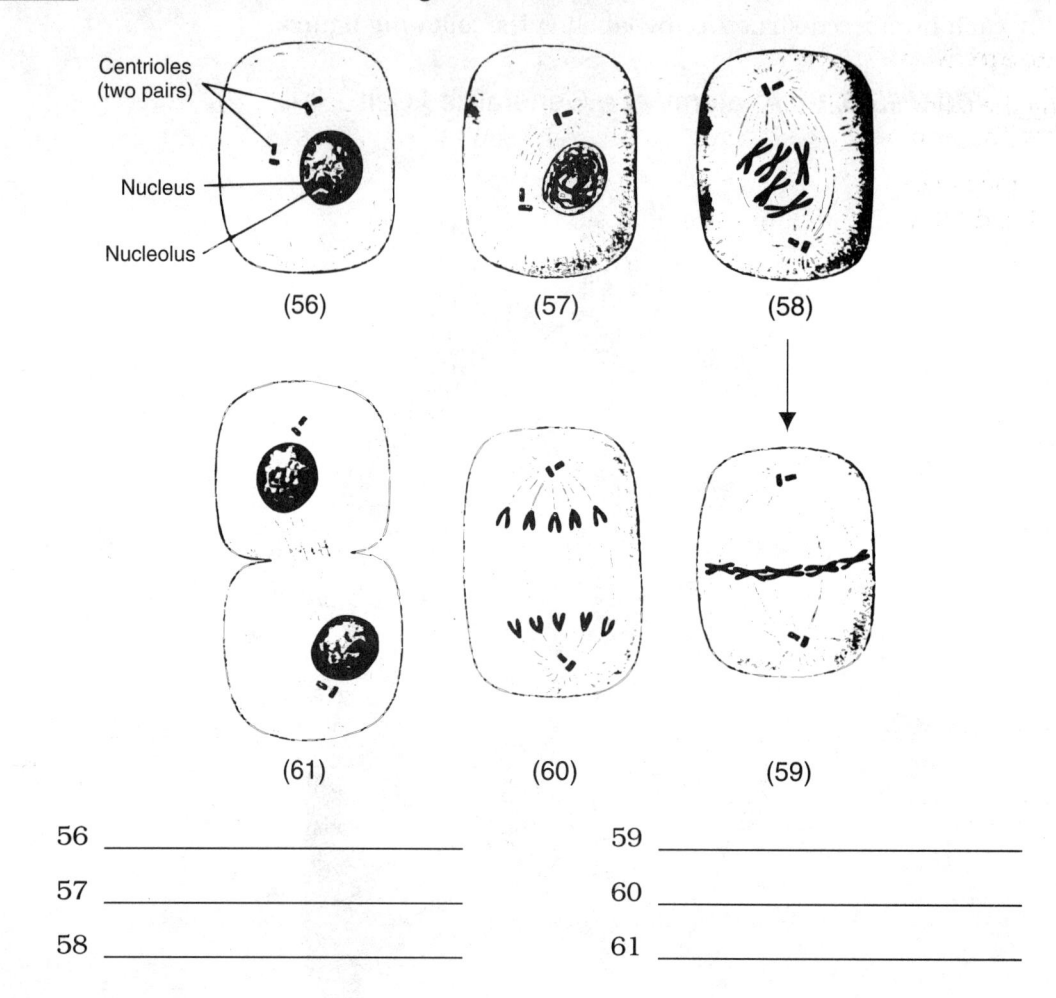

(56) — Centrioles (two pairs), Nucleus, Nucleolus

(57)

(58)

(61)

(60)

(59)

56 _____   59 _____
57 _____   60 _____
58 _____   61 _____

When you have successfully completed the exercises in L1 proceed to L2.

Level
-1-

LEVEL 2 CONCEPT SYNTHESIS

Concept Map I:

Using the following terms, fill in the numbered, blank spaces to complete the concept map. Follow the numbers which comply with the organization of the map.

- Ribosomes
- Nucleolus
- Membranous
- Centriole
- Lysosomes
- Lipid bilayer
- Proteins
- Organelles
- Fluid component

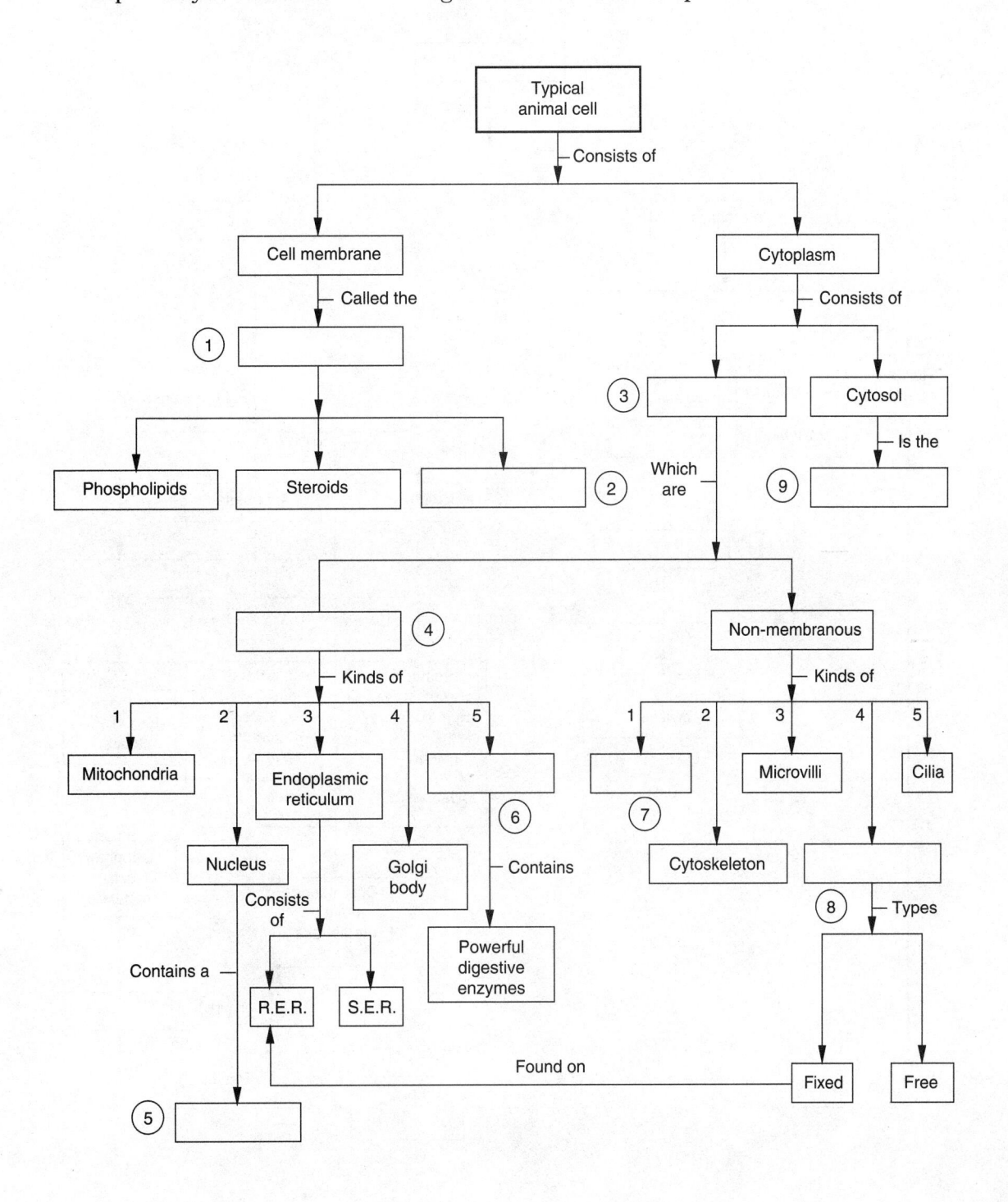

Chapter 3   The Cellular Level of Organization: Cell Structure

Concept Map II:

Using the following terms, fill in the numbered, blank spaces to complete the concept map. Follow the numbers which comply with the organization of the concept map.

Metaphase   Somatic cells   Telophase   Cytokinesis   Mitosis
DNA replication

Level 2 Concept Synthesis 41

Body Trek:

Using the terms below, fill in the blanks to complete the trek through the chemical organization of the human body.

Membrane proteins	Cell membrane	Matrix
ATP	Extracellullar fluid	Anchor proteins
Cell division	Endoplasmic reticulum	Cilia
Nucleoplasm	Golgi apparatus	Cristae
Intracellullar fluid	Organelles	Protein synthesis
Nucleus	Energy-producing enzymes	Protein synthesis
Mitochondria	Rough endoplasmic reticulum	
Chromosome	Ribosomes	Phospholipid
Channels	Nuclear envelope	Cytoskeleton
Nucleoli	Nuclear pores	

Robo is inhaled into the body via deep inspiration while its human host is sleeping. The micro-robot immediately lodges in the trachea among a group of pseudostratified, ciliated, columnar epithelial cells. Robo's initial maneuver is to get into a position for entry into one of the cells. The robot radios control command, "Might need a life jacket." There appears to be a watery "moat" around each cell, most likely the (16) _____. The robot's location seems to be in jeopardy because of the presence of small "finger-like" projections, the (17) _____, which are swaying back and forth and threatening to "wash" the robot farther down into the respiratory tract. The robot's mechanical arm extends and grabs hold of the outer boundary of a cell, the (18) _____. Robo is instructed to "look for" (19) _____ which form (20) _____ large enough for the robot to gain enty into the cell. As it passes through the opening, its chemical sensors pick up the presence of a (21) _____ bilayer with membrane proteins embedded in the membrane and (22) _____ attached to the inner membrane surface. Once inside, the trek through the cytosol or (23) _____ begins. Resistance to movement is greater inside the cell than outside because of the presence of dissolved materials. The first "observation" inside the cell is the presence of a protein framework, the (24) _____, which gives the cytoplasm strength and flexibility. Formed structures, the (25) _____, are in abundance, some attached and others freely floating in the cytosol. Structures such as the ribosomes, which are involved in (26) _____, and the centrioles, which direct strands of DNA during (27) _____, are noted quite easily as Robo treks through the cytosol. Small "cucumber-shaped" structures, the (28) _____, are "sighted;" however, the robot's entry capabilities are fully taxed owing to the unusual double membrane. After penetrating the outer membrane, an inner membrane containing numerous folds called (29) _____ block further entry. The inner membrane serves to increase the surface area exposed to the fluid contents or (30) _____. The presence of (31) _____, attached to folds would indicate that this is where the energy-storing molecule (32) _____ is generated. Robo senses the need for a quick "diffusion" through the outer membrane and back into the cytosol. The moving cytosol carries the micro-robot close to the center of the cell where it contacts the (33) _____, the control center of the cell. Robo is small enough to pass through tiny holes, the (34) _____, in the (35) _____ to gain entry into the structure. Once inside, the environment is awesome! Nuclear organelles called (36) _____ engage in activities which would indicate that they synthesize the components of the (37) _____ since RNA and ribosomal proteins are in abundance. The fluid content of the nucleus, the (38) _____ contains ions, enzymes, RNA, DNA, and their nucleotides. The DNA strands form complex structures called (39) _____, which contain information to synthesize thousands of different proteins and control the synthesis of RNA. Robo leaves the nucleus by way of the (40) _____ (ER). A portion of the ER, called the (41) _____, is responsible for the manufacture of proteins at specific sites along its surface. Some of the synthesized proteins are stored, while others will be transported via transport vesicles to the (42) _____, a system of flattened memrane discs. This structure functions in the synthesis and packaging of secretions and in cell membrane renewal. Robo's exit from the cell occurs through a secretory vesicle. The trek ends with the robot's entrance into the extracellular fluid and passage into the lumen of the trachea where it waits for a "cough" from its host to exit the respiratory tract and return to Mission Control.

Level =2=

[L2] Multiple Choice:

Place the letter corresponding to the correct answer in the space provided.

_____ 43. Isolating the cytoplasm from the surrounding fluid environment by the cell membrane is important because:

a. the cell organelles lose their shape if the membrane is destroyed
b. the nucleus needs protection to perform its vital functions
c. cytoplasm has a composition different from the extracellular fluid and the differences must be maintained
d. the cytoplasm contains organelles that need to be located in specific regions in order to function properly

_____ 44. Solutes cannot cross the lipid portion of a cell membrane because:

a. the lipid tails of phospholipid molecules will not associate with water molecules
b. most solutes are too large to get through the channels formed by membrane proteins
c. the heads are at the membrane surface and the tails are on the inside
d. communication between the interior of the cell and the extracellular fluid is cut off

_____ 45. Membranous organelles differ from nonmembranous organelles in that membranous organelles are:

a. always in contact with the cytosol
b. unable to perform functions essential to normal cell maintenance
c. usually found close to the nucleus of the cell
d. surrounded by lipid membranes that isolate them from the cytosol

_____ 46. The smooth ER (SER) has a variety of functions that center around the synthesis of:

a. lipids and carbohydrates
b. proteins and lipids
c. glycogen and proteins
d. carbohydrates and proteins

_____ 47. The reason lysosomes are sometimes called "cellular suicide packets" is:

a. the lysosome fuses with the membrane of other organelles
b. lysosomes fuse with endocytic vesicles with solid materials
c. the breakdown of lysosomal membranes can destroy a cell
d. lysosomes have structures which penetrate other cells

_____ 48. The energy-producing process in the mitochondria involves a series of reactions in which _____ is consumed and _____ is generated.

a. carbon dioxide; oxygen
b. water; oxygen
c. carbon dioxide; water
d. oxygen; carbon dioxide

Level 2   Concept Synthesis   43

_____ 49. The effect of diffusion in body fluids is that it:
   a. tends to increase the concentration gradient of the fluid
   b. tends to scatter the molecules and inactivate them
   c. tends to repel like charges and attract unlike charges
   d. tends to eliminate local concentration gradients

_____ 50. During osmosis water will always flow across a membrane toward the solution that has the:
   a. highest concentration of solvents
   b. highest concentration of solutes
   c. equal concentrations of solute
   d. equal concentrations of solvents

_____ 51. A solution that is hypotonic to cytoplasm has:
   a. a solute concentration lower than that of the cytoplasm
   b. a solute concentration higher than that of the cytoplasm
   c. a solute concentration that is equal to that of the cytoplasm
   d. an osmotic concentration higher than that of the intracellular fluid

_____ 52. Red blood cells are hemolyzed when the cells are placed in contact with:
   a. a hypotonic solution
   b. a hypertonic solution
   c. an isotonic solution
   d. a salt solution

_____ 53. One of the great advantages of moving materials by active transport is:
   a. carrier proteins are not necessary
   b. the process is not dependent on a concentration gradient
   c. the process has no energy cost
   d. a, b, and c are correct

_____ 54. The formation of a malignant tumor indicates that
   a. the cells are remaining within a connective tissue capsule
   b. the tumor cells resemble normal cells, but they are dividing faster
   c. mitotic rates of cells are no longer responding to normal control mechanisms
   d. metastasis is necessary and easy to control

[L2]   Completion:

Using the terms below, complete the following statements.

   cilia   microvilli   channels   diffusion
   isotonic   permeability   rough ER

55. Water molecules, small water-soluble compounds, and ions pass in and out of cells through _____.

56. Cells that are actively engaged in absorbing materials from the extracellular fluid, such as the cells of the digestive tract and the kidneys, contain cytoplasmic extensions called _____.

44 Chapter 3 The Cellular Level of Organization: Cell Structure

57. In the respiratory tract, sticky mucus and trapped dust particles are moved toward the throat and away from delicate respiratory surface because of the presence of _____.

58. Pancreatic cells that manufacture digestive enzymes contain an extensive _____.

59. The property that determines the cell membrane's effectiveness as a barrier is its _____.

60. A drop of ink spreading to color an entire glass of water demonstrates the process of _____.

61. If a solution has the same solute concentration as the cytoplasm and will not cause a net movement in or out of the cells, the solution is said to be _____.

[L2] Short Essay:

Briefly answer the following questions in the spaces provided.

62. Confirm your understanding of cell specialization by citing five (5) systems in the human body and naming a specialized cell found in each system.

63. List three (3) ways in which the cytosol differs chemically from the extracellular fluid.

64. What organelles would be necessary to construct a functional "typical" cell? (Assume the presence of cytosol and a cell membrane.)

65. What are the functional differences among centrioles, cilia, and flagella?

66. What two (2) major factors determine whether a substance can diffuse across a cell membrane?

Level 2

When you have successfully completed the exercises in L2 proceed to L3.

☐ LEVEL 3   CRITICAL THINKING/APPLICATION:

Using principles and concepts learned in Chapter 3, answer the following questions. Write your answers on a separate sheet of paper.

1. Using the principles of tonicity, explain why a lifeguard at an ocean beach will have more of a chance to save a drowning victim than a lifeguard at an inland freshwater lake.
2. One remedy for constipation is a saline laxative such as Epsom salts ($MgSO_4$). Why do such salts have a laxative effect?
3. In a hospital, a nurse gave a patient recovering from surgery a transfusion of 5% salt solution by mistake instead of a transfusion of physiological saline (0.9% salt). The patient almost immediately went into shock and soon after died. What caused the patient to enter into a state of shock?
4. If a prudent homemaker is preparing a tossed salad in the afternoon for the evening meal, the vegetables to be used will be placed in a bowl of cold water in order to keep these vegetables crisp. Osmotically speaking, explain why the vegetables remain crisp.

CHAPTER 4

The Tissue Level of Organization

■ Overview

Have you ever thought what it would be like to live on an island all alone? Your survival would depend on your ability to perform all the activities necessary to remain healthy and alive. In today's society surviving alone would be extremely difficult because of the important interrelationships and interdependence we have with others to support us in all aspects of life inherent in everyday living. So it is with individual cells in the multicellular body.

Individual cells of similar structure and function join together to form groups called tissues, which are identified on the basis of their origin, location, shape, and function. Many of the tissues are named according to the organ system in which they are found or the function which they perform such as neural tissue in the nervous system, muscle tissue in the muscular system or connective tissue that is involved with the structural framework of the body and supporting, surrounding, and interconnecting other tissue types.

The activities in Chapter 4 introduce the discipline of histology, the study of tissues, with emphasis on the four primary types: epithelium, connective, muscle, and nervous tissue. The questions and exercises are designed to help you organize and conceptualize the interrelationships and interdependence of individual cells that extend to the tissue level of cellular organization.

☐ LEVEL 1   REVIEW OF CHAPTER OBJECTIVES

1. Identify the four major tissues of the body and their roles.
2. Describe the types and functions of epithelial cells.
3. Describe the relationship between form and function for each epithelial type.
4. Compare the structures and functions of the various types of connective tissues.
5. Explain how epithelial and connective tissues combine to form four different types of membranes and specify the functions of each.
6. Describe the three types of muscle tissue and the special structural features of each type.
7. Discuss the basic structure and role of neural tissue.
8. Explain how tissues respond in a coordinated manner to maintain homeostasis.
9. Describe how aging affects tissues of the body.

[L1] Multiple Choice:

Place the letter corresponding to the correct answer in the space provided.

OBJ. 1 ____ 1. The four primary tissue types found in the human body are:
- a. squamous, cuboidal, columnar, glandular
- b. adipose, elastic, reticular, cartilage
- c. skeletal, cardiac, smooth, muscle
- d. epithelial, connective, muscle, neural

OBJ. 2 ____ 2. The type of tissue that covers exposed surfaces and lines internal passageways and body cavities is:
- a. muscle
- b. neural
- c. epithelial
- d. connective

OBJ. 2 ____ 3. The two types of layering recognized in epithelial tissues are:
- a. cuboidal and columnar
- b. squamous and cuboidal
- c. columnar and stratified
- d. simple and stratified

OBJ. 3 ____ 4. A single layer of epithelium covering a basement membrane is termed:
- a. simple epithelium
- b. stratified epithelium
- c. squamous epithelium
- d. cuboidal epithelium

OBJ. 3 ____ 5. Simple epithelial cells are characteristic of regions where:
- a. mechanical or chemical stresses occur
- b. support and flexibility are necessary
- c. padding and elasticity are necessary
- d. secretion and absorption occur

OBJ. 3 ____ 6. From a surface view, cells that look like fried eggs laid side by side are:
- a. squamous epithelium
- b. simple epithelium
- c. cuboidal epithelium
- d. columnar epithelium

OBJ. 3 ____ 7. Stratified epithelium has several cell layers above the basement membrane and is usually found in areas where:
- a. secretion and absorption occur
- b. mechanical or chemical stresses occur
- c. padding and elasticity are necessary
- d. storage and secretion occur

48 Chapter 4   The Tissue Level of Organization

OBJ. 3 ____ 8. Cells that form a neat row with nuclei near the center of each cell and that appear square in typical sectional views are:
   a. stratified epithelium
   b. squamous epithelium
   c. cuboidal epithelium
   d. columnar epithelium

OBJ. 3 ____ 9. The major structural difference between columnar epithelia and cuboidal epithelia is that the columnar epithelia:
   a. are hexagonal and the nuclei are near the center of each cell
   b. consist of several layers of cells above the basement membrane
   c. are thin and flat and occupy the thickest portion of the membrane
   d. are taller and slender and the nuclei are crowded into a narrow band close to the basement membrane

OBJ. 3 ____ 10. Simple squamous epithelium would be found in the following areas of the body:
   a. urinary tract and inner surface of circulatory system
   b. respiratory surface of lungs
   c. lining of body cavities
   d. a, b, and c are correct

OBJ. 3 ____ 11. Glandular epithelia contain cells that produce:
   a. exocrine secretions only
   b. exocrine or endocrine secretions
   c. endocrine secretions only
   d. secretions released from goblet cells only

OBJ. 4 ____ 12. The three basic components of all connective tissues are:
   a. free exposed surface, exocrine secretions, endocrine secretions
   b. fluid matrix, cartilage, osteocytes
   c. specialized cells, extracellular protein fibers, ground substance
   d. satellite cells, cardiocytes, osteocytes

OBJ. 4 ____ 13. The three classes of connective tissue based on structure and function are:
   a. fluid, supporting, and connective tissue proper
   b. cartilage, bone, and blood
   c. collagenic, reticular, and elastic
   d. adipose, reticular, and ground

OBJ. 4 ____ 14. The two major cell populations found in connective tissue proper are:
   a. fibroblasts and adipocytes
   b. mast cells and lymphocytes
   c. melanocytes and mesenchymal cells
   d. fixed cells and wandering cells

Level -1-

Level 1   Review of Chapter Objectives   49

OBJ. 4   ____ 15. Most of the volume in loose connective tissue is made up of:
    a. elastic fibers
    b. ground substance
    c. reticular fibers
    d. collagen fibers

OBJ. 4   ____ 16. The major purposes of adipose tissue in the body are:
    a. strength, flexibility, elasticity
    b. support, connection, conduction
    c. padding, cushioning, insulating
    d. absorption, compression, lubrication

OBJ. 4   ____ 17. The three major subdivisions of the extracellular fluid in the body are:
    a. blood, water, and saliva
    b. plasma, interstitial fluid, and lymph
    c. blood, urine, and saliva
    d. spinal fluid, cytosol, and blood

OBJ. 4   ____ 18. The two types of supporting connective tissue found in the body are:
    a. regular and irregular connective tissue
    b. collagen and reticular fibers
    c. proteoglycans and chondrocytes
    d. cartilage and bone

OBJ. 4   ____ 19. The three major types of cartilage found in the body are:
    a. collagen, reticular, and elastic
    b. regular, iregular, and dense
    c. hyaline, elastic, and fibrocartilage
    d. interstitial, appositional and calcified

OBJ. 4   ____ 20. The pads that lie between the vertebrae if the vertebral column contain:
    a. elastic fibers
    b. fibrocartilage
    c. hyaline cartilage
    d. bone

OBJ. 4   ____ 21. One difference between bone and cartilage is that:
    a. bone is highly vascular while cartilage is not
    b. bone repairs easily while cartilage does not
    c. oxygen demand is high in bone while it is low in cartilage
    d. a, b, and c are correct

OBJ. 5   ____ 22. Membranes which are associated with cavities that lack a direct opening to the outside are:
    a. serous membranes
    b. mucous membranes
    c. cutaneous membranes
    d. synovial membranes

| OBJ. 5 | ____ 23. The mucous membranes that are lined by simple epithelia perform the functions of:
  a. digestion and circulation
  b. respiration and excretion
  c. absorption and secretion
  d. a, b, and c are correct

| OBJ. 6 | ____ 24. Muscle tissue has the ability to:
  a. provide a framework for communication within the body
  b. carry impulses from one part of the body to another
  c. cover exposed surfaces of the body
  d. contract and produce active movement

| OBJ. 6 | ____ 25. The three types of muscle tissue found in the body are:
  a. elastic, hyaline, fibrous
  b. striated, nonstriated, fibrous
  c. voluntary, involuntary, nonstriated
  d. skeletal, cardiac, smooth

| OBJ. 7 | ____ 26. Neural tissue is specialized to:
  a. contract and produce movement
  b. carry electrical impulses from one part of the body to another
  c. provide structural support and fill internal spaces
  d. line internal passageways and body cavities

| OBJ. 7 | ____ 27. Structurally, neurons are unique because they are the only cell in the body that have:
  a. lacunae and canaliculi
  b. axons and dendrites
  c. satellite cells and neuroglia
  d. soma and stroma

| OBJ. 8 | ____ 28. The restoration of homeostasis after an injury involves two related processes, which are:
  a. necrosis and fibrous
  b. infection and immunization
  c. inflammation and regeneration
  d. isolation and reconstruction

| OBJ. 8 | ____ 29. Inflammation at an injury site produces the following responses:
  a. redness, warmth, and swelling
  b. bleeding, clotting, healing
  c. necrosis, fibrosis, scarring
  d. hematoma, shivering, retraction

| OBJ. 9 | ____ 30. One of the major effects of aging on connective tissues is:
  a. it becomes thinner and the individual bruises easily
  b. cartilage and bone soften and lose the ability to provide support
  c. cartilage becomes stiffer and less resilient and bones become brittle
  d. it becomes thicker and the tissue becomes harder

Level 1 Review of Chapter Objectives 51

[L1] Completion:

Using the terms below, complete the following statements.

areolar	exocytosis	infection	stratified epithelium
skeletal	mucous	osteoporosis	collagen
neuroglia	gap junction	connective	

OBJ. 1 31. The type of tissue that fills internal spaces is _____.

OBJ. 2 32. The type of tissue that makes up the surface of the skin is _____.

OBJ. 3 33. The junctional type that prevents the passage of water and solutes between cells is the _____.

OBJ. 3 34. In merocrine secretion, the product is released through the process of _____.

OBJ. 4 35. The most common fibers in connective tissue proper are _____ fibers.

OBJ. 4 36. The least specialized connective tissue in the adult body is _____.

OBJ. 5 37. The type of membrane that lines the digestive tract is _____.

OBJ. 6 38. The only type of muscle tissue that is under voluntary control is _____.

OBJ. 7 39. Neural tissue contains several different kinds of supporting cells called _____.

OBJ. 8 40. An inflammation resulting from a pathogen is known as a(n) _____.

OBJ. 8 41. The age-related reduction in bone strength in some women is known as _____.

[L1] Matching:

Match the terms in column "B" with the terms in column "A." Use letters for answers in the spaces provided.

	COLUMN "A"	COLUMN "B"
OBJ. 1 ___	42. Histology	A. Connect muscle to bone
OBJ. 2 ___	43. Covering epithelium	B. Connect bone to bone
OBJ. 2 ___	44. Glandular epithelium	C. Voluntary
OBJ. 3 ___	45. Microvilli	D. Repair process
OBJ. 4 ___	46. Tendons	E. Low dietary calcium levels
OBJ. 4 ___	47. Ligaments	F. Wandering cells
OBJ. 4 ___	48. Fibroblasts	G. Intercellular junction
OBJ. 4 ___	49. Mast cells	H. Epidermis
OBJ. 5 ___	50. Synovial membrane	I. Absorption
OBJ. 6 ___	51. Muscle tissue	J. Dendrites
OBJ. 6 ___	52. Skeletal muscle	K. Movement
OBJ. 7 ___	53. Synapse	L. Fixed cells
OBJ. 7 ___	54. Neuron	M. Exocrine
OBJ. 8 ___	55. Regeneration	N. Found in certain joints
OBJ. 9 ___	56. Osteoporosis	O. Study of tissues

52 Chapter 4 The Tissue Level of Organization

[L1] Drawing/Illustration Labeling:

Identify each numbered structure by labeling the following figures:

OBJ. 2 **FIGURE 4.1** Types of Epithelium

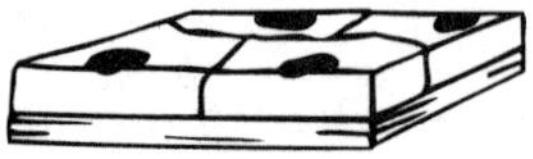

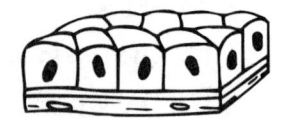

57 _____

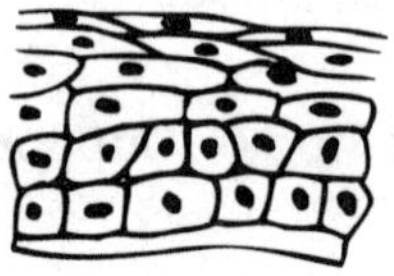

58 _____

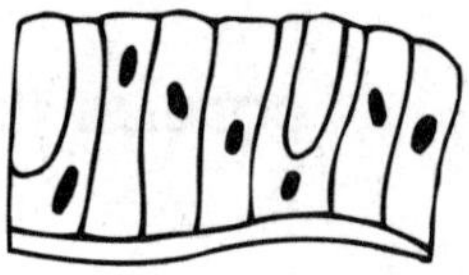

59 _____

60 _____

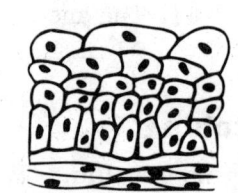

61 _____

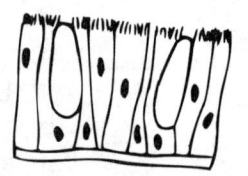

62 _____

Level 1 Review of Chapter Objectives 53

OBJ. 4 **FIGURE 4.2** Types of Connective Tissue

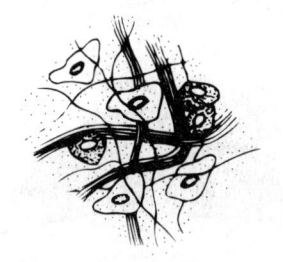

63 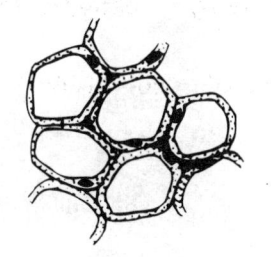 _____ 64 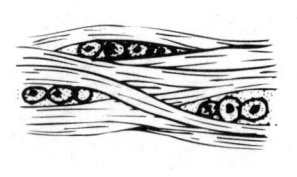 _____ 65 _____

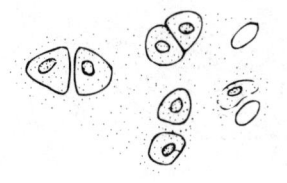

66 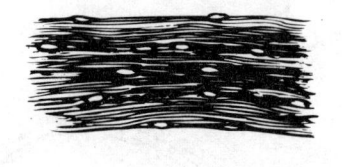 _____ 67 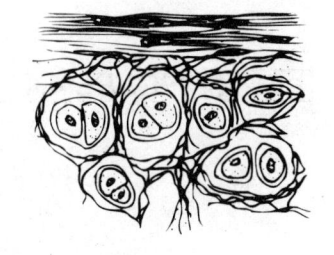 _____ 68 _____

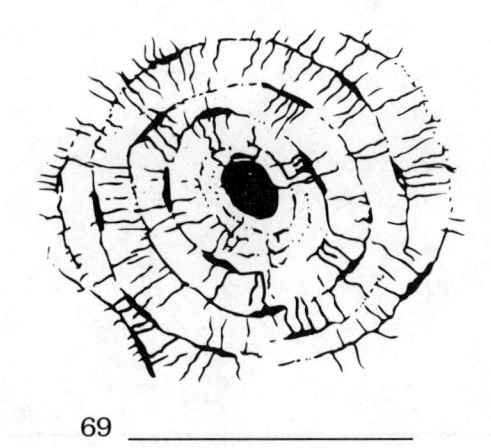

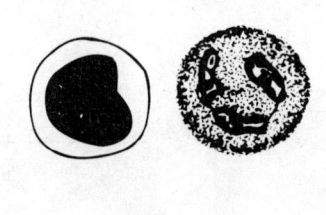

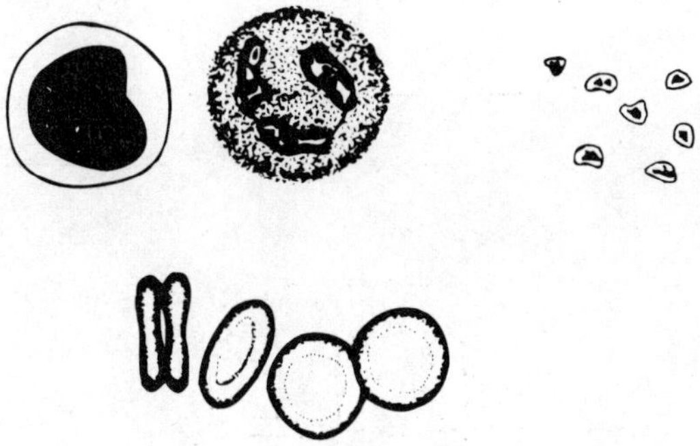

69 _____ 70 _____

54   Chapter 4   The Tissue Level of Organization

OBJ. 6   **FIGURE 4.3**   Types of Muscle Tissue

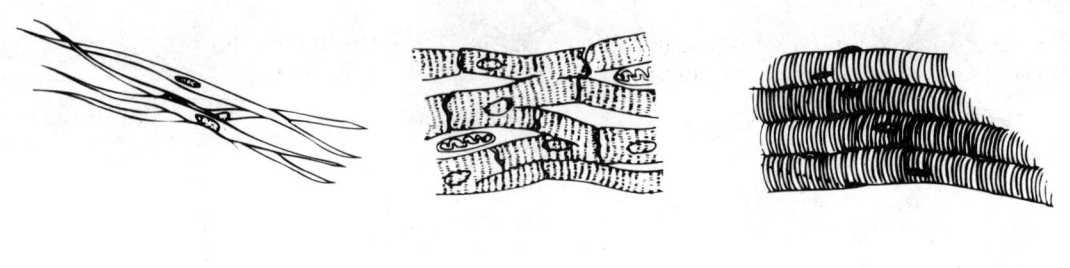

71 _____   72 _____   73 _____

OBJ. 7   **FIGURE 4.4**   Type of Nervous Tissue.

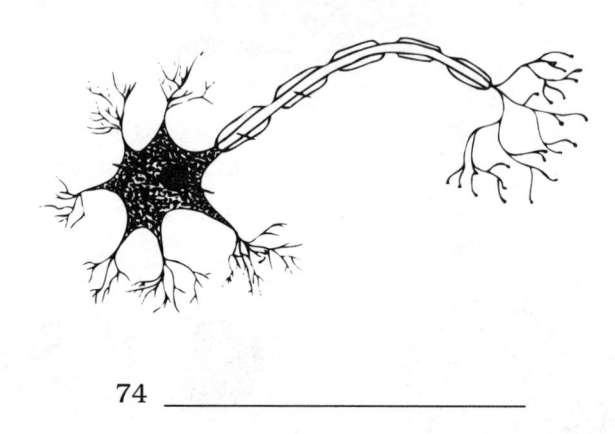

74 _____

When you have successfuly completed the exercises in L1 proceed to L2.

LEVEL 2 CONCEPT SYNTHESIS

Concept Map I:

Using the following terms fill in the numbered blank spaces to complete the concept map. Follow the numbers that comply with the organization of the map.

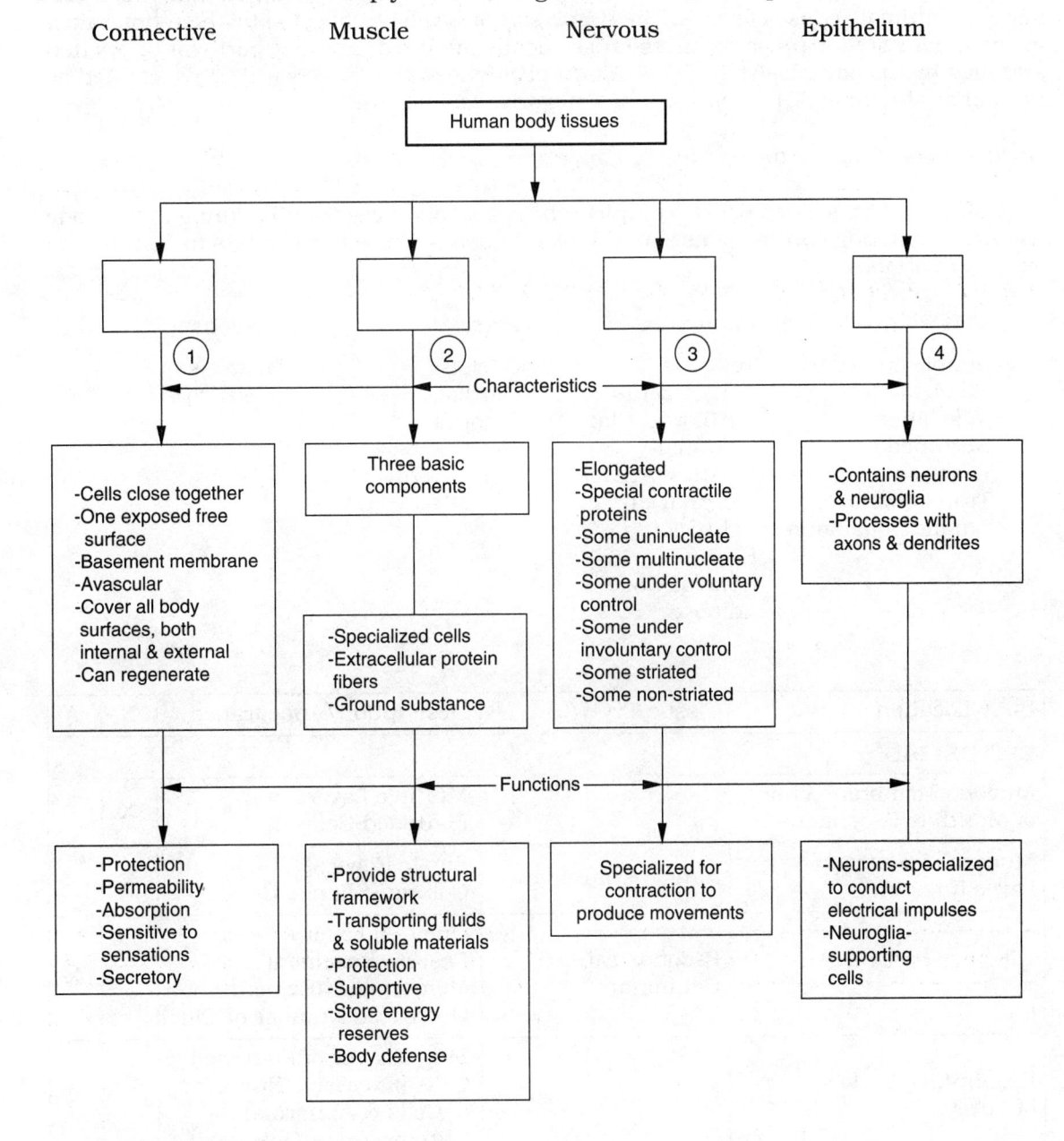

Connective   Muscle   Nervous   Epithelium

```
                    Human body tissues
                          |
    ┌─────────────┬───────┴───────┬─────────────┐
   (1)           (2)             (3)           (4)
            ←──────── Characteristics ────────→
```

Box 1 (Epithelium characteristics):
- Cells close together
- One exposed free surface
- Basement membrane
- Avascular
- Cover all body surfaces, both internal & external
- Can regenerate

Box 2 (Connective characteristics):
- Three basic components
- Specialized cells
- Extracellular protein fibers
- Ground substance

Box 3 (Muscle characteristics):
- Elongated
- Special contractile proteins
- Some uninucleate
- Some multinucleate
- Some under voluntary control
- Some under involuntary control
- Some striated
- Some non-striated

Box 4 (Nervous characteristics):
- Contains neurons & neuroglia
- Processes with axons & dendrites

←──────── Functions ────────→

Box 1 Functions (Epithelium):
- Protection
- Permeability
- Absorption
- Sensitive to sensations
- Secretory

Box 2 Functions (Connective):
- Provide structural framework
- Transporting fluids & soluble materials
- Protection
- Supportive
- Store energy reserves
- Body defense

Box 3 Functions (Muscle):
- Specialized for contraction to produce movements

Box 4 Functions (Nervous):
- Neurons-specialized to conduct electrical impulses
- Neuroglia-supporting cells

56 Chapter 4 The Tissue Level of Organization

Body Trek:

To complete the body trek to study tissues, the micro-robot will be used in an experimental procedure by a pathologist to view and collect tissue samples from a postmortem examination. Robo is equipped with a mini camera to scan body cavities and organs and will use its tiny arm with a blade to retrieve tissue samples for study. The procedure avoids the necessity of severe invasive activity but allows a complete "tissue autopsy" to determine the ultimate cause of death. The tissue samples will be collected by the robot, taken to the laboratory for preparation, microscopically analyzed, and a report will be written and filed by the pathologist and you. All descriptions of the tissues will be designated as normal or abnormal. The report will be categorized as follows:

Body location; tissue type; description/appearance; N; A.

Using the terms listed below, complete the report on pages 54–55 relating to the body tissues by entering your responses in the blank spaces. The letter N refers to normal; the letter A to abnormal.

Epithelia	*Connective*	*Muscle*	*Nervous*
Simple cuboidal	Tendons;	Skeletal	Neurons;
Trachea mucosa (ciliated)	Ligaments	Cardiac	Neuroglia
Stratified squamous	Cardiovascular system	Smooth	
Transitional	Elastic cartilage		
Simple Squamous	External ear; Epiglottis		
	Hyaline cartilage		
	Bone or Osseus		
	Adipose		

Body Location	Tissue Type	Description/Appearance	N	A
EPITHELIAL				
Mucous Membrane Lining of Mouth & Esophagus	(5)	Multiple Layers of Flattened Cells	X	
Mucosa of Stomach & Large Intestine	Simple Columnar	Single Rows of Column-Shaped Cells	X	
(6)	Pseudostratified Columnar	One Cell Layer – Cells Rest on Basement Membrane – (Evidence of Decreased Number of Cilia)		X
Respiratory Surface of Lungs	(7)	Single Layer of Flattened Cells (Excessive Number of Cells & Abnormal Chromosomes Observed)		X
Collecting Tubules of Kidney	(8)	Cube-Shape Neat Row of Single Cells	X	
Membrane Lining of Urinary Bladder	(9)	Cells with Ability to Slide Over One Another, Layered Appearance	X	

Level 2

Body Location	Tissue Type	Description/Appearance	N	A
CONNECTIVE				
Subcutaneous Tissue; Around Kidneys; Buttocks, Breasts	(10)	Closely Packed Fat Cells	X	
Widely Distributed Packages Organs; Forms Basement Membrane of Epithelial	Areolar (loose)	Three Types of Fibers; Many Cell Types	X	
(11)	Dense Fibrous	Fibroblasts in Matrix, Parallel Collagenic and Elastin Fibers	X	
Ends of Long Bones; Costal Cartilages of Ribs; Support Nose, Trachea, Larynx	(12)	Chondrocytes in Lacunae, Groups 2-4 Cells	X	
Intervertebral Disks Disks of Knee Joints	(13)	Chondrocytes in Lacunae, Dense arrangement of Fibers	X	
External Ear, Epiglottis	(14)	Chondrocytes in Lacunae Ligaments of Elastin Fibers	X	
Skeleton	(15)	Osteocytes in Lacunae, Well-Vascularized	X	
(16)	Blood	Liquid – Plasma RBCs, WBCs, Platelets	X	
MUSCLE				
Attached to Bones	(17)	Long; Cylindrical; Multinucleate	X	
Heart Wall	(18)	Cardiocytes; Intercalated Disks	X	
Walls of Hollow Organs;	(19)	Nonstriated; Uninucleate	X	
NERVOUS				
Brain; Spinal Cord; Peripheral Nervous System	Nervous	(20)	X	

This report confirms that death was due to metaplasia and anaplasia caused by excessive smoking. The cancer tumor cells in the lungs had extensive abnormal chromosomes.

[L2] Multiple Choice:

Place the letter corresponding to the correct answer in the space provided.

_____ 21. If epithelial cells are classified according to their cell shape, the classes would include:
- a. simple, stratified, pseudostratified
- b. squamous, cuboidal, columnar
- c. simple, squamous, stratified
- d. pseudostratified, stratified, columnar

_____ 22. Epithelial cells are differentiated from the other tissue types because they:
- a. always have a free surface exposed to the environment or to some internal chamber or passageway
- b. have few extracellular materials between adjacent epithelial cells
- c. do not contain blood vessels
- d. a, b, and c are correct

_____ 23. Certain epithelial cells are called pseudostratified columnar because:
- a. they have a layered appearance but all the cells contact the basement membrane
- b. they are stratified and all the cells do not contact the basement membrane
- c. their nuclei are all located the same distance from the cell surface
- d. they are a mixture of cell types

_____ 24. The two fluid connective tissues found in the human body are:
- a. mucous and matrix
- b. blood and lymph
- c. ground substance and hyaluronic acid
- d. collagen and plasma

_____ 25. During a weight loss program when nutrients are scarce, adipocytes:
- a. differentiate into mesenchymal cells
- b. are normally destroyed and disappear
- c. tend to enlarge and eventually divide
- d. deflate like collapsing balloons

_____ 26. Mucous membranes would be found primarily in the following systems:
- a. skeletal, muscular, endocrine, circulatory
- b. integumentary, lymphatic, nervous, endocrine
- c. digestive, respiratory, reproductive, urinary
- d. skeletal, lymphatic, circulatory, muscular

_____ 27. The pleura, peritoneum, and pericardium are examples of:
- a. mucous membranes
- b. body cavities
- c. visceral organs
- d. serous membranes

_____ 28. In contrast to serous or mucous membranes, the cutaneous membrane is:
    a. thin, permeable to water, and usually moist
    b. lubricated by goblet cells found in the epithelium
    c. thick, relatively waterproof, and usually dry
    d. enclosed by a fibrous connective capsule.

_____ 29. Of the following, the one that best defines inflammation is:
    a. the secretion of histamine to increase blood flow to the injured area
    b. a defense which involves the coordinated activities of several tissues
    c. a restoration process to heal the injured area
    d. the stimulation of macrophages to defend injured tissue

[L2] Completion:

Using the terms below, complete the following statements.

| endocrine | tight junctions | mucous | desmosomes |
| serous | exocrine | exfoliation | avascular |

30. Epithelium and cartilage, which lack a direct blood supply, are _____.
31. Glands of the female breast, which function to produce milk, are examples of a(n) _____ gland.
32. Hormone secretions produced by the pituitary gland are an example of a(n) _____ gland.
33. Cells of the epidermis adhere to one another due to their connection by _____.
34. Cells in which the outermost of the lipid layers of the cell membranes have fused are connected by _____.
35. Parotid salivary glands produce a watery fluid known as a(n) _____ secretion.
36. Sublingual salivary glands produce a thick fluid known as a(n) _____ secretion.
37. The process where cells are shed from an epithelial surface is called _____.

[L2] Short Essay:

Briefly answer the following questions in the spaces provided below.

38. Briefly descibe the four (4) primary tissue types in the body.

39. Summarize the four (4) essential functions of epithelium.

60 Chapter 4 The Tissue Level of Organization

40. What is the functional difference between microvilli and cilia on the exposed surfaces of epithelium tissue?

41. How do the processes of merocrine, apocrine and holocrine secretions differ?

42. What basic components are found in all connective tissues?

43. Describe the three basic types of fibers found in connective tissue.

44. What four (4) kinds of membranes consisting of epithelium and connective tissues that cover and protect other structures and tissues are found in the body?

45. Describe the three (3) types of muscle tissue found in the body.

46. What two types of cell populations make up nervous tissue, and what is the primary function of each type?

When you have successfully completed the exercises in L2 proceed to L3.

LEVEL 3   CRITICAL THINKING/APPLICATION

Using the principles and concepts learned about the tissue level of organization, answer the following questions. Write your answers on a separate sheet of paper.

1. Suppose you work in a hospital laboratory as a specialist in the Histology department. How do you perceive yourself as being an important part of a team of Allied Health Professionals involved in health care?
2. Exocrine glands secrete products that reach the surface by means of excretory ducts. What exocrine glands are found in the integumentary and digestive systems?
3. Why is the bacterium *Staphylococcus aureus* particularly dangerous when infection occurs in the connective tissues of the body?
4. The knee joint is quite susceptible to injury involving the tearing of cartilage pads within the knee joint. In most cases, why is surgery needed?

CHAPTER 5

The Integumentary System

■ Overview

The integumentary system consists of the skin and associated structures including hair, nails, and a variety of glands. The four primary tissue types making up the skin comprise what is considered to be the largest structurally integrated organ system in the human body.

Because the skin and its associated structures are readily seen by others, a lot of time is spent caring for the skin, to enhance its appearance and prevent skin disorders that may alter desirable structural features on and below the skin surface. The integument manifests many of the functions of living matter, including protection, excretion, secretion, absorption, synthesis, storage, sensitivity, and temperature regulation. Studying the important structural and functional relationships in the integument provides numerous examples which demonstrate patterns that apply to tissue interactions in other organ systems.

☐ LEVEL 1 REVIEW OF CHAPTER OBJECTIVES

1. Describe the main structural features of the integumentary system.
2. Describe the main structural features of the epidermis and explain their functional significance.
3. Explain what accounts for individual and racial differences in skin, such as skin color.
4. Describe how the integumentary system helps to regulate body temperature.
5. Discuss the effects of ultraviolet radiation on the skin and the role played by melanocytes.
6. Discuss the functions of the skin's accessory structures.
7. Explain the mechanisms that produce hair and determine hair texture and color.
8. Explain how the skin responds to injury and repairs itself.
9. Summarize the effects of the aging process on the skin.

Level 1 Review of Chapter Objectives 63

[L1] Multiple Choice:

Place the letter corresponding to the correct answer in the space provided.

OBJ. 1 ___ 1. The two functional components of the integument include:
   a. dermis and epidermis
   b. hair and skin
   c. cutaneous membrane and accessory structures
   d. keratin and melanocytes

OBJ. 1 ___ 2. Which of the following is a function of the integumentary system?
   a. sensory reception
   b. protection
   c. temperature regulation
   d. a, b and are correct

OBJ. 2 ___ 3. The layers of the epidermis, beginning with the deepest layer and proceeding outwardly, include the stratum:
   a. corneum, granulosum, spinosum, germinativum
   b. granulosum, spinosum, germinativum, corneum
   c. spinosum, germinativum, corneum, granulosum
   d. germinativum, spinosum, granulosum, corneum

OBJ. 2 ___ 4. The layers of the epidermis where mitotic divisions occur are:
   a. germinativum and spinosum
   b. corneum and germinativum
   c. spinosum and corneum
   d. mitosis occurs in all the layers

OBJ. 2 ___ 5. For a cell to move from the stratum germinivatum to the stratum corneum, it takes approximately:
   a. 6 to 8 weeks
   b. 5 to 7 days
   c. 8 to 10 weeks
   d. 2 to 4 weeks

OBJ. 3 ___ 6. Differences in skin color between individuals and races reflect disinct:
   a. numbers of melanocytes
   b. melanocyte distribution patterns
   c. levels of melanin synthesis
   d. U.V. responses and nuclear activity

OBJ. 3 ___ 7. The two basic factors interacting to produce skin color are:
   a. sunlight and ultraviolet radiation
   b. the presence of carotene and melanin
   c. melanocyte production and oxygen supply
   d. circulatory supply and pigment concentration and composition

64 Chapter 5 The Integumentary System

[OBJ. 4] ____ 8. When the body temperature becomes abnormally high, thermoregulatory homeostasis is maintained by:
   a. an increase in sweat gland activity and blood flow to the skin
   b. a decrease in blood flow to the skin and sweat gland activity
   c. an increase in blood flow to the skin and a decrease in sweat gland activity
   d. an increase in sweat gland activity and a decrease in blood flow to the skin

[OBJ. 5] ____ 9. Skin exposure to small amounts of ultraviolet radiation serves to:
   a. produce a tan that is beneficial to the skin
   b. convert a steroid related to cholesterol into vitamin D
   c. induce growth of cancerous tissue in the skin
   d. induce melanocyte production

[OBJ. 6] ____ 10. The two major components of the dermis are:
   a. capillaries and nerves
   b. dermal papillae and a subcutaneous layer
   c. sensory receptors and accessory structures
   d. papillary and deep reticular layers

[OBJ. 6] ____ 11. From the following selections, choose the one that identifies what the dermis contains to communicate with other organ systems.
   a. blood vessels
   b. lymphatics
   c. nerve fibers
   d. a, b, and c are correct

[OBJ. 6] ____ 12. Special smooth muscles in the dermis that, when contracted, produce "goose bumps" are called:
   a. tissue papillae
   b. arrector pili
   c. root sheaths
   d. cuticular papillae

[OBJ. 6] ____ 13. Accessory structures of the skin include:
   a. dermis, epidermis, subcutaneous layer
   b. cutaneous and subcutaneous layers
   c. hair follicles, sebaceous and sweat glands
   d. a, b, and c are correct

[OBJ. 6] ____ 14. Nail production occurs at the epithelial fold not visible from the surface called the:
   a. nail bed
   b. cuticle
   c. nail root
   d. lunula

[OBJ. 7] ____ 15. Hair production occurs in the:
   a. reticular layers of the dermis
   b. papillary layer of the dermis
   c. cutaneous layer
   d. stratum germinativum of the epidermis

Level -1-

OBJ. 7 ___ 16. Except for red hair, the natural factor responsible for varying shades of hair color is:
   a. number of melanocytes
   b. amount of carotene production
   c. the type of pigment present
   d. a, b, and c

OBJ. 8 ___ 17. Excessive exposure of the skin to U.V. radiation may cause redness, edema, blisters, and pain. The presence of blisters classifies the burn as:
   a. first degree
   b. second degree
   c. third degree
   d. fourth degree

OBJ. 8 ___ 18. The immediate response by the skin to an injury is:
   a. bleeding occurs and mast cells trigger an inflammatory response
   b. the epidermal cells are immediately replaced
   c. fibroblasts in the dermis create scar tissue
   d. the formation of a scab

OBJ. 8 ___ 19. The practical limit to the healing process of the skin is the formation of inflexible, fibrous, noncellular:
   a. scabs
   b. skin grafts
   c. ground substance
   d. scar tissue

OBJ. 9 ___ 20. Dangerously high body temperatures occur sometimes in the elderly due to:
   a. reduction in the number of Langerhans cells
   b. decreased blood supply to the dermis
   c. decreased sweat gland activity
   d. b and c are correct

OBJ. 9 ___ 21. A factor which causes increased skin damage and infection in the elderly is:
   a. decreased sensitivity of the immune system
   b. decreased vitamin D production
   c. a decline in melanocyte activity
   d. a decline in glandular activity

OBJ. 9 ___ 22. Hair turns gray or white due to:
   a. a decline in glandular activity
   b. a decrease in the number of immune system cells
   c. decreased melanocyte activity
   d. decreased blood supply to the dermis

66 Chapter 5 The Integumentary System

[L1] Completion:

Using the terms below, complete the following statements.

follicle	skin	cyanosis	sebaceous glands
glandular	menanocyte	stratum corneum	sebum
dermal blood supply	stratum lucidum	melanin	decrease

OBJ. 1   23. Specialized glands of the _____ in the female breast produce milk.

OBJ. 2   24. In areas where the skin is thick, such as the palms of the hands and the soles of the feet, the cells are flattened, densely packed, and opaque in color. This layer is called the _____.

OBJ. 2   25. Keratin, a fibrous protein, would be found primarily in the _____.

OBJ. 3   26. The peptide secreted by the pituitary gland which increases the rate of melanin synthesis is _____.

OBJ. 4   27. If the body temperature drops below normal, heat is conserved by a(n) _____ in the diameter of dermal blood vessels.

OBJ. 5   28. The pigment which absorbs ultraviolet radiation before it can damage mitochondrial DNA is _____.

OBJ. 6   29. The secretion which lubricates and inhibits the growth of bacteria on the skin is called _____.

OBJ. 7   30. Hair follicles are often associated with _____.

OBJ. 7   31. Hair develops from a group of epidermal cells at the base of a tube-like depression called a(n) _____.

OBJ. 8   32. During a sustained reduction in circulatory supply, the skin takes on a bluish coloration called _____.

OBJ. 9   33. In older Caucasians, the skin becomes very pale because of a decline in _____ activity.

OBJ. 9   34. In older adults, dry and scaly skin is usually a result of a decrease in _____ activity.

[L1] Matching:

Match the terms in column "B" with the terms in column "A." Use letters for answers in the spaces provided.

                                                                                 COLUMN "A"   COLUMN "B"

OBJ. 1   ____ 35. Adipose tissue   A. Vitamin D

OBJ. 2   ____ 36. Epidermis   B. Second degree burn

OBJ. 3   ____ 37. Melanin   C. Thinning hair

OBJ. 4   ____ 38. Thermoregulation   D. Sweat glands

OBJ. 5   ____ 39. Ultraviolet radiation   E. Nails

OBJ. 6   ____ 40. Accessory structures   F. Loss of elastic fibers

OBJ. 6   ____ 41. Dermis   G. Blood vessel and nerve supply

OBJ. 7   ____ 42. Inactive follicle   H. Stratified squamous epithelium

OBJ. 8   ____ 43. Blisters   I. Skin pigment

OBJ. 9   ____ 44. Wrinkles   J. Subcutaneous

Level -1-

Level 1 Review of Chapter Objectives 67

[L1] Drawing/Illustration Labeling:

Identify each numbered structure by labeling the following figure:

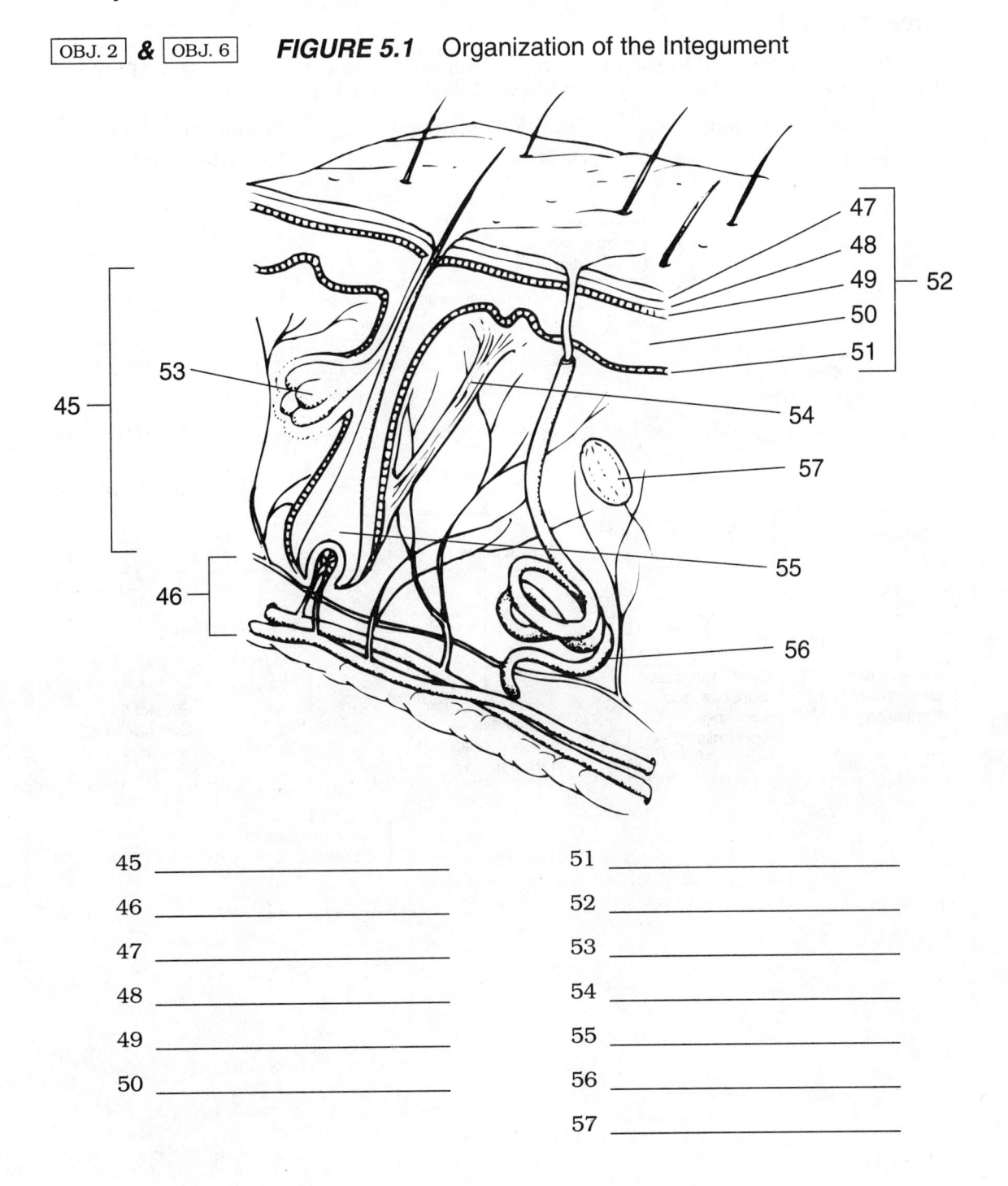

OBJ. 2 & OBJ. 6   **FIGURE 5.1** Organization of the Integument

45 _____	51 _____
46 _____	52 _____
47 _____	53 _____
48 _____	54 _____
49 _____	55 _____
50 _____	56 _____
	57 _____

When you have successfully completed the exercises in L1 proceed to L2.

Chapter 5 The Integumentary System

☐ LEVEL 2 CONCEPT SYNTHESIS

Concept Map I:

Using the terms below, fill in the numbered, blank spaces to complete the concept map. Follow the numbers which comply with the organization of the map.

- Sensory reception
- Lubrication
- Vitamin D synthesis
- Dermis
- Produce secretions
- Exocrine glands

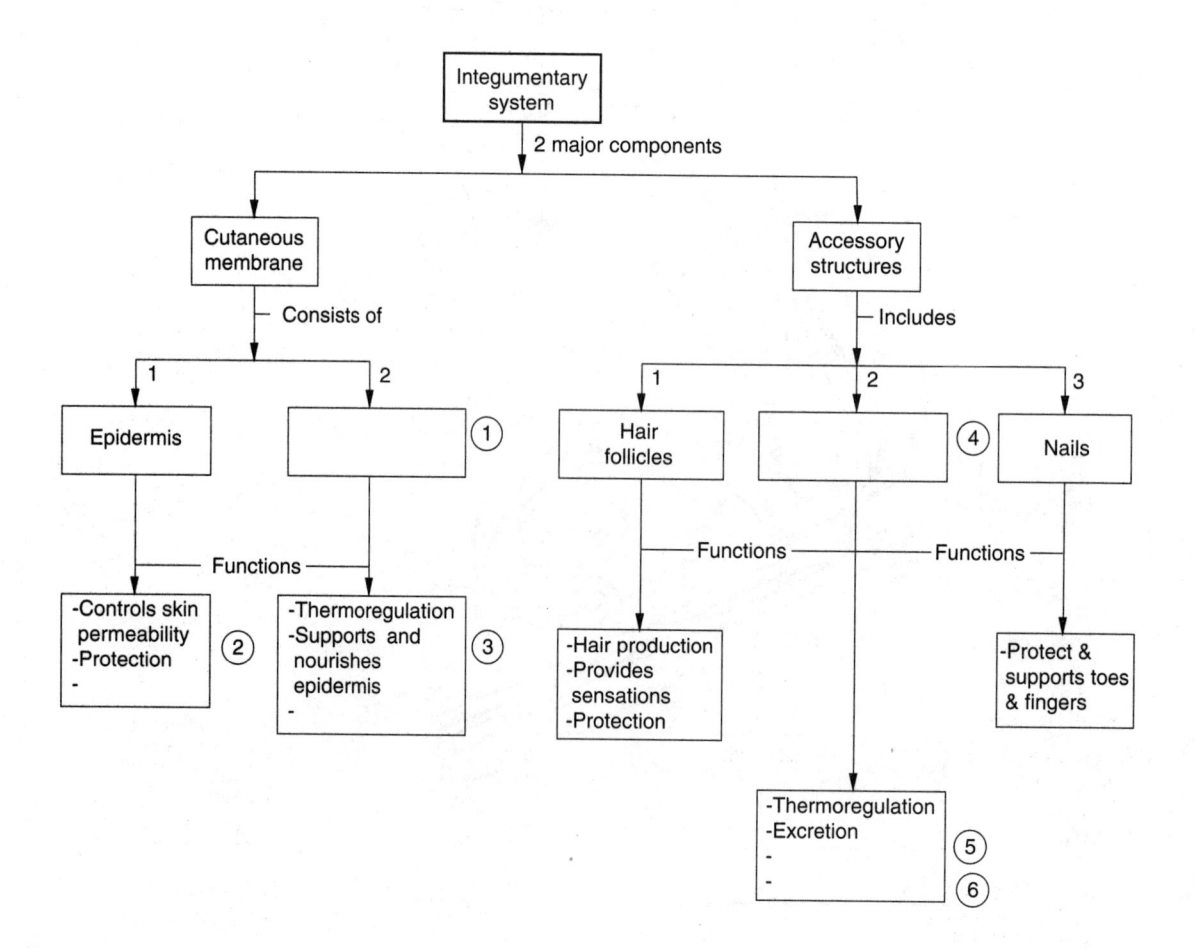

Concept Map II:

Using the terms below, fill in the numbered, blank spaces to complete the concept map. Follow the numbers which comply with the organization of the map.

- Nerves
- Fat
- Epidermis
- Connective tissue
- Collagen
- Granulosum
- Skin
- Papillary Layer

Concept map structure:

- Integument — Is the — (7) _____
- (7) Consists of:
  - Cutaneous membrane — 2 components:
    - (8) _____ — Consists of — Stratified squamous Epithelium — composed of four layers (deepest to surface):
      - Stratum germinivatum
      - Stratum spinosum
      - Stratum _____ (9)
      - Stratum corneum
    - Dermis — 2 regions:
      - Superficial — Called — (10) _____
      - Deeper — Reticular layer
    - Consists of:
      - Loose, connective tissue capillaries & _____ (11)
      - Dense connective tissue, & _____ fibers (12)
  - Subcutaneous layer — Consists of:
    - Loose, _____ tissue and (13) _____ cells (14)
    - Area used for — Subcutaneous injections

Level 2

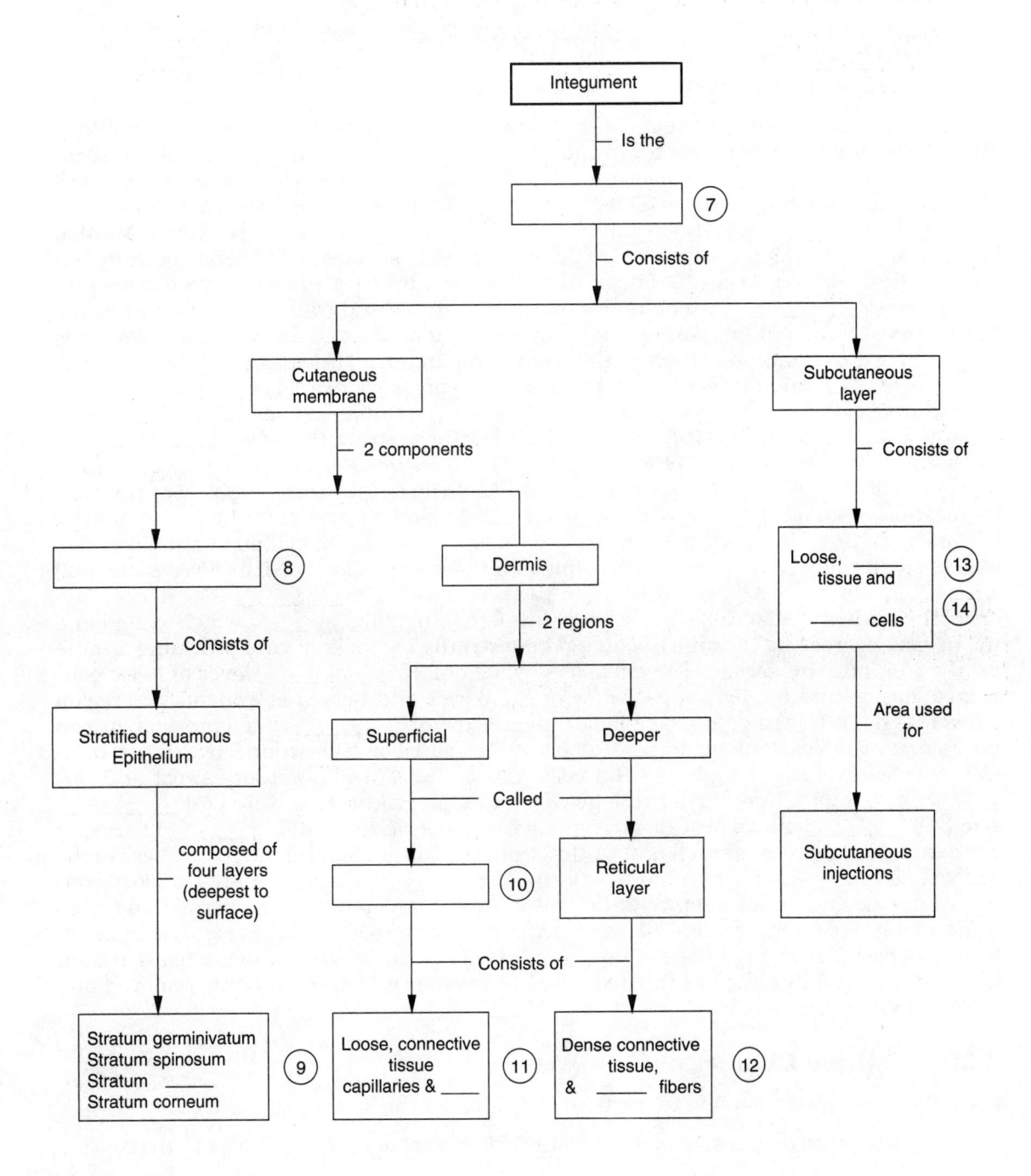

70 Chapter 5 The Integumentary System

Body Trek:

Using the terms below, fill in the blanks to complete the trek through the integument.

Stratum lucidum	Stratum granulosum	Sebaceous
Collagen	Desmosomes	Epidermal ridges
Mitosis	Papillary	Cuticle
Elastin	Stratum spinosum	Keratin
Dermal papillae	Lunula	Subcutaneous
Stratum germinativum	Reticular layer	

The body trek begins as the micro-robot is placed on the nail body of the thumbnail. Turning around and advancing toward the proximal end of the nail plate, a pale crescent known as the (15) _____ comes into view. This area serves as the "entrance" to a part of the stratum corneum which is folded and extends over the exposed nail nearest the root, forming the (16) _____. Robo expresses confusion as the message relayed to Mission Control says, "I thought I would be trekking on a living surface, but I sense nothing but layers of dead, flattened cells." A chemical analysis confirms the presence of a fibrous protein called (17) _____, which makes the cells durable and water resistant and allows them to exist for about two weeks until they are shed or washed away. Robo treks along the "dead" surface until it arrives at the palm of the hand, a "thick" area of the skin. The robot's descent is carefully controlled because of the presence of a "glassy" (18) _____, a clear layer of flattened, densely packed cells. Robo continues his descent and arrives at "grainy" layers of cells, the (19) _____. Below these strata the layers are several cells thick and bound together by (20) _____. Some of the cells act as if they are in the process of dividing. Due to the arrangement and activity of these cells, Robo confirms that its location is the (21) _____. The deeper Robo probes, the more lively the activity becomes. In the deepest stratum of the epidermis, the dominant cell population consists of actively dividing cells which are replenishing those strata above. This layer is the (22) _____, which are actively involved in the process of (23) _____. The deeper layers of the epidermis that Robo has trekked through form (24) _____ which extend into the dermis, increasing the area of contact between the two regions and providing a route for the trek into the dermis. The dermis consists of a (25) _____ layer of loose connective tissue, and the first appearance of capillaries and nerves is evident. The region derives its name from nipple-shaped mounds called (26) _____ which project between the epidermal ridges. Probing deeper, Robo senses an area of dense connective tissue, bundles of collagen fibers, lymphatics, fat cells, muscle cells, and accessory sweat and (27) _____ glands. These structures give rise to a layer known as the (28) _____. The (29) _____ fibers provide strength, while the scattered (30) _____ fibers give the dermis the ability to stretch and contract during normal movements. The fibers of the deepest dermal layer are continuous with the (31) _____ layer, an area of loose connective tissue and an abundance of fat cells. Sensory receptors in the dermal and deep epidermal layers interfere with Robo's movements and the search for an exit is imminent. Mission Control instructs Robo to find a hair follicle on the dorsal side of the hand, mount the hair shaft, and proceed to the distal end of the hair where the robot is removed and re-energized for the next trek.

[L2] Multiple Choice:

Place the letter corresponding to the correct answer in the space provided.

_____ 32. Third degree burns differ from first and second degree burns in that:

    a. the epidermis, dermis, and subcutaneous layers are destroyed

    b. they are more painful

    c. fluid accumulates between the dermis and epidermis

    d. the burn is restricted to the superficial layers of the skin

Level 2   Concept Synthesis   71

_____ 33. Nails on the fingers and toes function in which of the following ways:

    a. protect the exposed finger or toe tip
    b. limit the distortion of the finger or toe tip during mechanical stress
    c. allows a better grasp of objects
    d. a, b and c are correct

_____ 34. Wounds are classified as open or closed. From the following choices, select the one which does not include only open wounds.

    a. abrasions, avulsions, incisions, lacerations
    b. lacerations, incisions, avulsions, contusions
    c. punctures, abrasions, incisions, avulsions
    d. avulsions, lacerations, incisions, punctures

_____ 35. Because freshwater is hypotonic to body fluids, sitting in a freshwater bath causes:

    a. water to leave the epidermis and dehydrate the tissue
    b. water from the interstitial fluid to penetrate the surface and evaporate
    c. water to enter the epidermis and cause the epithelial cells to swell
    d. complete cleansing because the bacteria on the surface drown

_____ 36. As a person ages, the sensitivity of the immune component of their integumentary system decreases due to which of the following?

    a. the skin thins and becomes more susceptible to infections
    b. the number of Langerhans cells declines
    c. the skin is more easily damaged
    d. a, b and c are correct

_____ 37. The integumentary system is responsible for synthesizing vitamin D. Vitamin D, in turn, is essential to the skeletal system for which of the following reasons?

    a. for excretion of certain hormones in the urine
    b. for excretion of acidic ions in the urine
    c. for calcium absorption from the digestive system
    d. for normal clotting of integumentary blood vessels

_____ 38. Which of the following cells is responsible for triggering an inflammation reaction in the skin?

    a. mast cells
    b. melanocytes
    c. macrophages
    d. a and c are correct

Chapter 5 The Integumentary System

[L2] Completion:

Using the terms below, complete the following statements.

    Epidermal ridges   Malignant melanomas   Melanocytes
    Liposomes   Lipid-soluble carriers   Dandruff

39. _____ are responsible for the whorl patterns known as "fingerprints."
40. Drugs administered via _____ are capable of penetrating the skin.
41. _____ containing DNA fragments have been used experimentally to alter the cell membranes of skin cancer cells.
42. The type of skin cancer that occurs due to malignancies and metastacies of the melanocytes is _____.
43. The condition known as albinism occurs when _____ are incapable of producing normal amounts of pigment.
44. Excessive shedding of cells from the outer layer of the skin is known as _____.

[L2] Short Essay:

Briefly answer the following questions in the spaces provided below.

45. A friend says to you, "Don't worry about what you say to her; she is thick-skinned." Anatomically speaking, what areas of the body would your friend be referring to? Why are these areas thicker?

46. A hypodermic needle is used to introduce drugs into the loose connective tissue of the subcutaneous layer. Beginning on the surface of the skin in the region of the thigh, list, in order, the layers of tissue the needle would penetrate to reach the hypodermis.

47. The general public associates a tan with good health. What is wrong with this assessment?

48. Many shampoo advertisements list the ingredients, such as honey, kelp extracts, beer, vitamins and other nutrients as being beneficial to the hair. Why could this be considered false advertisement?

When you have successfully completed the exercises in L2 proceed to L3.

☐ LEVEL 3 CRITICAL THINKING/APPLICATION

Using principles and concepts learned about the integumentary system, answer the following questions. Write your answers on a separate sheet of paper.

1. Even though the stratum corneum is water resistant, it is not waterproof. When the skin is immersed in water, osmotic forces may move water in or out of the epithelium. Long-term exposure to seawater endangers survivors of a shipwreck by accelerating dehydration. How and why does this occur?
2. A young Caucasian girl is frightened during a violent thunderstorm during which lightning strikes nearby. Her parents notice that she is pale, in fact, she has "turned white." Why has her skin color changed to this "whitish" appearance?
3. Someone asks you, "Is hair really important to the human body?" What responses would you give to show the functional necessities of hair?
4. Individuals who participate in endurance sports must continually provide the body with fluids. Explain why this is necessary.
5. Why do calluses form on the palms of the hands when doing manual labor?
6. Bacterial invasion of the superficial layers of the skin is quite common. Why is it difficult to reach the underlying connective tissues? (Cite at least six (6) features of the skin that help protect the body from invasion by bacteria.)

CHAPTER 6

The Skeletal System

■ Overview

The human skeletal system is composed of 206 bones, which can be grouped into two major subdivisions: the axial and the appendicular skeletons. These names indicate the location and major function of the subdivisions. The axial skeleton consists of 80 individual bones and provides the human body with its primary vertical axis. It consists of the skull, vertebral column and the thoracic cage. The appendicular skeleton, on the other hand, consists of 126 bones and includes not only the two arm and two leg appendages but also the groups of bones which provide attachment of the appendages to the axial skeleton. These attachments include the pectoral and pelvic girdles.

This chapter includes a wide variety of information on the structural and functional aspects of the skeletal system, including the microscopic structure of osseous, or bone, material; the developmental processes which form bones; the study of the individual bones and their marking of the axial and appendicular skeletons; and the joints which articulate the bones of the skeleton.

☐ LEVEL 1   REVIEW OF CHAPTER OBJECTIVES

1. Describe the functions of the skeletal system.
2. Compare the structures and functions of compact and spongy bones.
3. Discuss the processes by which bones develop and grow and account for variations in their internal structure.
4. Describe the remodeling and repair of the skeleton and discuss homeostatic mechanisms responsible for regulating mineral deposition and turnover.
5. Name the components of the axial and appendicular skeletons and their functions.
6. Identify the bones of the skull.
7. Discuss the differences in structure and function of the various vertebrae.
8. Relate the structural differences between the pectoral and pelvic girdles to their various functional roles.
9. Distinguish among different types of joints and link structural features to joint functions.
10. Describe the dynamic movements of the skeleton and the structure of representative articulations.
11. Explain the relationship between joint structure and mobility, using specific examples.
12. Discuss the functional relationships between the skeletal system and other body systems.

[L1] Multiple Choice:

Place the letter corresponding to the correct answer in the space provided.

OBJ. 1 _____ 1. The function(s) of the skeletal system is (are) that:
   a. it is a storage area for calcium and lipids
   b. it is involved in blood cell formation
   c. it provides structural support for the body
   d. a, b, and c are correct

OBJ. 1 _____ 2. Storage of lipids that represent an important energy reserve in bone occur in areas of:
   a. red marrow
   b. yellow marrow
   c. bone matrix
   d. a, b, and c are correct

OBJ. 2 _____ 3. Mature bone cells found in lacunae are called:
   a. osteoblasts
   b. osteocytes
   c. osteoclasts
   d. stem cells

OBJ. 2 _____ 4. One of the basic histological differences between compact bone and spongy bone is that in compact bone:
   a. the basic functional unit is the Haversian system
   b. osteocytes are not present
   c. there are plates called trabeculae present
   d. osteons are not present

OBJ. 2 _____ 5. Spongy bone, unlike compact bone, resembles a network of bony plates separated spaces that are normally filled with:
   a. osteocytes
   b. lacunae
   c. bone marrow
   d. lamella

OBJ. 2 _____ 6. Spongy bone is found primarily at the _____ of long bones.
   a. bone surfaces, except inside joint capsules
   b. the epiphyses of long bones, where they articulate with other skeletal elements
   c. axis of the diaphysis
   d. exterior region of the bone shaft to withstand forces applied at either end

OBJ. 2 _____ 7. Compact bone is usually found where:
   a. bones are not heavily stressed
   b. stresses arrive from many directions
   c. trabeculae are aligned with extensive crossbracings
   d. stresses arrive from a limited range of directions

76 Chapter 6 The Skeletal System

OBJ. 3 ___ 8. The process during which bones begin development as cartilage models and the cartilage is later replaced by bone is called:
   a. intramembranous ossification
   b. endochondral ossification
   c. articular ossification
   d. secondary ossification

OBJ. 3 ___ 9. On the diaphysis side of the epiphyseal plate is the:
   a. location of the secondary ossification centers
   b. region where collagen fibers are being added to the osteons
   c. region where cartilage is being replaced by bone
   d. location where osteoblasts are being produced

OBJ. 3 ___ 10. The bony skeleton begins to form about _____ after fertilization, and usually does not stop growing until about age _____.
   a. 6 weeks; 25
   b. 3 weeks; 18
   c. 10 weeks; 20
   d. 3 months; 30

OBJ. 3 ___ 11. The process of replacing other tissue with bone is called
   a. calcification
   b. ossification
   c. remodeling
   d. b and c are correct

OBJ. 4 ___ 12. Of the following selections the one that best describes a homeostatic mechanism of the skeleton is:
   a. as new bone forms through the activity of osteoblasts, older bone is destroyed by osteoclasts
   b. mineral absorption from the mother's blood stream during prenatal development
   c. Vitamin D stimulating the absorption and transport of calcium and phosphate ions
   d. a, b, and c are correct

OBJ. 4 ___ 13. The major effect that exercise has on bones is that:
   a. it provides oxygen for bone development
   b. it enhances the process of ossification
   c. it serves to maintain and increase bone mass
   d. it accelerates the healing process when a fracture occurs

OBJ. 4 ___ 14. In a greenstick fracture:
   a. only one side of the shaft is broken
   b. the shaft bone is broken across its long axis
   c. the bone protrudes through the skin
   d. the bone is shattered into small fragments

Level -1-

Level 1 Review of Chapter Objectives 77

OBJ. 5 ___ 15. The axial skeleon can be recognized because it:
- a. includes the bones of the arms and legs
- b. forms the longitudinal axis of the body
- c. includes bones of the pectoral and pelvic girdle
- d. a, b, and c are correct

OBJ. 5 ___ 16. What percentage of the bones in the body comprise the axial skeleton?
- a. 60 %
- b. 80 %
- c. 20 %
- d. 40 %

OBJ. 5 ___ 17. The axial skeleton creates a framework that supports and protects organ systems in the:
- a. dorsal and ventral body cavities
- b. pleural cavity
- c. abdominal cavity
- d. pericardial cavity

OBJ. 5 ___ 18. The first seven pairs of ribs are called true ribs, while the lower five pairs are called false ribs because:
- a. the fused cartilages merge with the costal cartilage
- b. they do not attach directly to the sternum
- c. the last two pairs have no connection with the sternum
- d. they differ in shape from the true ribs

OBJ. 5 ___ 19. The skeleton of the chest or thorax consists of:
- a. cervical vertebrae, ribs, sternum
- b. cervical vertebrae, ribs, thoracic vertebrae
- c. cervical vertebrae, ribs, pectoral girdle
- d. thoracic vertebrae, ribs, sternum

OBJ. 5 ___ 20. The three components of the adult sternum are the:
- a. pneumothorax, hemothorax, tuberculum
- b. manubrium, body, xiphoid process
- c. head, capitulum, tuberculum
- d. a, b, and c are correct

OBJ. 5 ___ 21. The bones that compose the appendicular division of the skeleton consist of:
- a. the bones which form the longitudinal axis of the body
- b. the rib cage and the vertebral column
- c. the skull and the arms and legs
- d. the pectoral and pelvic girdles, and the upper and lower limbs

78 Chapter 6 The Skeletal System

OBJ. 5 ___ 22. One of the major functional differences between the appendicular and axial divisions is that the appendicular division:
- a. adjusts the position of the head, neck and trunk
- b. protects organ systems in the dorsal and ventral body cavities
- c. makes you an active, mobile individual
- d. assists directly in respiratory movements

OBJ. 5 ___ 23. A composite structure that includes portions of both the appendicular and axial skeletons is the:
- a. pelvis
- b. pectoral girdle
- c. pelvic girdle
- d. a, b, and c are correct

OBJ. 5 ___ 24. The parallel bones that support the forearm are the:
- a. humerus and femur
- b. ulna and radius
- c. tibia and fibula
- d. scapula and clavicle

OBJ. 5 ___ 25. The largest medial bone of the lower leg is the:
- a. femur
- b. fibula
- c. tibia
- d. humerus

OBJ. 6 ___ 26. The bones of the cranium that exclusively represent single, unpaired bones are the:
- a. occipital, parietal, frontal, temporal
- b. occipital, frontal, sphenoid, ethmoid
- c. frontal, temporal, parietal, sphenoid
- d. ethmoid, frontal, parietal, temporal

OBJ. 6 ___ 27. The paired bones of the cranium are the:
- a. ethmoid and sphenoid
- b. frontal and occipital
- c. occipital and parietal
- d. parietal and temporal

OBJ. 6 ___ 28. The single, unpaired bones that compose the skeletal part of the face are the:
- a. mandible and vomer
- b. nasal and lacrimal
- c. mandible and maxilla
- d. nasal and palantine

OBJ. 6 ___ 29. The sutures that articulate the bones of the skull are the:
- a. parietal, occipital, frontal, temporal
- b. lacrimal, sinusoidal, coronal
- c. posterior, anterior, lateral, dorsal
- d. lambdoidal, sagittal, coronal, squamosal

Level -1-

Level 1 Review of Chapter Objectives 79

OBJ. 6 ___ 30. The bones that make up the orbit include:
   a. lacrimal, zygomatic, maxilla
   b. ethmoid, temporal, zygomatic
   c. lacrimal, ethmoid, sphenoid
   d. temporal, frontal, sphenoid

OBJ. 6 ___ 31. Foramina, located on the bones of the skull, serve primarily as passageways for:
   a. secretions
   b. sound and sight
   c. nerves and blood vessels
   d. muscle fibers and nerve fibers

OBJ. 6 ___ 32. The lines, tubercles, crests, ridges, and other processes on the bones represent areas which are used primarily for:
   a. attachment of muscles to bones
   b. attachment of bone to bone
   c. joint articulation
   d. increasing the surface area of bones

OBJ. 6 ___ 33. The sinuses of the skull are found in which bones?
   a. sphenoid, ethmoid, vomer, lacrimal
   b. sphenoid, frontal, ethmoid, maxillary
   c. ethmoid, frontal, lacrimal, maxillary
   d. lacrimal, vomer, ethmoid, frontal

OBJ. 6 ___ 34. The nasal complex consists of which bones?
   a. frontal, sphenoid, ethmoid bones
   b. maxilla, lacrimal, ethmoidal concha
   c. inferior concha
   d. a, b, and c are correct

OBJ. 6 ___ 35. At birth, the bones of the skull can be distorted without damage because of the:
   a. cranial foramina
   b. fontanels
   c. alveolar process
   d. cranial ligaments

OBJ. 7 ___ 36. The primary spinal curves that appear late in fetal development:
   a. help shift the trunk weight over the legs
   b. accommodate the lumbar and cervical regions
   c. become accentuated as the toddler walks
   d. accommodate the thoracic and abdominopelvic organs

OBJ. 7 ___ 37. An abnormal lateral curvature of the spine is called:
   a. kyphosis
   b. lordosis
   c. scoliosis
   d. amphiarthrosis

80   Chapter 6   The Skeletal System

OBJ. 7 ____ 38. The vertebrae that indirectly effect changes in the volume of the rib cage are the:
   a. thoracic
   b. cervical
   c. lumbar
   d. sacral

OBJ. 7 ____ 39. The most massive and least mobile of the vertebra are
   a. the thoracic
   b. the cervical
   c. the lumbar
   d. the sacral

OBJ. 7 ____ 40. Of the following selections, the one which correctly identifies the sequence of the vertebra from superior to inferior is:
   a. thoracic, cervical, lumbar, coccyx, sacral
   b. cervical, lumbar, thoracic, sacral, coccyx
   c. cervical, thoracic, lumbar, sacral, coccyx
   d. cervical, thoracic, sacral, lumbar, coccyx

OBJ. 7 ____ 41. Vertebra C1 and C2 have specific names, which are:
   a. sacrum and coccyx
   b. atlas and axis
   c. cervical and costal
   d. b and c are correct

OBJ. 7 ____ 42. The sacrum consists of five fused elements which afford protection for which organs?
   a. reproductive, digestive, excretory
   b. respiratory, reproductive, endocrine
   c. urinary, respiratory, digestive
   d. endocrine, respiratory, urinary

OBJ. 8 ____ 43. The bones of the pectoral girdle include:
   a. clavicle and scapula
   b. ilium and ischium
   c. humerus and femur
   d. ulna and radius

OBJ. 8 ____ 44. The largest posterior process on the scapula is the:
   a. corocoid process
   b. acromion process
   c. olecranon fossa
   d. styloid process

OBJ. 8 ____ 45. The bones of the pelvic girdle include the:
   a. tibia and fibula
   b. ilium, pubis, ischium
   c. ilium, ischium, acetabulum
   d. b and c are correct

OBJ. 8 ___ 46. The primary function of the pectoral girdle is to:

    a. protect the organs of the thorax

    b. provide areas for articulation with the vertebral column

    c. position the shoulder joint and provide a base for arm movement

    d. support and maintain the position of the skull

OBJ. 8 ___ 47. The two specific areas of the skeleton that are generally used to identify significant differences between men and women are the:

    a. arms and legs

    b. ribs and vertebral column

    c. skull and pelvis

    d. a, b, and c are correct

OBJ. 9 ___ 48. Joints, or articulations, are classified on the basis of their degree of movement. From the following selections choose the one which identifies, in correct order, the following joints on the basis of: no movement, slight movement, and free movement:

    a. amphiarthrosis, diarthrosis, synarthorsis

    b. diarthrosis, synarthrosis, amphiarthrosis

    c. amphiarthrosis, synarthrosis, diarthrosis

    d. synarthrosis, amphiarthrosis, diarthrosis

OBJ. 9 ___ 49. The amphiarthrotic articulation that limits movements between the two pubic bones is the:

    a. pubic symphysis

    b. obturator foramen

    c. greater sciatic notch

    d. pubic tubercle

OBJ. 9 ___ 50. The type of synarthrosis that bonds each tooth to the surrounding bony socket is a:

    a. synchrondrosis

    b. syndesmosis

    c. gomphosis

    d. symphysis

OBJ. 9 ___ 51. The function(s) of synovial fluid include:

    a. nourishes the chondrocytes

    b. provides lubrication

    c. acts as a shock absorber

    d. a, b, and c are correct

OBJ. 9 ___ 52. The primary function(s) of menisci include:

    a. to subdivide a synovial cavity

    b. to channel the flow of synovial fluid

    c. to allow for variatons in the shapes of articulating surfaces

    d. a, b, and c are correct

Chapter 6 The Skeletal System

OBJ. 10 ____ 53. Flexion is defined as movement that:
   a. increases the angle between articulating bones
   b. decreases the angle between articulating bones
   c. moves a limb from the midline of the body
   d. moves a limb toward the midline of the body

OBJ. 10 ____ 54. The movement that allows you to gaze at the ceiling:
   a. rotation
   b. circumduction
   c. hyperextension
   d. elevation

OBJ. 10 ____ 55. The reason that the elbow and knee are called hinged joints is:
   a. the articulating surfaces are able to slide across one another
   b. all combinations of movement are possible
   c. they permit angular movement in a single plane
   d. sliding and rotation are prevented and angular motion is restricted to two directions

OBJ. 10 ____ 56. The shoulder and hip joints are examples of:
   a. hinge joints
   b. ball and socket joints
   c. pivot joints
   d. gliding joints

OBJ. 10 ____ 57. Movements of the vertebral column are limited to:
   a. flexion and extension
   b. lateral flexion
   c. rotation
   d. a, b, and c are correct

OBJ. 10 ____ 58. The joint that permits the greatest range of motion of any joint in the body is:
   a. hip joint
   b. shoulder joint
   c. elbow joint
   d. a and b are correct

OBJ. 10 ____ 59. The elbow joint is quite stable because:
   a. the body surfaces of the humerus and ulna interlock
   b. the articular capsule is very thick
   c. the capsule is reinforced by stout ligaments
   d. a, b, and c are correct

OBJ. 10 ____ 60. The knee joint functions as a:
   a. hinge joint
   b. ball and socket joint
   c. saddle joint
   d. gliding joint

| OBJ. 10 | ___ 61. The reason the points of contact in the knee joint are constantly changing is:

    a. there is no single unified capsule or common synovial cavity
    b. the cartilage menisci conform to the shape of the surface of the femur
    c. the rounded femoral condyles roll across the top of the tibia
    d. a, b, and c are correct

| OBJ. 11 | ___ 62. The popliteal ligaments extend between the femur and the heads of the tibia and fibula reinforcing the:

    a. anterior surface of the knee joint
    b. lateral surface of the knee joint
    c. inside of the joint capsule
    d. back of the knee joint

| OBJ. 11 | ___ 63. The iliofemoral, pubofemoral and ischiofemoral ligaments are involved in reinforcement and stabilization of the:

    a. shoulder joint
    b. hip joint
    c. knee joint
    d. elbow joint

| OBJ. 11 | ___ 64. The subscromial bursa and the subcoracoid bursa reduce friction at the:

    a. elbow joint
    b. hip joint
    c. shoulder joint
    d. knee joint

| OBJ. 12 | ___ 65. The system which is responsible for synthesizing Vitamin D which, in turn, is important for the uptake of the calcium stored in bones is the:

    a. digestive system
    b. integumentary system
    c. muscular system
    d. endocrine system

| OBJ. 12 | ___ 66. Which of the following hormones is necessary for growth and maintenance of the skeletal system?

    a. growth hormone
    b. sex hormones
    c. thyroid hormone
    d. a, b, and c are correct

84 Chapter 6 The Skeletal System

[L1] Completion:

Using the terms below, complete the following statements.

osteon	minerals	ossification	support	epiphysis
calcium	remodeling	axial	muscles	intramembranous
endochondral	primary	costal	cranium	foramen magnum
cervical	paranasal	secondary	pectoral girdle	malleolus
clavicle	acetabulum	glenoid fossa	coxae	synovial
symphysis	scapulohumeral	bursae	knee	supination
gliding	red bone marrow	floating	suture	fontanels

OBJ. 1 67. Of the five major functions of the skeleton, the two that depend on the dynamic nature of bone are storage and _____.

OBJ. 2 68. The basic functional unit of compact is the _____.

OBJ. 2 69. The expanded region of a long bone consisting of spongy bone is called the _____.

OBJ. 3 70. When osteoblasts differentiate within connective tissue the process is called _____ ossification.

OBJ. 3 71. The type of ossification that begins with the formation of a hyaline cartilage model is _____.

OBJ. 3 72. The process which refers specifically to the formation of bone is termed _____.

OBJ. 3 73. The major mineral associated with the development and mineralization of bone is _____.

OBJ. 4 74. The organic and mineral components of the bone matrix are continually being recycled and renewed through the process of _____.

OBJ. 4 75. The ability of bone to adapt to new stresses results from the turnover and recycling of _____.

OBJ. 5 76. The part of the skeletal system that forms the longitudinal axis of the body is the _____ division.

OBJ. 5 77. The bones of the skeleton provide an extensive surface area for the attachment of _____.

OBJ. 5 78. The cartilaginous extensions that connect the ribs to the sternum are the _____.

OBJ. 5 79. The last two pairs of ribs that do not articulate with the sternum are called _____ ribs.

OBJ. 5 80. The process that the tibia and fibula have in common that acts as a shield for the ankle is the _____.

OBJ. 5 81. At the hip joint to either side, the head of the femur articulates with the _____.

OBJ. 6 82. The part of the skull that provides protection for the brain is the _____.

OBJ. 6 83. The opening that connects the cranial cavity with the canal enclosed by the vertebral column is the _____.

OBJ. 6 84. The airspaces connected to the nasal cavities are the _____.

OBJ. 6 85. At birth, the cranial bones are connected by areas of fibrous connective tissues called _____.

Level -1-

OBJ. 7 86. The spinal curves that assist in allowing a child to walk and run are called _____ curves.

Level 1 Review of Chapter Objectives

OBJ. 7   87. The spinal curves that develop first during development are called _____ curves.

OBJ. 7   88. The vertebrae that stabilize relative positions of the brain and spinal cord are the _____ vertebrae.

OBJ. 8   89. The only direct connection between the pectoral girdle and the axial skeleton is the _____.

OBJ. 8   90. The shoulder area and its component bones comprise a region referred to as the _____.

OBJ. 8   91. The scapula articulates with the proximal end of the humerus at the _____.

OBJ. 8   92. The pelvic girdle consists of six bones collectively referred to as the _____.

OBJ. 9   93. A synarthrotic joint found only between the bones of the skull is a _____.

OBJ. 9   94. The amphiarthrotic joint where bones are separated by a wedge or pad of fibro-cartilage is a _____.

OBJ. 9   95. Small, synovial-filled pockets that form where a tendon or ligament rubs against other tissues are called _____.

OBJ. 10 96. Movement in the wrist and hand in which the palm is turned forward is _____.

OBJ. 10 97. Diarthrotic joints that permit a wide range of motion are called _____.

OBJ. 10 98. The joints between the superior and inferior articulations of adjacent vertebrae are _____.

OBJ. 10 99. The joint that permits the greatest range of motion of any joint in the body is the _____ joint.

OBJ. 11 100. The joint that resembles three separate joints with no single unified capsule or common synovial cavity is the _____.

OBJ. 12 101. The location where lymphocytes are produced is the _____.

[L1] Matching:

Match the terms in column "B" with the terms in column "A." Use letters for answers in the spaces provided.

		COLUMN "A"		COLUMN "B"
OBJ. 1	___ 102.	Red blood cell formation	A.	Remodeling
OBJ. 2	___ 103.	Spongy bone	B.	Nonarticulating
OBJ. 3	___ 104.	Osteogenesis	C.	Ball and socket
OBJ. 4	___ 105.	Bone maintenance	D.	Calcium
OBJ. 5	___ 106.	Hyoid	E.	C1 through C7
OBJ. 6	___ 107.	Air-filled chambers	F.	Muscle to bone
OBJ. 7	___ 108.	Cervical vertebrae	G.	Red bone marrow
OBJ. 8	___ 109.	Shoulder	H.	Knee
OBJ. 9	___ 110.	Tendon	I.	Trabeculae
OBJ. 10	___ 111.	Pronation-Supination	J.	Forearm
OBJ. 11	___ 112.	Suprapatellar bursae	K.	Paranasal sinuses
OBJ. 12	___ 113.	Necessary for muscle contraction	L.	Bone formation

Chapter 6 The Skeletal System

[L1] Drawing/Illustration Labeling:

Identify each numbered structure by labeling the following figures.

OBJ. 5
OBJ. 6

FIGURE 6.1 Anterior View of the Skull

114 _____	120 _____
115 _____	121 _____
116 _____	122 _____
117 _____	123 _____
118 _____	124 _____
119 _____	125 _____

OBJ. 5
OBJ. 6

FIGURE 6.2 Lateral View of the Skull

126 _____	134 _____
127 _____	135 _____
128 _____	136 _____
129 _____	137 _____
130 _____	138 _____
131 _____	139 _____
132 _____	140 _____
133 _____	

OBJ. 5
OBJ. 6

FIGURE 6.3 Inferior View of the Skull

141 _____	145 _____
142 _____	146 _____
143 _____	147 _____
144 _____	148 _____

Level 1

Level 1 Review of Chapter Objectives 87

OBJ. 5
OBJ. 7

FIGURE 6.4   The Vertebral Column

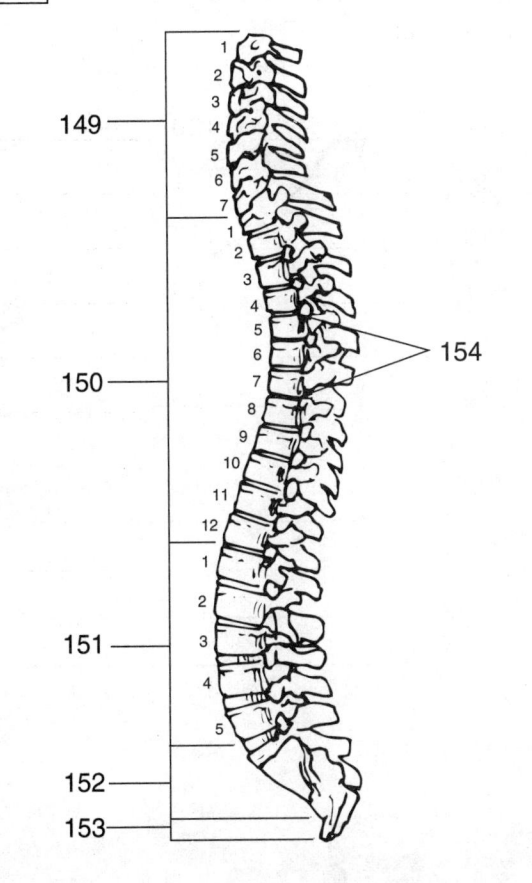

149 _____
150 _____
151 _____
152 _____
153 _____
154 _____

OBJ. 5   ***FIGURE 6.5***   The Ribs

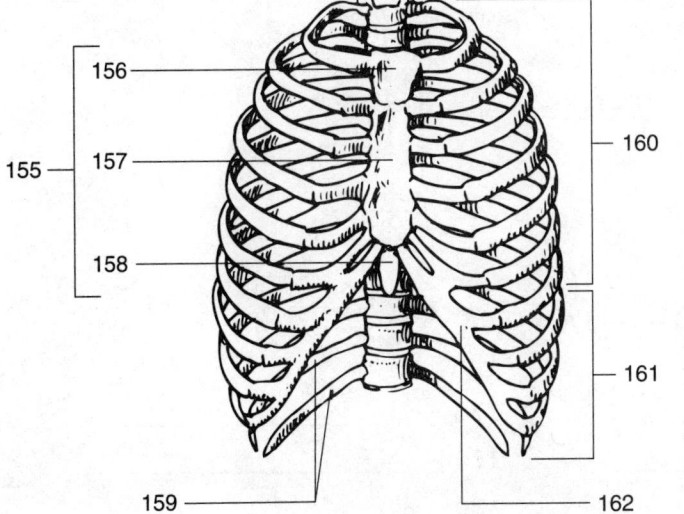

155 _____
156 _____
157 _____
158 _____
159 _____
160 _____
161 _____
162 _____

88 Chapter 6 The Skeletal System

FIGURE 6.6 The Scapula

Lateral view

Posterior view

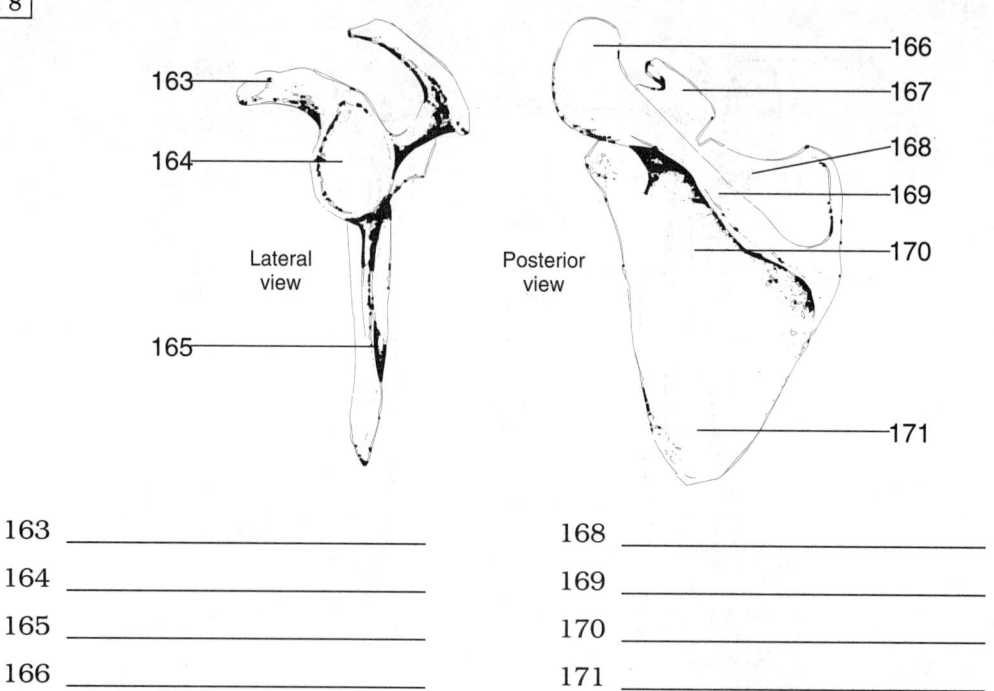

163 _____
164 _____
165 _____
166 _____
167 _____

168 _____
169 _____
170 _____
171 _____

FIGURE 6.7 The Humerus

Anterior view

Posterior view

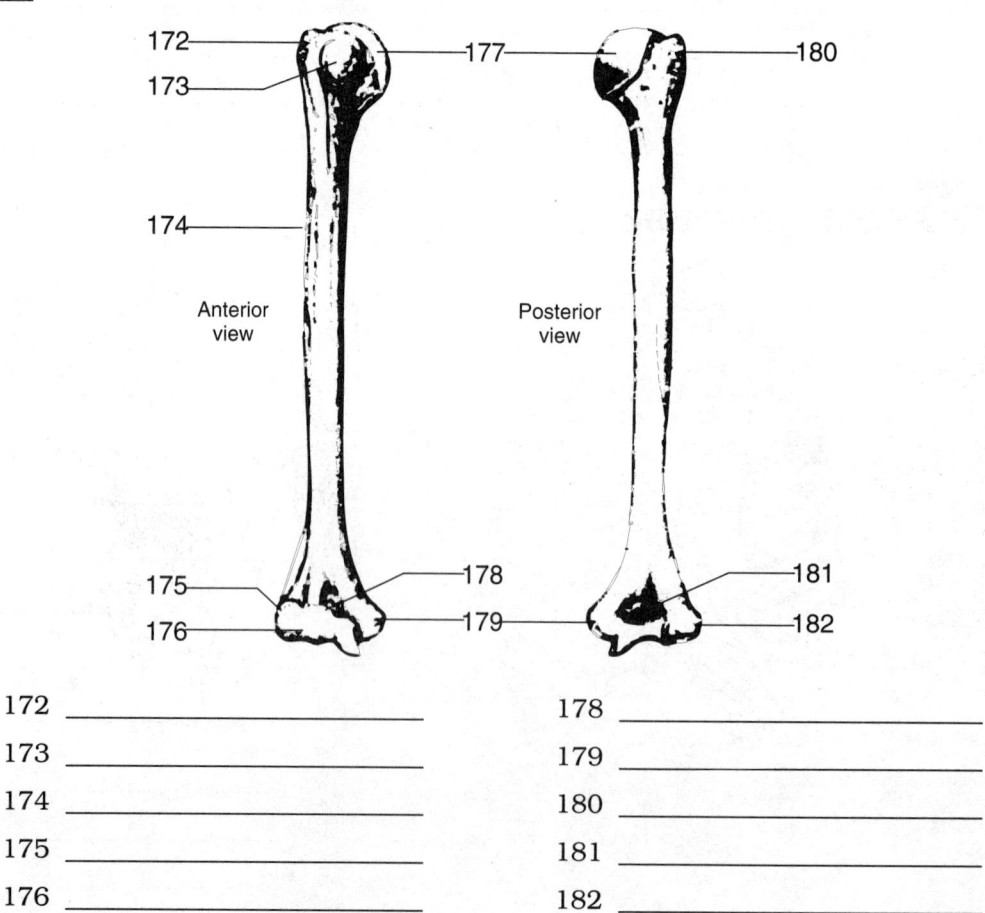

172 _____
173 _____
174 _____
175 _____
176 _____
177 _____

178 _____
179 _____
180 _____
181 _____
182 _____

Level 1 Review of Chapter Objectives 89

OBJ. 5 **FIGURE 6.8** The Radius and Ulna

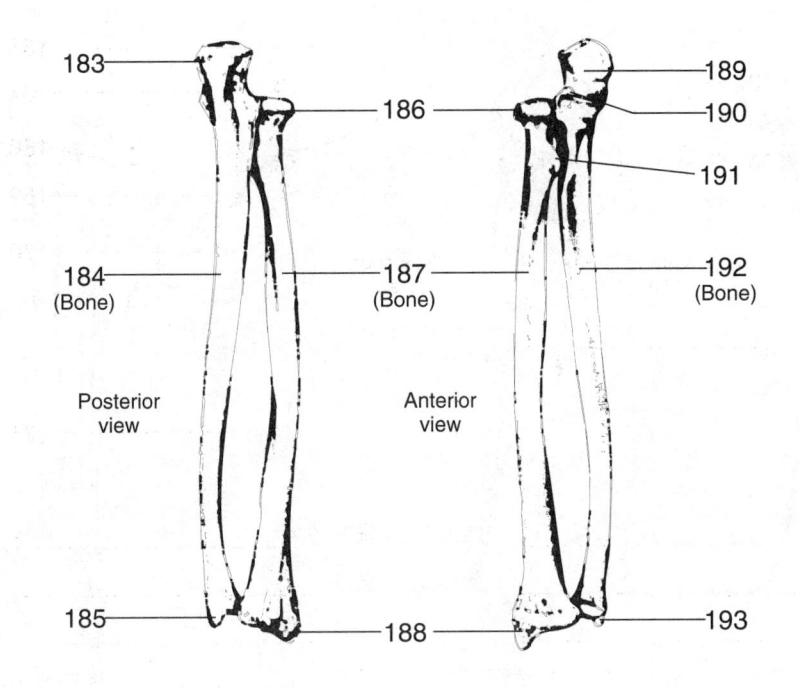

Posterior view

Anterior view

183 _____
184 _____
185 _____
186 _____
187 _____
188 _____

189 _____
190 _____
191 _____
192 _____
193 _____

OBJ. 5
OBJ. 8 **FIGURE 6.9** The Pelvis

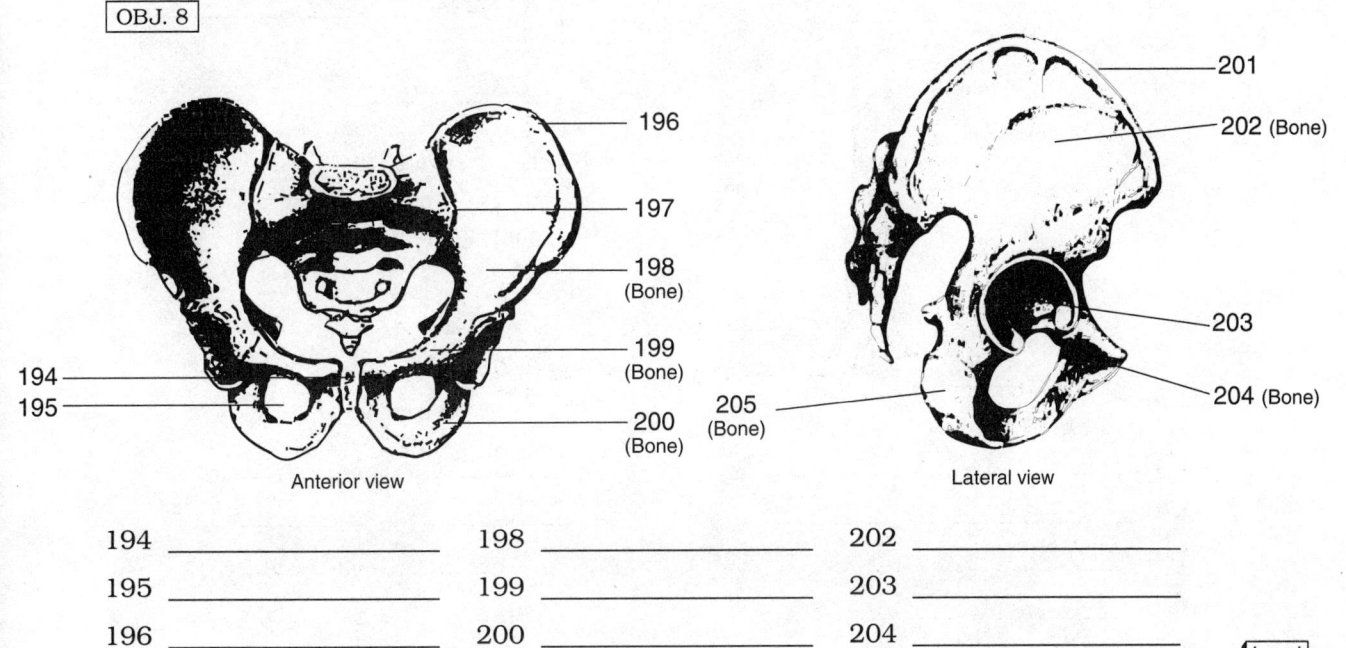

Anterior view

Lateral view

194 _____
195 _____
196 _____
197 _____

198 _____
199 _____
200 _____
201 _____

202 _____
203 _____
204 _____
205 _____

Level
-1-

90 Chapter 6 The Skeletal System

OBJ. 5 / OBJ. 8   **FIGURE 6.10**   The Femur & The Tibia and Fibula

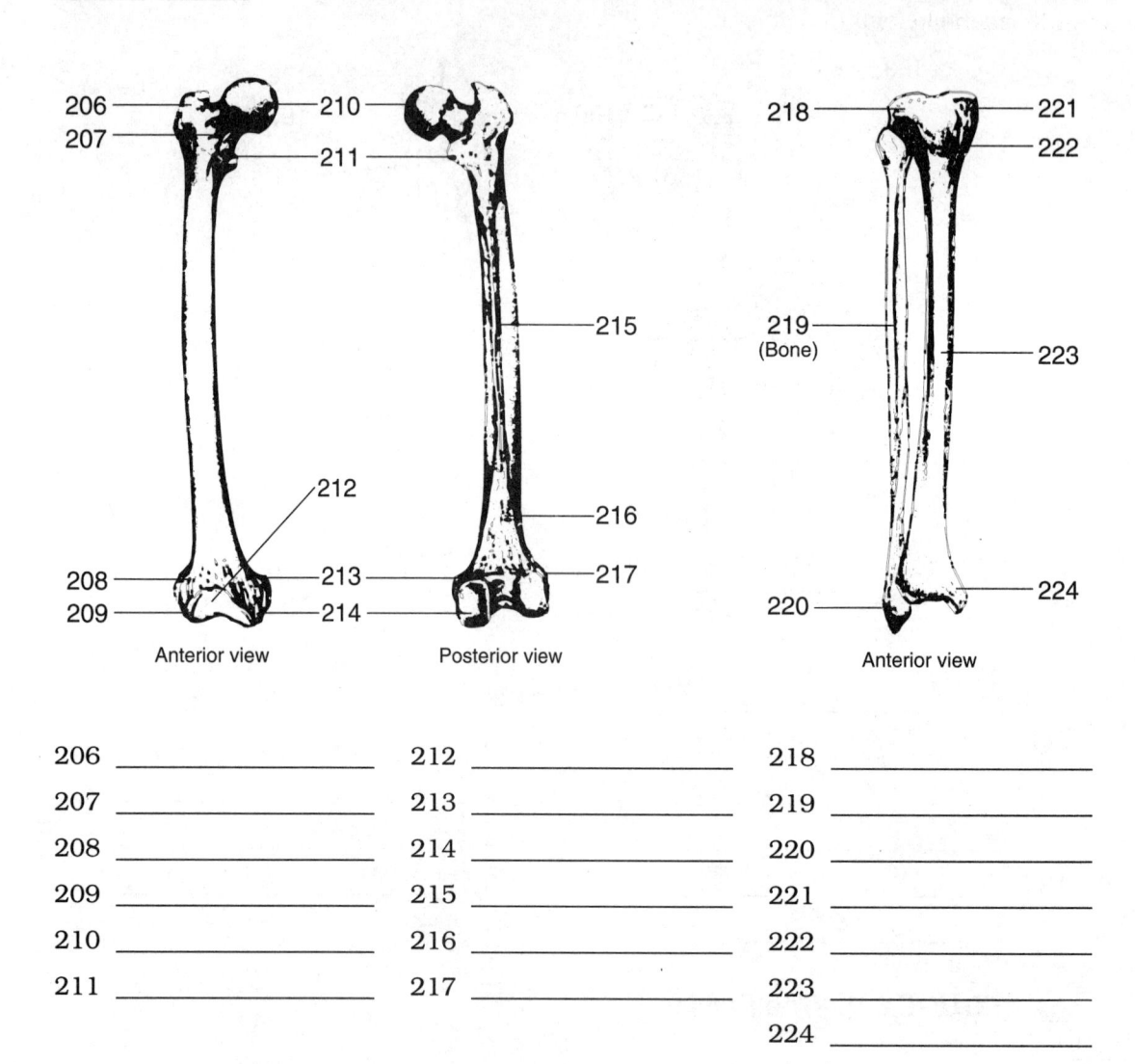

Anterior view   Posterior view   Anterior view

206 _____	212 _____	218 _____
207 _____	213 _____	219 _____
208 _____	214 _____	220 _____
209 _____	215 _____	221 _____
210 _____	216 _____	222 _____
211 _____	217 _____	223 _____
		224 _____

Level -1-

Level 1   Review of Chapter Objectives   91

OBJ. 10   **FIGURE 6.11**   Movements of the Skeleton

Identify each skeletal movement.

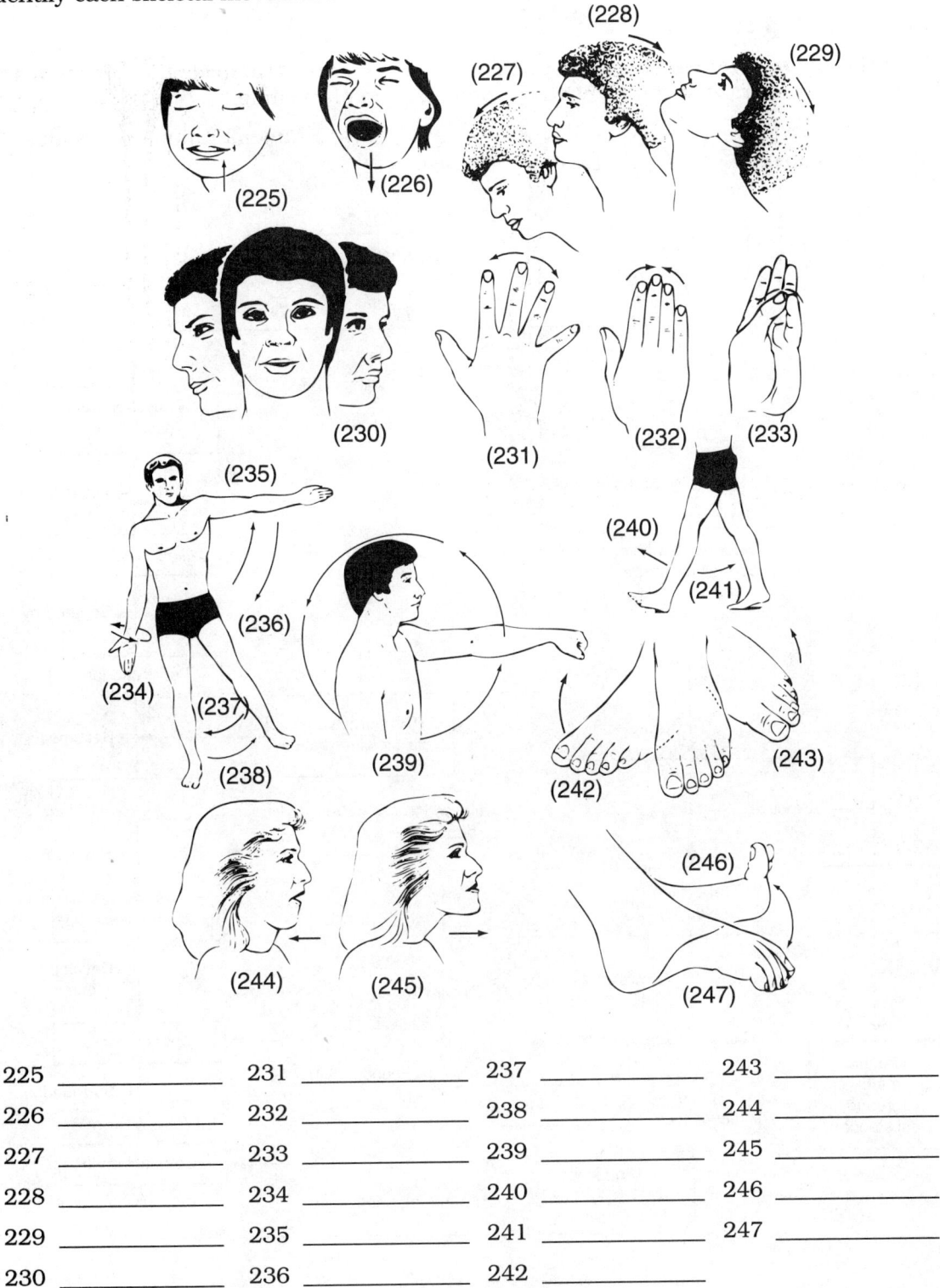

225 _____	231 _____	237 _____	243 _____
226 _____	232 _____	238 _____	244 _____
227 _____	233 _____	239 _____	245 _____
228 _____	234 _____	240 _____	246 _____
229 _____	235 _____	241 _____	247 _____
230 _____	236 _____	242 _____	

When you have successfully completed the exercises in L1 proceed to L2.

92 Chapter 6 The Skeletal System

☐ LEVEL 2—CONCEPT SYNTHESIS

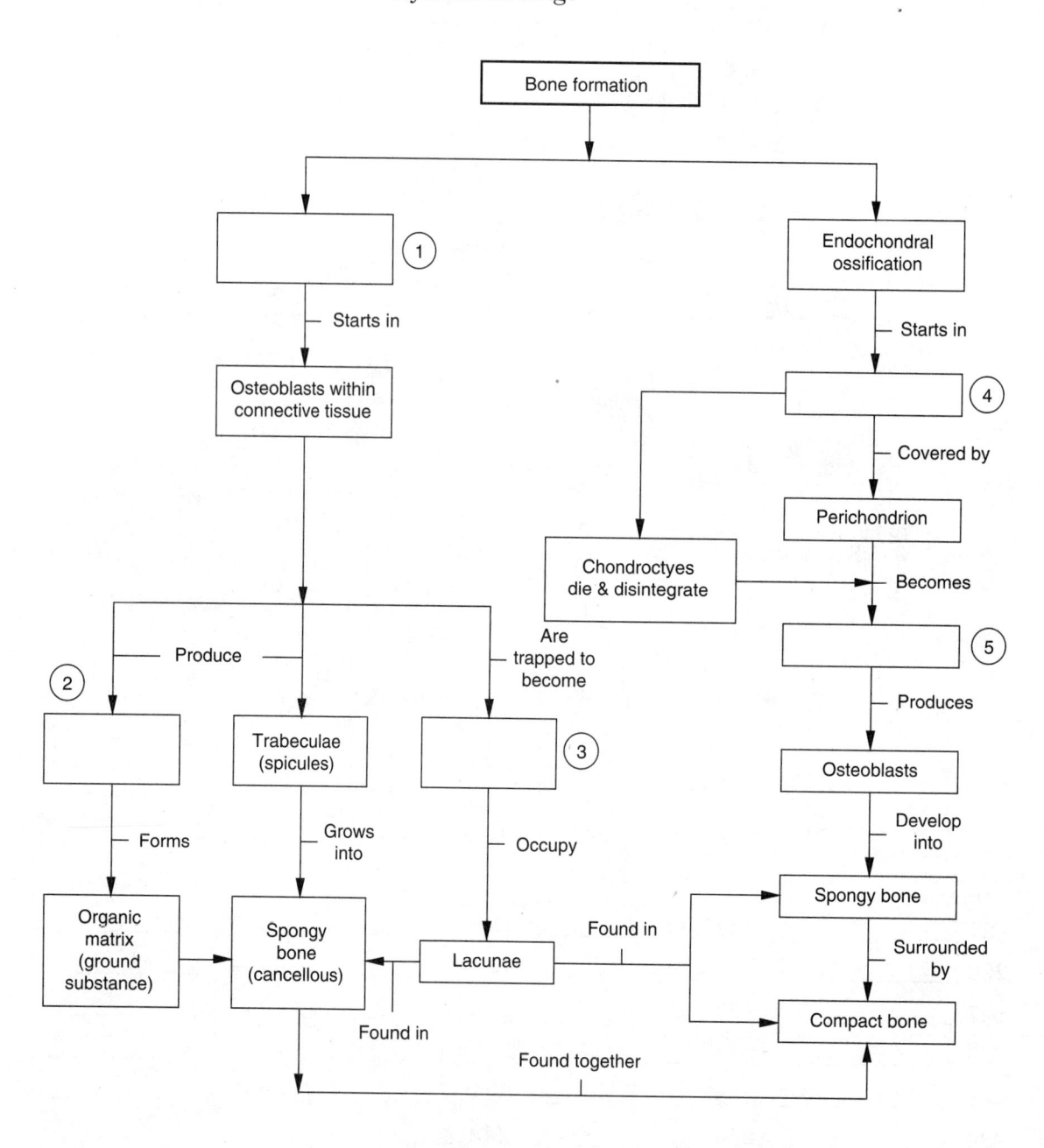

Concept Map I:

Using the following terms, fill in the numbered, blank spaces to complete the concept map. Follow the numbers that comply with the organization of the map.

- Osteocytes
- Periosteum
- Collagen
- Hyaline cartilage
- Intramembranous ossification

```
                        Bone formation
                       /              \
              [  1  ]                Endochondral
                 |                   ossification
              Starts in                 |
                 |                   Starts in
              Osteoblasts within        |
              connective tissue      [  4  ]
                 |                       |
                 |                   Covered by
                 |                       |
                 |                   Perichondrion
                 |                       |
                 |         Chondrocytes  |
                 |         die &        Becomes
                 |         disintegrate  |
                 |                       |
    Produce      |        Are         [  5  ]
    /            |        trapped to     |
   /             |        become      Produces
 [ 2 ]     Trabeculae   [ 3 ]            |
   |       (spicules)     |          Osteoblasts
  Forms        |         Occupy          |
   |         Grows         |          Develop
   |         into          |          into
 Organic       |           |             |
 matrix        |           |         Spongy bone
 (ground    Spongy     Lacunae  Found in |
 substance) bone   ←                    Surrounded
            (cancellous)                 by
                  |        Found in      |
                  |                  Compact bone
                  |     Found together   ↑
                  └──────────────────────┘
```

Level
=2=

Level 2 Concept Synthesis

Concept Map II:

Using the following terms, fill in the numbered, blank spaces to complete the concept map. Follow the numbers that comply with the organization of the map.

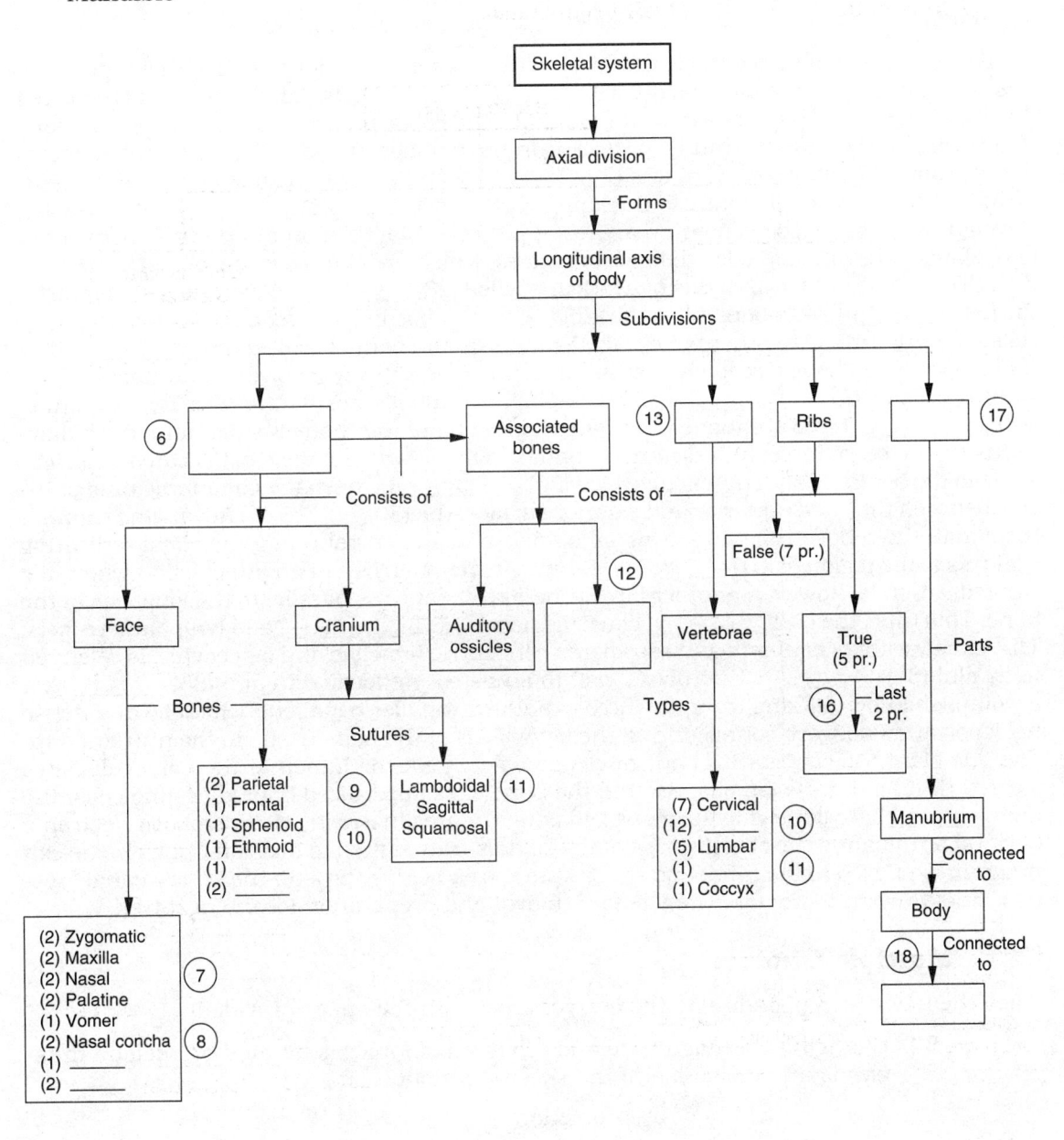

- Floating ribs, 2 pair
- Vertebral column
- Occipital
- Mandible
- Temporal
- Lacrimal
- Xiphoid process
- Hyoid
- Coronal
- Sternum
- Sacral
- Thoracic
- Skull

94 Chapter 6 The Skeletal System

Body Trek

Using the terms below, fill in the blanks to complete the trek through the long bone in the upper arm, the humerus.

Red marrow	Endosteum	Lacuna	Trabeculae
Canaliculi	Volkmann's Canal	Osteoclasts	Blood vessels
Compact bone	Compound	Osteon	Osteocytes
Lamella	Yellow marrow	Haversian canal	
Periosteum	Red blood cells	Cancellous or spongy	

For this trek Robo will enter the interior of the humerus, the long bone in the upper arm. The entry point is accessible due to a (19)_____ fracture in which the bone has projected through the skin at the distal end of the shaft. The robot proceeds to an area of the bone that is undisturbed by the trauma occurring in the damaged region. The micro-robot enters the medullary cavity which contains (20)_____ and moves proximally through a "sea" of fat to a region where it contacts the lining of the cavity, the (21)_____. After passing through the lining, Robo senses an area that projects images of an interlocking network of long plates or beams riddled with holes or spaces, which are characteristic of (22)_____ bone. The structural forms of this network are called (23)_____, which consist of matrix, the (24)_____, with bone cells, the (25)_____, located between the layers. The bone cells communicate with other bone cells through small channels called (26)_____. The "holes" or spaces have a reddish glow and appear to be actively involved in producing disk-shaped cells or (27)_____, which establish the robot's position in a cavity containing (28)_____. Robo's extended arm grabs onto one of the "bony beams" and, after moving along the beam for a short distance, contact is made with a large canal located at a right angle to the bone's shaft. This canal, called (29)_____, is the major communicating pathway between the bone's interior and exterior surface, the (30)_____. Advancing through the canal, the robot's sensors are signaling dense tissue surrounding the canal indicating that this is the region of (31)_____. Suddenly, Robo arrives at an intersection where the canal dead-ends; however, another large tube-like canal runs parallel to the long axis of the bone. This tube, the (32)_____, contains nerves, (33)_____, and lymphatic vessels. This canal, with its contents and associated concentric lamellae and osteocytes, is referrred to as a(n) (34)_____. The robot's visit to an osteocyte located in a(n) (35)_____ is accomplished by trekking from the large canal into smaller canaliculi which form a dense transportation network connecting all the living cells of the bony tissue to the nutrient supply. The giant osteocytes with dark nuclei completely fill the lumen at the bone cells sites located throughout the lamella. Around the bone sites specialized bone-digesting cells, the (36)_____, are liquefying the matrix, making the area insensitive to the robot's electronic devices, terminating the effectiveness of the signals transmitted to Mission Control. The exit program is relayed to the robot and the "reverse" trek begins through the bone's canal "system" and a return to the fracture site for removal and preparation for the next trek.

[L2] Multiple Choice:

Place the letter corresponding to the correct answer in the space provided.

_____ 37. Changing the magnitude and direction of forces generated by skeletal muscles is an illustration of the skeletal function of:

        a. protection
        b. leverage
        c. energy reserve
        d. storage

_____ 38. The outer surface of the bone, the periosteum:

        a. isolates the bone from surrounding tissue
        b. provides a route for circulatory and nerve supply
        c. actively participates in bone growth and repair
        d. a, b, and c are correct

Level 2   Concept Synthesis   95

_____ 39. The calcification of cartilage results in the production of:
- a. spongy bone
- b. ossified cartilage
- c. compact bone
- d. calcified cartilage

_____ 40. In human beings, the major factor determining the size and proportion of the body is:
- a. the growth of the skeleton
- b. the amount of food eaten
- c. the size of the musculature
- d. thyroid metabolism

_____ 41. Healing of a fracture, even after severe damage, depends on the survival of:
- a. the bone's mineral strength and its resistance to stress
- b. the circulatory supply and the cellular components of the endosteum and periosteum
- c. osteoblasts within the spongy and compact bone
- d. the cartilaginous callus which protects the fractured area

_____ 42. The three (3) organs regulating the calcium ion concentration in body fluids are:
- a. heart, liver, lungs
- b. liver, kidneys, stomach
- c. pancreas, heart, lungs
- d. bones, intestinal tract, kidneys

_____ 43. Appositional bone growth at the outer surface results in:
- a. an increase in the diameter of a growing bone
- b. an increase in the overall length of a bone
- c. a thickening of the cartilages that support the bones
- d. an increased hardening of the periosteum

_____ 44. The area of the greatest degree of flexibility along the vertebral column is found from:
- a. C3 through C7
- b. T1 through T6
- c. T7 through T12
- d. L1 through L5

_____ 45. Intervertebral discs are found in between all vertebrae except:
- a. between C1 and C1, and T12 and L1
- b. within the sacrum and coccyx
- c. between L5 and the sacrum
- d. between C1 and C2; and within the sacrum and coccyx

96 Chapter 6 The Skeletal System

_____ 46. Part of loss in height that accompanies aging results from:
    a. degeneration of osseous tissue in the diaphysis of long bones
    b. degeneration of skeletal muscles attached to bones
    c. the decreasing size and resiliency of intervertebral discs
    d. the reduction in number of vertebrae due to aging

_____ 47. The framework of the sphenoid which protects the pituitary gland is the:
    a. crista galli
    b. cribriform plate
    c. sella turcica
    d. frontal squama

_____ 48. The growth of the cranium is usually associated with:
    a. the expansion of the brain
    b. the development of the fontanels
    c. the closure of the sutures
    d. the time of birth

_____ 49. The unique compromise of the articulations in the appendicular skeleton is:
    a. the stronger the joint, the less restricted the range of motion
    b. the weaker the joint, the more restricted the range of motion
    c. the stronger the joint, the more restricted the range of motion
    d. the strength of the joint and range of motion are unrelated

_____ 50. If you run your fingers along the superior surface of the shoulder joint, you will feel a process called the:
    a. coracoid
    b. acromion
    c. coronoid
    d. styloid

_____ 51. The four proximal carpals are:
    a. trapezium, trapezoid, capitate, hamate
    b. trapezium, triquetrum, capitate, lunate
    c. scaphoid, trapezium, lunate, capitate
    d. scaphoid, lunate, triquetrum, pisiform

_____ 52. The distal carpals are:
    a. scaphoid, lunate, triquetrum, pisiform
    b. trapezium, trapezoid, capitate, hamate
    c. trapezium, scaphoid, trapezoid, lunate
    d. scaphoid, capitate, triquetrum, hamate

Level 2

_____ 53. The only ankle bone that articulates with the tibia and fibula is the:
   a. calcaneus
   b. talus
   c. navicular
   d. cuboid

[L2] Completion:

Using the terms below, complete the following statements:

osteopenia	bursitis	kyphosis	lordosis	hyperextension
arthroscopy	arthritis	endochondral	depressed	intramembranous
scoliosis	articular cartilage			

54. Dermal bones, such as several bones of the skull, the lower jaw, and the collarbone, are a result of _____ ossification.
55. Limb bone development is a good example of the process of _____ ossification.
56. Fragile limbs, a reduction in height, and the loss of teeth are a part of the aging process referred to as _____.
57. A common type of skull fracture is a _____.
58. A normal thoracic curvature which becomes exaggerated, producing a "roundback" appearance, is a _____.
59. An exaggerated lumbar curvature or "swayback" appearance is a _____.
60. An abnormal lateral curvature which usually appears in adolescence during periods of rapid growth is _____.
61. Inflammation of a bursae results in _____.
62. The technique which uses fiber optics to permit exploration of a joint without major surgery is _____.
63. Rheumatic diseases that affect synovial joints result in the development of _____.
64. Arthritis always involves damage to the _____.
65. A movement that allows you to gaze at the ceiling is _____.

[L2] Short Essay:

Briefly answer the following questions in the spaces provided below.

66. How does the process of calcification differ from ossification?

67. Differentiate between the beginning stage of intramembraneous and endochondral ossification.

Chapter 6 The Skeletal System

68. What are the fundamental relationships between the skeletal system and other body systems?

69. What are the primary functions of the axial skeleton?

70. What are the primary functions of the appendicular skeleton?

71. How are muscles and bones physiologically linked?

72. What are the six (6) types of joints in human body? Give an example of each.

73. How does the stability of the elbow joint compare with that of the hip? Why?

When you have successfully completed the exercises in L2 proceed to L3.

☐ LEVEL 3   CRITICAL THINKING/APPLICATION

Using principles and concepts learned in chapter 6, answer the following questions. Write your answers on a separate sheet of paper.

1. Why is an individual who experiences premature puberty not as tall as expected at age 18?
2. Good nutrition and exercise are extemely important in bone development, growth and maintenance. If you were an astronaut, what vitamin supplements and what type of exercise would you need to be sure that the skeletal system retained its integrity while in a weightless environment in space?
3. During a car accident you become a victim of whiplash. You experience pains in the neck and across the upper part of the back. Why?
4. A clinical diagnosis has been made that substantiates the presence of a herniated disc and a severe case of sciatica. What is the relationship between the two conditions?
5. As a teacher of anatomy what structural characteristics would you identify for the students to substantiate that the hip joint is stronger and more stable that the shoulder joint?
6. Two patients sustain hip fractures. In one case, a pin is inserted into the joint and the injury heals well. In the other, the fracture fails to heal. Identify the types of fractures that are probably involved. Why did the second patient's fracture fail to heal and what steps can be taken to restore normal function?

CHAPTER 7

The Muscular System

■ Overview

It would would be impossible for human life to exist without muscle tissue. This is because many functional processes and all our dynamic interactions, both internally and externally, with our environment depend on movement. In the human body, muscle tissue is necessary for movement to take place. The body consists of various types of muscle tissue, including cardiac, which is found in the heart; smooth, which forms a substantial part of the walls of hollow organs; and skeletal, which is attached to the skeleton. Smooth and cardiac muscles are involuntary and are responsible for transport of materials within the body. Skeletal muscle is voluntary and allows us to maneuver and manipulate in the environment; it also supports soft tissues, guards entrances and exits, and serves to maintain body temperature.

The study of the muscular system must also include the skeletal muscles that make up about 40 percent of the body mass and that can be controlled voluntarily. It is virtually impossible to master all the facts involved with the approximately 700 muscles that have been identified in the human body. A representative number of muscles from all parts of the body are selected and surveyed. The survey includes the gross anatomy of muscles, anatomical arrangements, muscle attachments, and muscular performance relative to basic mechanical laws.

The Study Guide exercises for Chapter 7 have a dual purpose: first, to present the basic structural and functional characteristics of skeletal muscle tissue. Emphasis is placed on muscle cell structure, muscle contraction and muscle mechanics, the energetics of muscle activity, muscle performance, and integration with other systems. Second, to focus on organizing the muscles into small numbers of anatomical and functional groups, the general appearance of the muscles, and the factors that interact to determine the effects of muscle contraction.

☐ LEVEL 1   REVIEW OF CHAPTER OBJECTIVES

1. Describe the properties and functions of muscle tissue.
2. Describe the organization of muscle at the tissue level.
3. Identify the structural components of a sarcomere.
4. Explain the key steps involved in the contraction of a skeletal muscle fiber.
5. Compare the different types of muscle contractions.

6. Describe the mechanisms by which muscle fibers obtain and use energy to power contractions.
7. Relate the types of muscle fibers to muscle performance.
8. Distinguish between aerobic and anaerobic endurance and explain their implications for muscular performance.
9. Contrast skeletal, cardiac, and smooth muscle in terms of structure and function.
10. Identify the principal axial muscles of the body, together with their origins and insertions.
11. Identify the principal appendicular muscles of the body, together with their origins and insertions
12. Describe the effects of exercise and aging on muscle tissue.
13. Discuss the functional relationships between the muscular system and other body systems.

[L1] Multiple Choice:

Place the letter corresponding to the correct answer in the space provided.

OBJ. 1 _____ 1. Muscle tissue consists of cells that are highly specialized for the function of:
    a. excitability
    b. contractibility
    c. extensibility
    d. a, b, and c are correct

OBJ. 1 _____ 2. The three types of muscle tissue are:
    a. epimysium, perimysium, endomysium
    b. skeletal, cardiac, smooth
    c. elastic, collagen, fibrous
    d. voluntary, involuntary, resting

OBJ. 1 _____ 3. Skeletal muscles move the body by:
    a. using the energy of ATP to form ADP
    b. serving as a series of levers and pullies attached to bones of the skeleton
    c. means of neural stimulation
    d. pulling on the bones of the skeleton

OBJ. 2 _____ 4. Skeletal muscles are often called voluntary muscles because:
    a. ATP activates skeletal muscles for contraction
    b. the skeletal muscles contain neuromuscular junctions
    c. they contract when stimulated by motor neurons of the central nervous system
    d. connective tissue harnesses generated forces voluntarily

OBJ. 2 _____ 5. The smallest functional unit of the muscle fiber is:
    a. thick filaments
    b. thin filaments
    c. Z line
    d. sarcomere

Chapter 7 The Muscular System

OBJ. 2 ____ 6. Nerves and blood vessels are contained within the connective tissues of the:

    a. epimysium and endomysium
    b. the endomysium only
    c. epimysium and perimysium
    d. the perimysium only

OBJ. 3 ____ 7. The thin filaments consist of:

    a. a pair of protein strands together to form chains of actin molecules
    b. a helical array of actin molecules
    c. a pair of protein strands wound together to form chains of myosin molecules
    d. a helical array of myosin molecules

OBJ. 3 ____ 8. The thick filaments consist of:

    a. a pair of protein strands wound together to form chains of myosin molecules
    b. a helical array of myosin molecules
    c. a pair of protein strands wound together to form chains of actin molecules
    d. a helical array of actin molecules

OBJ. 4 ____ 9. All of the muscle fibers controlled by a single motor neuron constitute a:

    a. motor unit
    b. sarcomere
    c. neuromuscular junction
    d. cross-bridge

OBJ. 4 ____ 10. The reason there is less precise control over leg muscles compared to the muscles of the eye is:

    a. single muscle fibers are controlled by many motor neurons
    b. many muscle fibers are controlled by many motor neurons
    c. a single muscle fiber is controlled by a single motor neuron
    d. many muscle fibers are controlled by a single motor neuron

OBJ. 4 ____ 11. The sliding filament theory explains that the physical change that takes place during contraction is:

    a. the thick filaments are sliding toward the center of the sarcomere alongside the thin filaments
    b. the thick and thin filaments are sliding toward the center of the sarcomere together
    c. the Z lines are sliding toward the H zone
    d. the thin filaments are sliding toward the center of the sarcomere alongside the thick filaments

Level -1-

Level 1 Review of Chapter Objectives 103

OBJ. 4 ___ 12. Troponin and tropomyosin are two proteins that can prevent the contractile process by:
- a. combining with calcium to prevent active site binding
- b. causing the release of calcium from the sacs of the sarcoplasmic reticulum
- c. covering the active site and blocking the actin-myosin interaction
- d. inactivating the myosin to prevent crossbridging

OBJ. 4 ___ 13. In order for an active site to be available for the cross-bridge binding, the presence of _____ is required.
- a. actin
- b. myosin
- c. actin and myosin
- d. calcium

OBJ. 5 ___ 14. In an isotonic contraction:
- a. the tension in the muscle varies as it shortens
- b. the muscle length doesn't change due to the resistance
- c. the cross-bridges must produce enough tension to overcome the resistance
- d. tension in the muscle decreases as the resistance increases

OBJ. 5 ___ 15. In an isometric contraction:
- a. tension rises but the length of the muscle remains constant
- b. the tension rises and the muscle shortens
- c. the tension produced by the muscle is greater than the resistance
- d. the tension of the muscle increases as the resistance decreases

OBJ. 6 ___ 16. Mitochondrial activities are relatively efficient, but their rate of ATP generation is limited by:
- a. the presence of enzymes
- b. the availability of carbon dioxide and water
- c. the energy demands of other organelles
- d. the availability of oxygen

OBJ. 7 ___ 17. Extensive blood vessels, mitochondria, and myoglobin are found in the greatest concentration in:
- a. fast fibers
- b. slow fibers
- c. intermediate fibers
- d. type II fibers

104 Chapter 7   The Muscular System

OBJ. 8 ___ 18. The length of time a muscle can continue to contract while supported by mitochondrial activities is referred to as:
   a. anaerobic endurance
   b. aerobic endurance
   c. hypertrophy
   d. recruitment

OBJ. 8 ___ 19. Altering the characteristics of muscle fibers and improving the performance of the cardiovascular system results in improving:
   a. thermoregulatory adjustment
   b. hypertrophy
   c. anaerobic endurance
   d. aerobic endurance

OBJ. 9 ___ 20. The property of cardiac muscle that allows it to contract without neural stimulation is called:
   a. pacesetting
   b. automaticity
   c. plasticity
   d. a, b, and c are correct

OBJ. 9 ___ 21. The type of muscle tissue that does not contain sarcomeres is:
   a. cardiac
   b. skeletal
   c. smooth
   d. a and c are correct

OBJ. 9 ___ 22. Smooth muscle contractions in the respiratory passageways would cause:
   a. increased resistance to air flow
   b. decreased resistance to air flow
   c. immediate death
   d. resistance to air flow will not be affected

OBJ. 10 ___ 23. The movable attachment of muscle to bone or other connective tissue is referred to as the:
   a. origin
   b. insertion
   c. rotator
   d. joint

OBJ. 10 ___ 24. A muscle whose contraction is chiefly responsible for producing a particular movement is called:
   a. a synergist
   b. an antagonist
   c. an originator
   d. a prime mover

Level -1-

Level 1   Review of Chapter Objectives   105

OBJ. 10 ___ 25. Muscles are classified functionally as synergists when:
   a. muscles perform opposite tasks and are located on opposite sides of the limb
   b. muscles contract together and are coordinated in affecting a particular movement
   c. a muscle is responsible for a particular movement
   d. the movement involves flexion and extension

OBJ. 10 ___ 26. From the following selections choose the one that includes only muscles of facial expression:
   a. masseter, nasalis, auricularis, digastricus
   b. splenius, masseter, longissimus, platysma
   c. quadratus, frontalis, orbicularis oris, nasalis
   d. buccinator, orbicularis oris, orbicularis oculi

OBJ. 10 ___ 27. The superficial muscles of the spine are identified by subdivisions that include:
   a. cervicis, thoracis, lumborum
   b. iliocostalis, longissimus, spinalis
   c. longissimus, transversus, longus
   d. capitis, splenius, spinalis

OBJ. 10 ___ 28. The oblique series of muscles located between the vertebral spine and the ventral midline include:
   a. spinalis, diaphragm, rectus abdominis, external obliques
   b. subclavius, trapezius, capitis, iliocostalis
   c. scalenes, intercostals, obliques, transversus
   d. internal obliques, transversus, diaphragm

OBJ. 10 ___ 29. From the following selections choose the one that includes only muscles that move the shoulder girdle:
   a. teres major, deltoid, pectoralis major, triceps
   b. triceps, longissimus, masseter, biceps
   c. trapezius, sternocleidomastoid, pectoralis minor, subclavius
   d. internal oblique, triceps, deltoid, pectoralis minor

OBJ. 10 ___ 30. From the following selections choose the one that includes only muscles that move the upper arm:
   a. deltoid, teres major, latissimus dorsi, pectoralis major
   b. trapezius, pectoralis minor, triceps, biceps brachii
   c. rhomboideus, serratus anterior, trapezius
   d. brachialis, pronator, supinator, pectoralis minor

OBJ. 11 ___ 31. The muscles that arise on the humerus and the forearm and rotate the radius without producing either flexion or extension of the elbow are the:
   a. pronator teres and supinator
   b. brachialis and deltoid
   c. triceps and biceps brachii
   d. carpi ulnaris and brachialis

Level
-1-

[OBJ. 11] ___ 32. The terms that describe the actions of the muscles that move the palm and fingers are:

    a. depressor, levator, pronator, rotator
    b. tensor, supinator, levator, pronator
    c. rotator, tensor, extensor, adductor
    d. adductor, abductor, extensor, flexor

[OBJ. 11] ___ 33. The reason we use the word "bicep" to describe a particular muscle is:

    a. there are two areas in the body where biceps are found
    b. there are two muscles in the body with the same characteristics
    c. there are two tendons of origin
    d. the man who named it was an Italian by the name of Biceppe Longo

[OBJ. 11] ___ 34. The muscle groups that are responsible for movement of the thigh include:

    a. abductor, flexor, extensor
    b. adductor, gluteal, lateral rotator
    c. depressor, levator, rotator
    d. procerus, capitis, pterygoid

[OBJ. 11] ___ 35. The flexors that move the lower leg commonly known as the hamstrings include:

    a. rectus femoris, vastus intermedius, vastus lateralis, vastus medialis
    b. sartorius, rectus femoris, gracilis, vastus medialis
    c. piriformis, lateral rotators, obturator, sartorius
    d. biceps femoris, semimembranosus, semitendinosus

[OBJ. 11] ___ 36. The extensors that move the lower leg commonly known as the quadriceps include:

    a. piriformis, lateral rotator, obturator, sartorius
    b. semimembranosus, semitendinosus, gracilis, sartorius
    c. popliteus, gracilis, rectus femoris, biceps femoris
    d. rectus femoris, vastus intermedius, vastus lateralis, vastus medialis

[OBJ. 11] ___ 37. Major muscles that produce plantar flexion involved with movement of the lower leg are the:

    a. tibialis anterior, gluteus, sartorius
    b. flexor hallucis, obturator, gracilis
    c. gastrocnemius, soleus, tibialis posterior
    d. sartorius, soleus, flexor hallucis

[OBJ. 11] ___ 38. The actions that the arm muscles produce that are not evident in the action of the leg muscles are:

    a. abduction and adduction
    b. flexion and extension
    c. pronation and supination
    d. rotation and adduction

Level -1-

Level 1   Review of Chapter Objectives   107

OBJ. 11   ___ 39. The most common functional role of the muscles of both the forearm and the upper leg involves the action of:
- a. flexion and extension
- b. adduction and abduction
- c. rotation and supination
- d. pronation and supination

OBJ. 12   ___ 40. Fibrosis, the deposition of fibrous material, in aging muscle tissue makes the muscle:
- a. harder and results in increased tolerance for exercise
- b. less flexible, and the collagen fibers can restrict movement and circulation
- c. more elastic but less flexible
- d. more flexible and more subject to injury

OBJ. 13   ___ 41. Calcium ions for muscle contraction is stored in which body system?
- a. digestive
- b. endocrine
- c. integumentary
- d. skeletal

[L1]   Completion:

Using the terms below, complete the following statements.

endurance	epimysium	twitch	atrophy	rectus femoris
origin	ATP	sarcolemma	tendon	sarcomeres
pacemaker	diaphragm	fascicles	deltoid	red muscles
contraction	white muscles	recruitment	synergist	hypertrophy
T tubules	oxygen debt	troponin	cross-bridges	endocrine

OBJ. 1   42. The cells that make up muscle tissues are highly specialized for the process of _____.

OBJ. 2   43. The dense layer of collagen fibers surrounding a muscle is called the _____.

OBJ. 2   44. Bundles of muscle fibers are called _____.

OBJ. 2   45. The dense regular connective tissue that attaches skeletal muscle to bones is known as a _____.

OBJ. 2   46. The cell membrane that surrounds the cytoplasm of a muscle fiber is called the _____.

OBJ. 2   47. Structures that help distribute the command to contract throughout the muscle fiber are called _____.

OBJ. 2   48. Muscle cells contain contractible units called _____.

OBJ. 3   49. Because they connect thick and thin filaments, the myosin heads are also known as _____.

OBJ. 4   50. The smooth but steady increase in muscular tension produced by increasing the number of active motor units is called _____.

OBJ. 4   51. Active site exposure during the contraction process occurs when calcium binds to _____.

OBJ. 5   52. A single stimulus-contraction-relaxation sequence in a muscle fiber is a _____.

108 Chapter 7 The Muscular System

OBJ. 6   53. When muscles are actively contracting, the process requires large amounts of energy in the form of _____.

OBJ. 7   54. Muscles dominated by fast fibers are sometimes referred to as _____.

OBJ. 7   55. Muscles dominated by slow fibers are sometimes referred to as _____.

OBJ. 8   56. The amount of oxygen used in the recovery period to restore normal pre-exertion conditions is referred to as _____.

OBJ. 8   57. The amount of time for which the individual can perform a particular activity is referred to as _____.

OBJ. 9   58. The timing of contractions in cardiac muscle tissues is determined by specialized muscle fibers called _____ cells.

OBJ. 10   59. The stationary, immovable, or less movable attachment of a muscle is the _____.

OBJ. 10   60. A muscle that assists the prime mover in performing a particular action is a _____.

OBJ. 10   61. The muscle that separates the thoracic and abdominopelvic cavities is the _____.

OBJ. 11   62. The major abductor of the arm is the _____.

OBJ. 11   63. The large quadricep muscle that extends the leg and flexes the thigh is the _____.

OBJ. 12   64. A reduction in muscle size, tone and power is called _____.

OBJ. 12   65. Muscle enlargement due to repeated stimulation to near maximal tension is referred to as _____.

OBJ. 13   66. The hormone calcitonin is produced by the _____ system.

[L1] Matching:

Match the terms in column "B" with the terms in column "A." Use letters for answers in the spaces provided.

COLUMN "A"   **COLUMN "B"**

OBJ. 1   ____ 67. Skeletal muscle   A. Thick filaments
OBJ. 2   ____ 68. Fascicles   B. Resting tension
OBJ. 3   ____ 69. Striations   C. Cardiac muscle fibers
OBJ. 3   ____ 70. Myosin   D. Muscle bundles
OBJ. 4   ____ 71. Cross-bridging   E. Lactic acid
OBJ. 5   ____ 72. Muscle tone   F. Red muscles
OBJ. 6   ____ 73. Energy reserve   G. Fibrosis
OBJ. 7   ____ 74. Slow fibers   H. Smooth muscle cell
OBJ. 8   ____ 75. Anaerobic glycolysis   I. Produce skeletal movements
OBJ. 9   ____ 76. Intercalated discs   J. Actin-myosin interaction
OBJ. 9   ____ 77. No striations   K. Skeletal muscle cell
OBJ. 10   ____ 78. Stationary muscle attachment   L. Creatine phosphate
OBJ. 10   ____ 79. Movable muscle attachment   M. Gastrocnemius
OBJ. 10   ____ 80. Oppose action of prime mover   N. Insertion
OBJ. 10   ____ 81. Pectoralis major   O. Origin
OBJ. 11   ____ 82. Supports shoulder girdle   P. Flexes the arm
OBJ. 11   ____ 83. "Calf" muscle   Q. Rotator cuff
OBJ. 12   ____ 84. Aging   R. Antagonist

Level -1-

Level 1 Review of Chapter Objectives

[L1] Drawing/Illustration Labeling:

Identify each numbered structure by labeling the following figures:

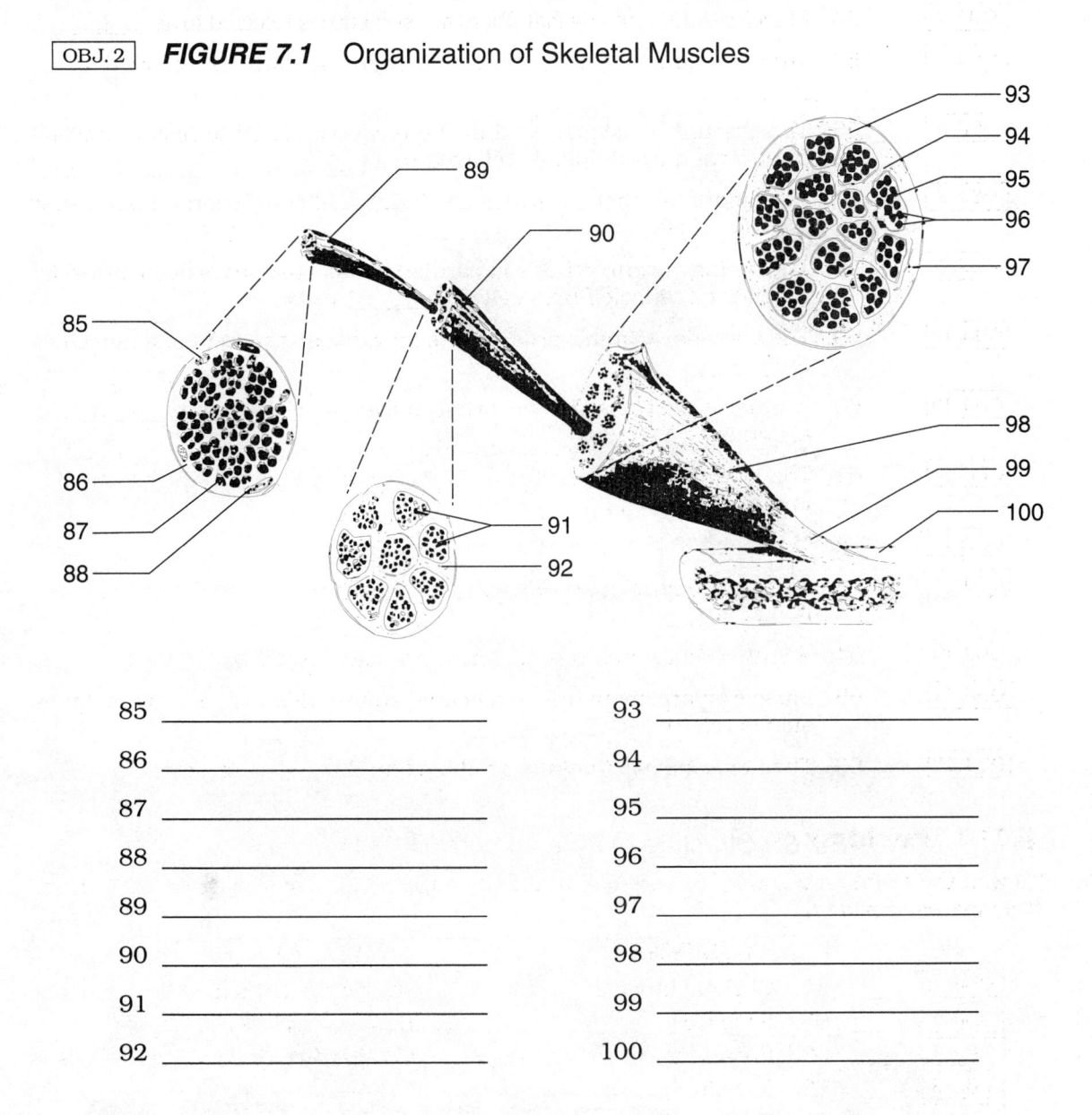

OBJ. 2 **FIGURE 7.1** Organization of Skeletal Muscles

85 _____
86 _____
87 _____
88 _____
89 _____
90 _____
91 _____
92 _____

93 _____
94 _____
95 _____
96 _____
97 _____
98 _____
99 _____
100 _____

110 Chapter 7 The Muscular System

OBJ. 2 **FIGURE 7.2** The Histological Organization of Skeletal Muscle

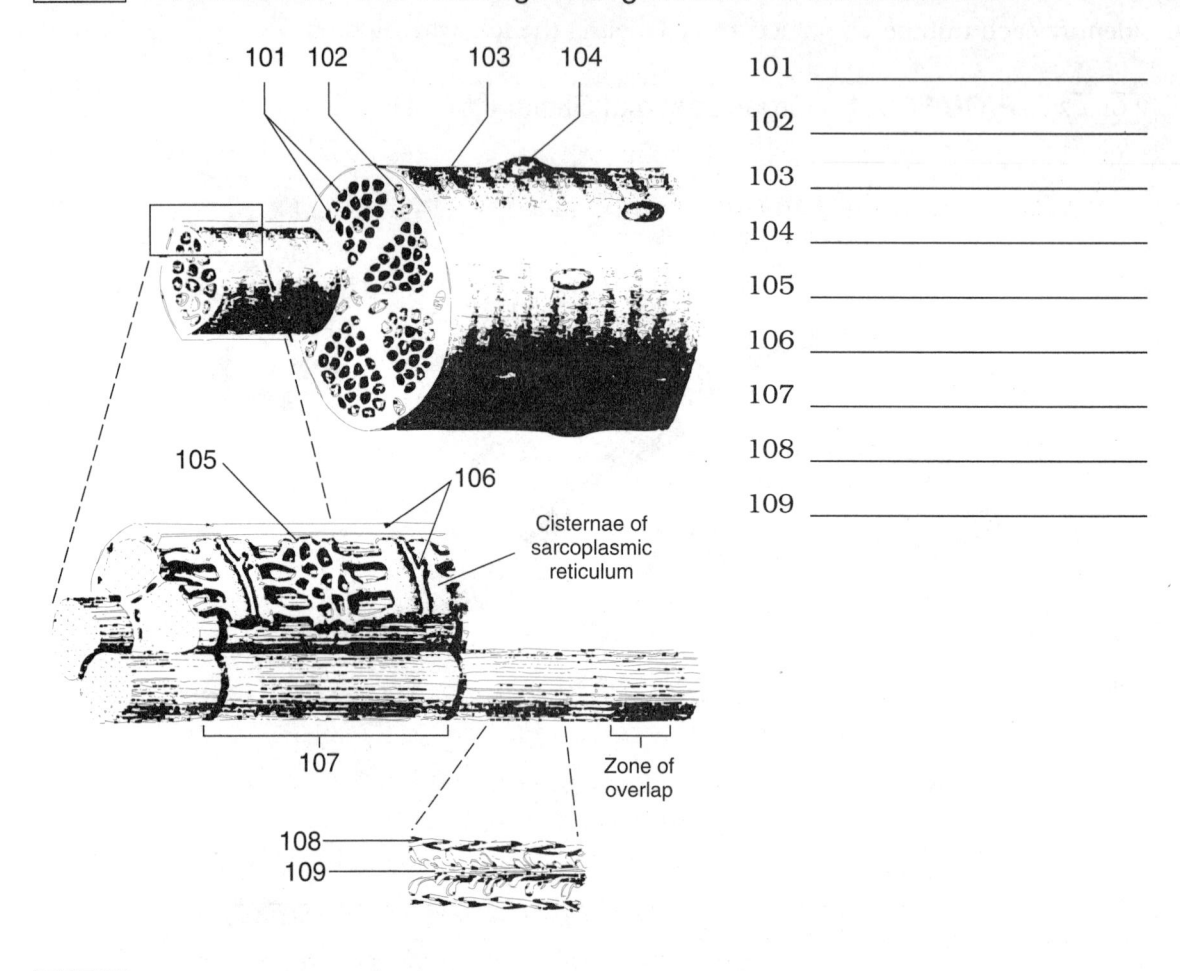

101 _____
102 _____
103 _____
104 _____
105 _____
106 _____
107 _____
108 _____
109 _____

OBJ. 3 **FIGURE 7.3** Structure of a Sarcomere

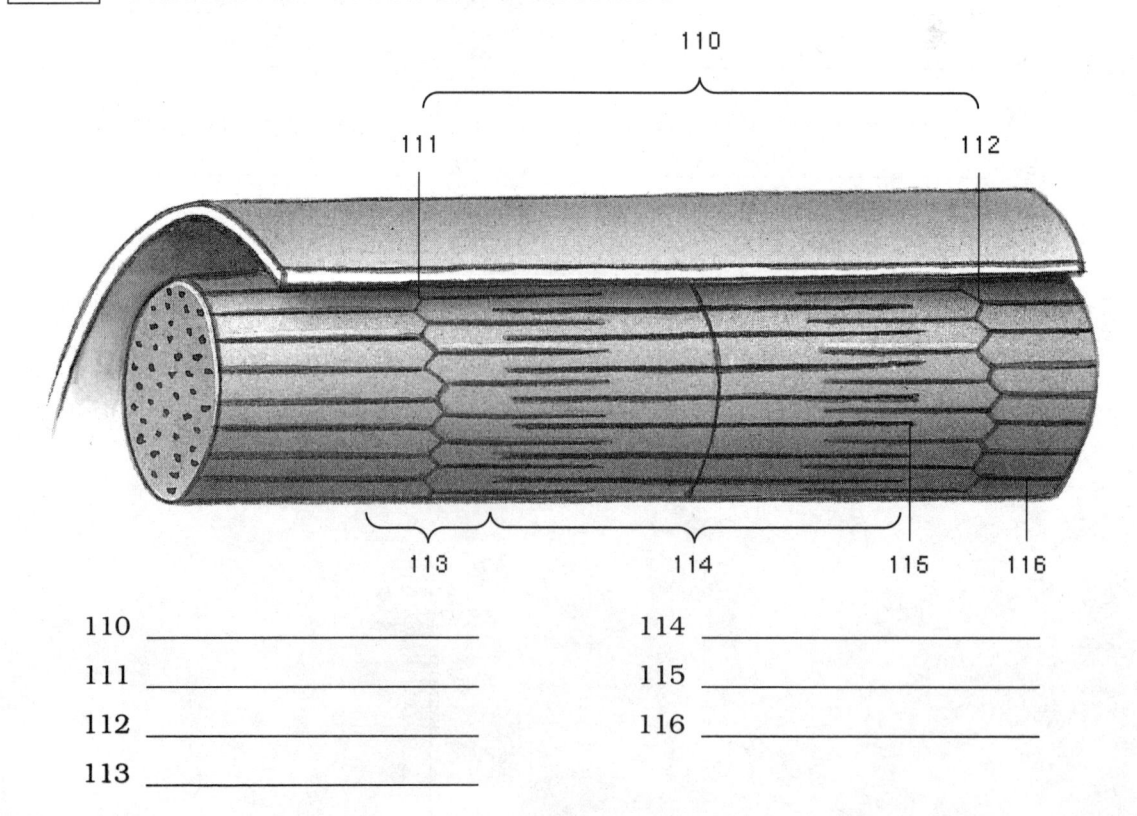

110 _____
111 _____
112 _____
113 _____

114 _____
115 _____
116 _____

Level -1-

Level 1 Review of Chapter Objectives 111

OBJ. 9   FIGURE 7.4   Types of Muscle Tissue

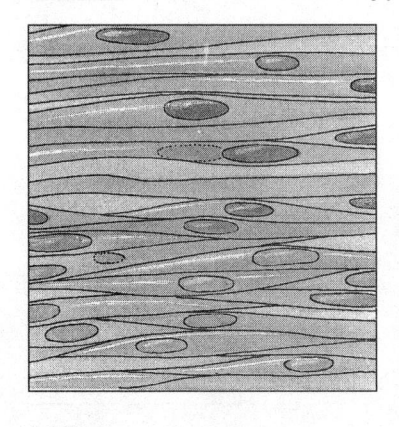

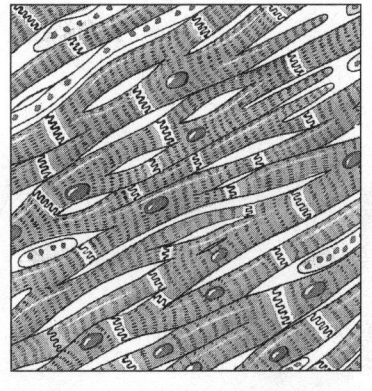

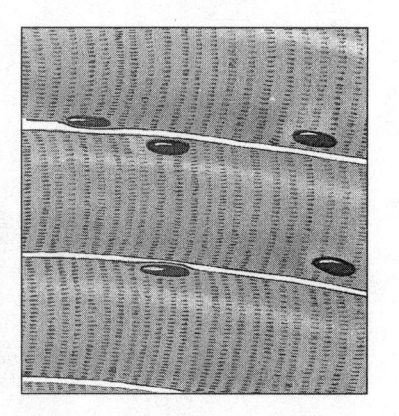

117 _____   118 _____   119 _____

OBJ. 10
OBJ. 11   FIGURE 7.5   Major Superficial Skeletal Muscles (anterior view)

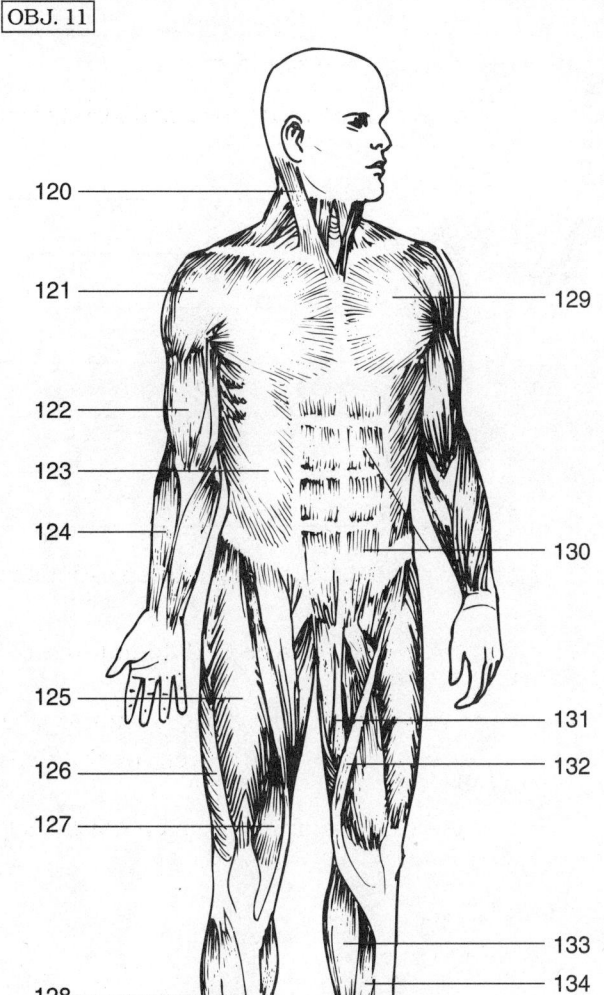

120 _____
121 _____
122 _____
123 _____
124 _____
125 _____
126 _____
127 _____
128 _____
129 _____
130 _____
131 _____
132 _____
133 _____
134 _____

Anterior view

112　Chapter 7　The Muscular System

OBJ. 10
OBJ. 11
FIGURE 7.6　Major Superficial Skeletal Muscles (posterior view)

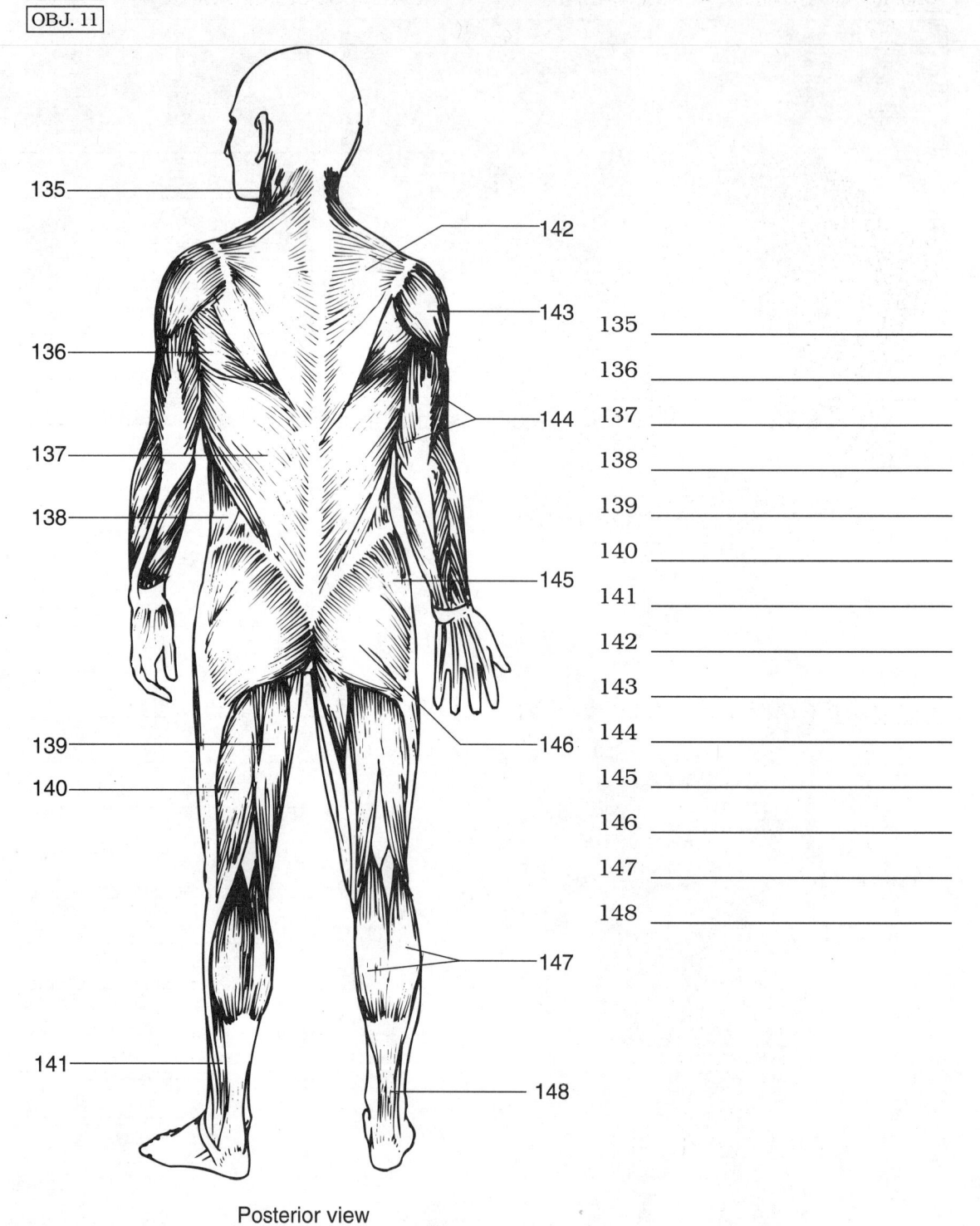

135 _____
136 _____
137 _____
138 _____
139 _____
140 _____
141 _____
142 _____
143 _____
144 _____
145 _____
146 _____
147 _____
148 _____

Posterior view

Level 1

Level 1   Review of Chapter Objectives   113

OBJ. 10   **FIGURE 7.7**   Superficial View of Facial Muscles (lateral view)

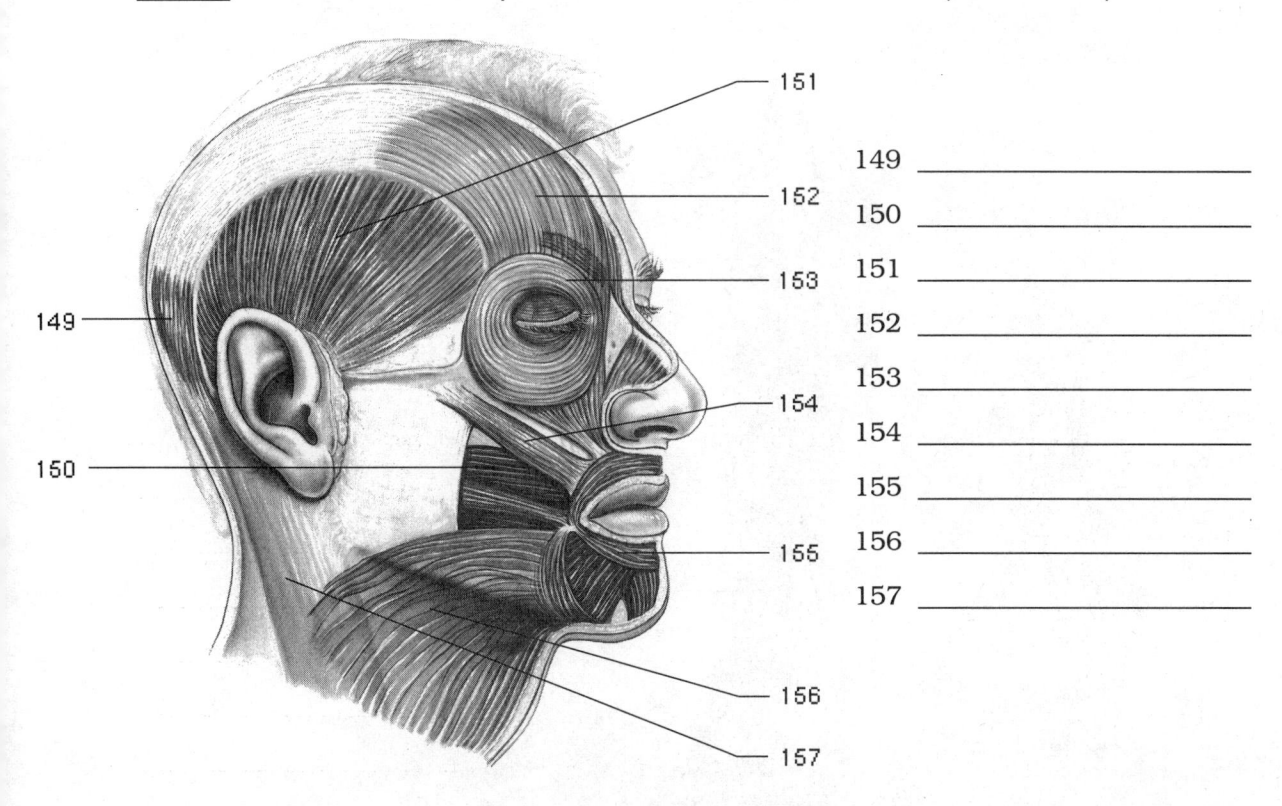

149 _____
150 _____
151 _____
152 _____
153 _____
154 _____
155 _____
156 _____
157 _____

OBJ. 11   **FIGURE 7.8**   Superficial Muscles of the Forearm (anterior view)

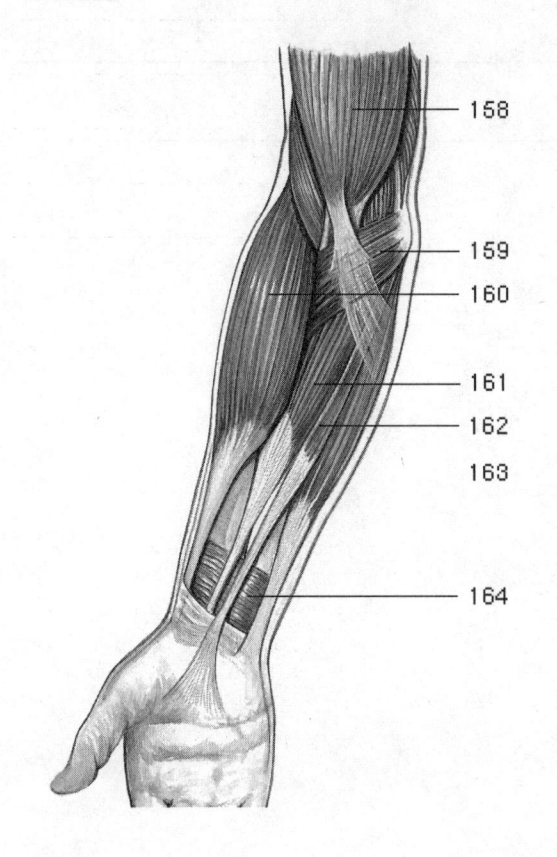

158 _____
159 _____
160 _____
161 _____
162 _____
163 _____
164 _____

Level
-1-

114 Chapter 7 The Muscular System

OBJ. 11 **FIGURE 7.9** Superficial Muscles of the Lower Leg (lateral view)

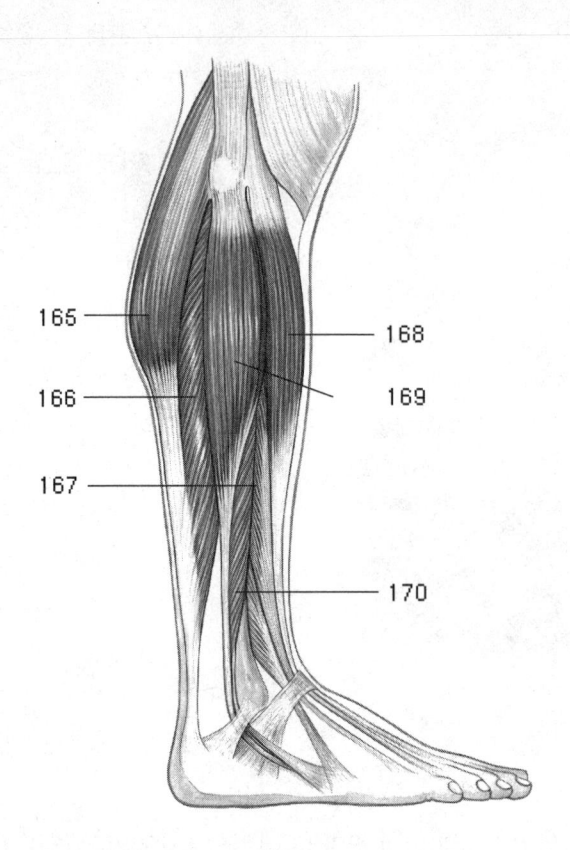

| 165 _____ | 166 _____ | 167 _____ |
| 168 _____ | 169 _____ | 170 _____ |

Level
-1-

Level 1   Review of Chapter Objectives   115

OBJ. 11   Superficial Muscles of the Thigh

FIGURE 7.10   (anterior view)   **FIGURE 7.11**   (posterior view)

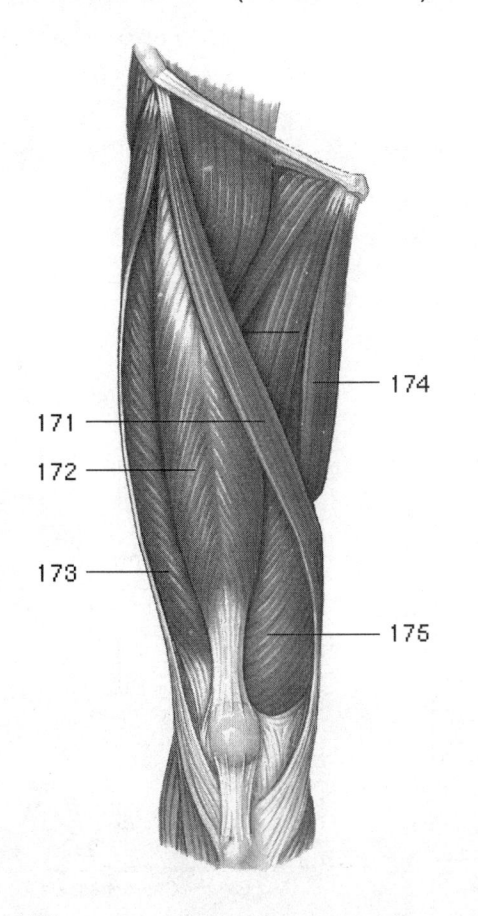

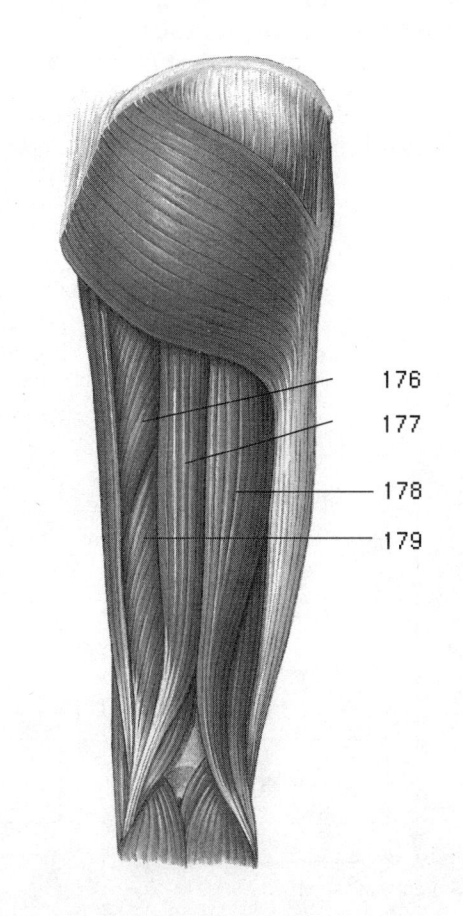

171 _____   176 _____
172 _____   177 _____
173 _____   178 _____
174 _____   179 _____
175 _____

When you have successfully completed the exercises in L1 proceed to L2.

Level
-1-

Chapter 7 The Muscular System

☐ LEVEL 2—CONCEPT SYNTHESIS

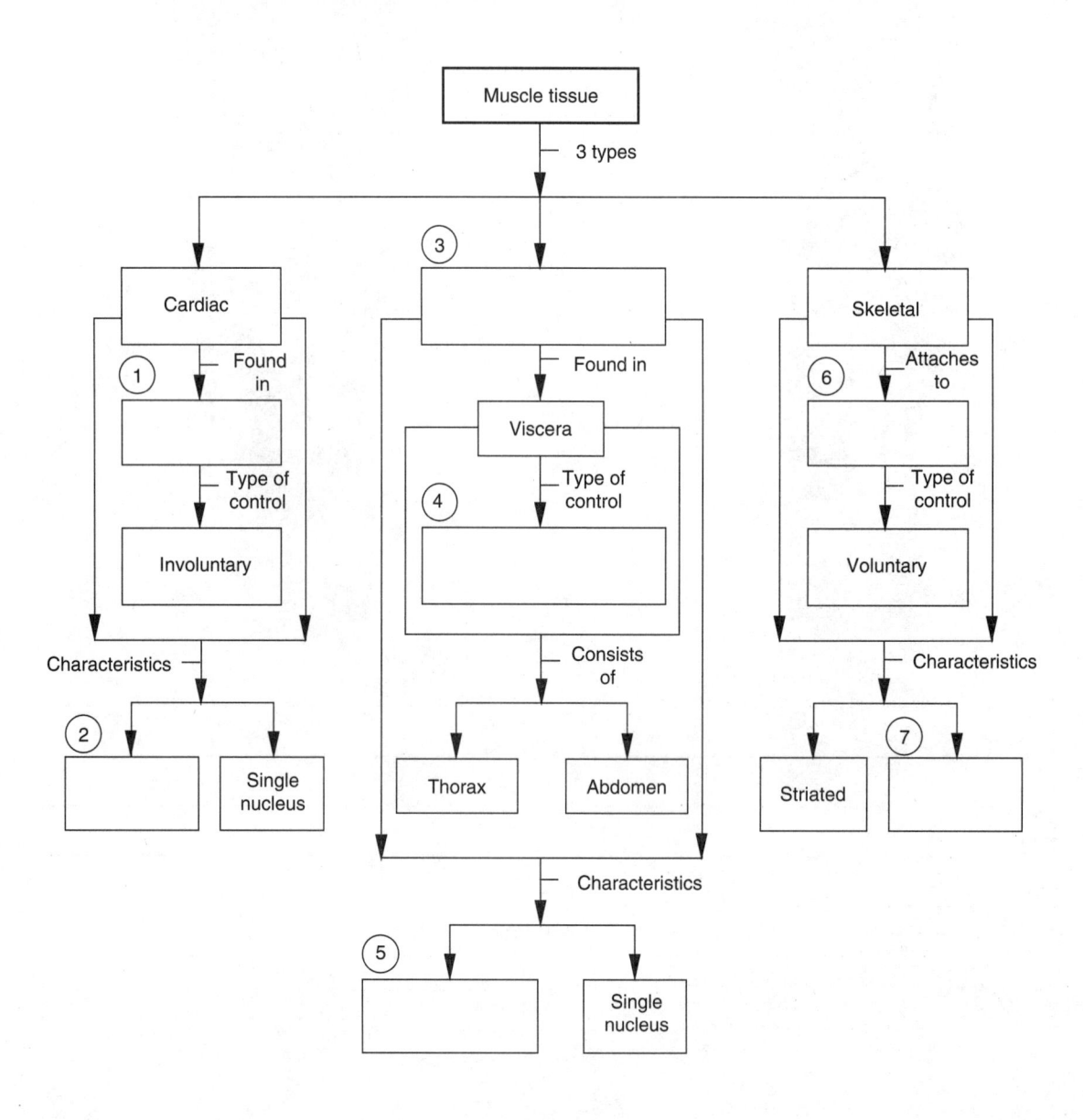

Concept Map I

Using the following terms, fill in the numbered, blank spaces to complete the concept map. Follow the numbers that comply with the organization of the map.

| Smooth | Involuntary | Striated | Heart |
| Multinucleated | Bones | Non-striated | |

```
                        Muscle tissue
                             │
                           3 types
        ┌────────────────────┼────────────────────┐
        ▼                    ▼                    ▼
     Cardiac              ( 3 )               Skeletal
        │                    │                    │
      Found              Found in            Attaches
    (1)  in                  │             (6)   to
        ▼                 Viscera                 ▼
     [    ]                  │                 [    ]
        │                Type of                  │
     Type of            (4) control            Type of
     control              [      ]             control
        ▼                                         ▼
   Involuntary                                Voluntary
        │                    │                    │
  Characteristics       Consists of         Characteristics
     ┌──┴──┐              ┌──┴──┐              ┌──┴──┐
    (2)    ▼              ▼     ▼              ▼    (7)
    [  ] Single        Thorax Abdomen       Striated [  ]
         nucleus
                             │
                       Characteristics
                          ┌──┴──┐
                         (5)    ▼
                         [  ] Single
                              nucleus
```

Level 2

Concept Map II

Using the following terms, fill in the numbered, blank spaces to complete the concept map. Follow the numbers that comply with the organization of the map.

    Cross-bridging (heads of myosin attach to turned-on thin filaments)
    Energy + ADP + Phosphate
    Release of Ca^{++} from sacs of sarcoplasmic reticulum
    Shortening (i.e., contraction of myofibrils and muscle fibers they compose)

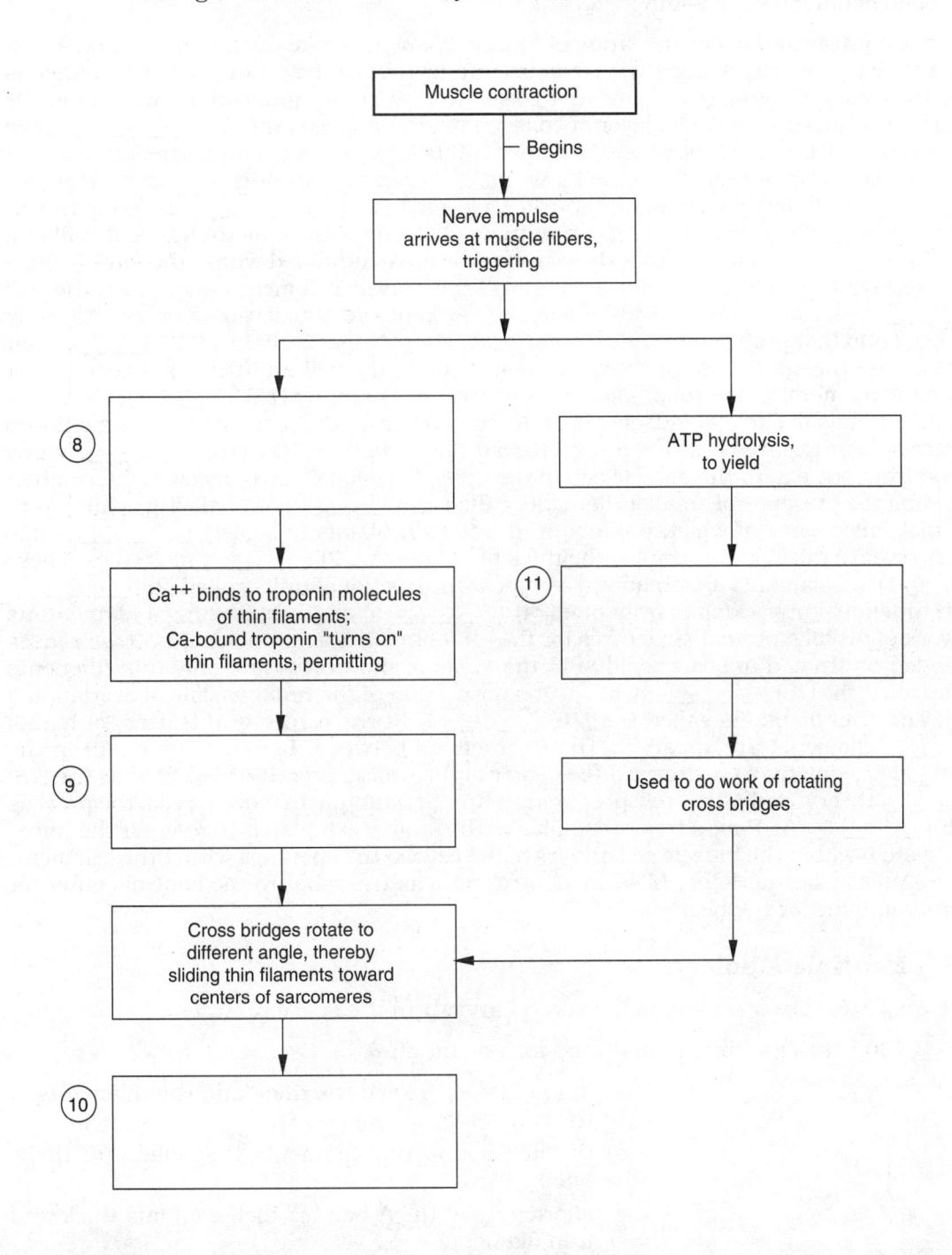

```
                    ┌─────────────────────┐
                    │ Muscle contraction  │
                    └──────────┬──────────┘
                               │ Begins
                               ▼
                    ┌─────────────────────┐
                    │   Nerve impulse     │
                    │ arrives at muscle   │
                    │  fibers, triggering │
                    └──────────┬──────────┘
                               │
                   ┌───────────┴───────────┐
                   ▼                       ▼
        ┌──────────────────┐      ┌──────────────────┐
    (8) │                  │      │  ATP hydrolysis, │
        │                  │      │     to yield     │
        └─────────┬────────┘      └─────────┬────────┘
                  ▼                         ▼
        ┌──────────────────┐           ┌─────────┐
        │ Ca++ binds to    │       (11)│         │
        │ troponin molecules│          │         │
        │ of thin filaments;│          └────┬────┘
        │ Ca-bound troponin │               │
        │ "turns on" thin   │               ▼
        │ filaments,        │      ┌──────────────────┐
        │ permitting        │      │ Used to do work  │
        └─────────┬─────────┘      │ of rotating      │
                  ▼                │ cross bridges    │
        ┌──────────────────┐       └────────┬─────────┘
    (9) │                  │                │
        └─────────┬────────┘                │
                  ▼                         │
        ┌──────────────────┐                │
        │ Cross bridges    │◄───────────────┘
        │ rotate to        │
        │ different angle, │
        │ thereby sliding  │
        │ thin filaments   │
        │ toward centers   │
        │ of sarcomeres    │
        └─────────┬────────┘
                  ▼
        ┌──────────────────┐
   (10) │                  │
        └──────────────────┘
```

Chapter 7 The Muscular System

Body Trek:

Using the terms below, fill in the blanks to complete the trek through the muscle tissue.

thick	nuclei	fascicles	actin
contraction	Z line	endomysium	A band
myosin	sarcomeres	sarcolemma	T tubules
myofibrils	I band	myofilaments	perimysium
epimysium	sliding filament		

Robo's programming for the study of muscle tissue will take the micro-robot on a trek into a skeletal muscle. A large syringe is used to introduce the robot via a subcutaneous injection into the deep fascia connective tissue until it comes into contact with a muscle that is surrounded by a dense layer of collagen fibers known as the (12) _____. Once inside the muscle, the robot senses the appearance of a series of compartments consisting of collagen, elastic fibers, blood vessels, and nerves, all surrounded by the (13) _____. The individual compartments are referred to as (14) _____. Probing deeper, there appears to be a network of loose connective tissue with numerous reticular fibers, the (15) _____, which surrounds each muscle fiber contained within the muscle bundle. Robo's entrance into the muscle by way of the muscle cell membrane, called the (16) _____, is facilitated by a series of openings to "pipe-like" structures that are regularly arranged and that project into the muscle fibers. These "pipes" are the (17) _____ that serve as the transport system between the outside of the cell and the cell interior. Just inside the membrane, the robot picks up the presence of many (18) _____, a characteristic common to skeletal muscle fibers. Robo's trek from the pipe-like environment into the sarcoplasm exposes neatly arranged thread-like structures, the (19) _____, which extend from one end of the muscle cell to the other. Mission Control receives information regarding the presence of smaller filaments called (20) _____, consisting of large protein molecules some of which are arranged into thin filaments or (21) _____, while others reveal a thicker appearance, the thick filaments or (22) _____ molecules. These thick and thin filaments are organized as repeating functional units called (23) _____. Each functional unit extends from one (24) _____ to another, forming a filamentous network of disklike protein structures for the attachment of actin molecules. Robo senses a banded or striated appearance due to the areas of the unit where only thin filaments exist, called the (25) _____, while a greater portion of the unit consists of overlapping thick and thin filaments called the (26) _____. In the center of this area, only (27) _____ filaments are apparent. The interactions between the filaments result in the sliding of the thin filaments toward the center of the unit, a process referred to as the (28) _____ theory, and ultimately producing a function unique to muscle cells, the process of (29) _____. As Robo's trek is completed, the robot's exit plan is to re-enter the "pipe-like" system within the muscle cell and leave the cell via the openings within the cell membrane. After retrieving Robo, Mission Control returns the robot to the control center for re-programming for the next task.

[L2] Multiple Choice:

Place the letter corresponding to the correct answer in the space provided.

_____ 30. Muscle contraction occurs as a result of:

    a. interactions between the thick and thin filaments of the sarcomere

    b. the interconnecting filaments that make up the Z lines

    c. shortening of the A band, which contains thick and thin filaments

    d. shortening of the I band, which contains thin filaments only

Level 2   Concept Synthesis   119

_____ 31. The process of cross-bridging, which occurs at an active site, involves a series of sequential-cyclic reactions that include:
    a. attach, return, pivot, detach
    b. attach, pivot, detach, return
    c. attach, detach, pivot, return
    d. attach, return, detach, pivot

_____ 32. When Ca^{++} binds to troponin, it produces a change by:
    a. initiating activity at the neuromuscular junction
    b. causing the actin-myosin interaction to occur
    c. decreasing the calcium concentration at the sarcomere
    d. exposing the active site on the thin filaments

_____ 33. The phases of a single twitch in sequential order include:
    a. contraction phase, latent phase, relaxation phase
    b. latent period, relaxation phase, contraction phase
    c. latent period, contraction phase, relaxation phase
    d. relaxation phase, latent phase, contraction phase

_____ 34. After contraction, a muscle fiber returns to its original length through:
    a. the active mechanism for fiber elongation
    b. elastic forces and the movement of opposing muscles
    c. the tension produced by the initial length of the muscle fiber
    d. involvement of all the sarcomeres along the myofibrils

_____ 35. The total force exerted by a muscle as a whole depends on:
    a. the rate of stimulation
    b. how many motor units are activated
    c. the number of calcium ions released
    d. a, b, and c are correct

_____ 36. The primary energy reserves found in skeletal muscle cells are:
    a. carbohydrates, fats, proteins
    b. DNA, RNA, ATP
    c. ATP, creatine phosphate, glycogen
    d. ATP, ADP, AMP

_____ 37. The two mechanisms used to generate ATP from glucose are:
    a. aerobic respiration and anaerobic glycolysis
    b. ADP and creatine phosphate
    c. cytoplasm and mitochondria
    d. a, b, and c are correct

_____ 38. In anaerobic glycolysis, glucose is broken down to pyruvic acid, which is converted to:
    a. glycogen
    b. lactic acid
    c. acetyl-CoA
    d. citric acid

_____ 39. The maintenance of normal body temperature is dependent on:
   a. the temperature of the environment
   b. the pH of the blood
   c. the production of energy by muscles
   d. the amount of energy produced by anaerobic glycolysis

_____ 40. An example of an activity that requires anaerobic endurance:
   a. a 50-yard dash
   b. a 3-mile run
   c. a 10-mile bicycle ride
   d. running a marathon

_____ 41. Athletes training to develop anaerobic endurance perform:
   a. few, long, relaxing workouts
   b. a combination of weight training and marathon running
   c. frequent, brief, intensive workouts
   d. stretching, flexibility, and relaxation exercises

_____ 42. The major support that the muscular system gets from the cardiovascular system is:
   a. direct response by controlling the heart rate and the respiratory rate
   b. constriction of blood vessels and decrease in heart rate for thermoregulatory control
   c. nutrient and oxygen delivery and carbon dioxide removal
   d. decreased volume of blood and rate of flow for maximal muscle contraction

_____ 43. The two factors that interact to determine the effects of individual skeletal muscle contraction are:
   a. the degree to which the muscle is stretched and the amount of tension produced
   b. the anatomical arrangement of the muscle fibers and the way the muscle attaches to the skeletal system
   c. the strength of the stimulus and the speed at which the stimulus is applied
   d. the length of the fibers and the metabolic condition of the muscle

_____ 44. When a muscle is stretched too far, the muscle loses power because:
   a. the overlap between myofilaments is reduced
   b. the amount of tension is increased due to over-stretching
   c. the sarcomere is stretched and the tension increases
   d. a, b, and c are correct

_____ 45. When a muscle contracts and its fibers shorten:
   a. the origin moves toward the insertion
   b. the origin and the insertion move in opposite directions
   c. the origin and insertion move in the same direction
   d. the insertion moves toward the origin

_____ 46. The structural commonality of the rectus femoris and rectus abdominis is that they are:
- a. parallel muscles whose fibers run along the long axis of the body
- b. both found in the region of the rectum
- c. muscles whose fibers are arranged to control peristalsis in the rectum
- d. attached to bones involved in similar functional activities

_____ 47. If you are engaging in an activity in which the action involves the use of the levator scapulae you are:
- a. shrugging your shoulders
- b. raising your hand
- c. breathing deeply
- d. looking up toward the sky

_____ 48. The biceps muscle makes a prominent bulge when:
- a. extending the forearm pronated
- b. flexing the forearm supinated
- c. extending the forearm supinated
- d. flexing the forearm pronated

[L2] Completion:

Using the terms below, complete the following statements.

fatigue	isotonic	quadriceps	innervation
tetanus	sartorius	motor unit	biomechanics
muscle tone	perineum	hamstrings	

49. Resting tension in a skeletal muscle is called _____.
50. The condition that results when a muscle is stimulated but cannot respond is referred to as _____.
51. A single cranial or spinal motor neuron and the muscle fibers it innervates comprise a _____.
52. At sufficiently high electrical frequencies, the overlapping twitches result in one strong, steady contraction referred to as _____.
53. When the muscle shortens but its tension remains the same, the contraction is _____.
54. The analysis of biological systems in mechanical terms is the study of _____.
55. The term used to refer to the identity of the nerve that controls a muscle is _____.
56. The muscle that is active when crossing the legs is the _____.
57. The muscles of the pelvic floor that extend between the sacrum and pelvic girdle form the muscular _____.
58. The flexors of the legs are commonly referred to as the _____.
59. The extensors of the legs are commonly referred to as the _____.

Chapter 7 The Muscular System

[L2] Short Essay:

Briefly answer the following questions in the spaces provided below.

60. What are the five (5) functions performed by skeletal muscle?

61. Draw an illustration of a sarcomere and label the parts according to the unit organization.

62. Cite the five (5) interlocking steps involved in the contraction process.

63. What is the relationship among fatigue, anaerobic glycolysis, and oxygen debt?

64. Why do fast fibers fatigue more rapidly than slow fibers?

65. What are the four (4) groups of muscles that comprise the axial musculature?

66. What two (2) major groups of muscles comprise the appendicular musculature?

When you have successfully completed the exercises in L2 proceed to L3.

☐ LEVEL 3 CRITICAL THINKING/APPLICATION

Using the principles and concepts learned about skeletal muscle tissue, answer the following questions. Write your answers on a separate sheet of paper.

1. Suppose you are assigned the responsibility of developing training programs tailored to increase both aerobic and anaerobic endurance. What types of activities would be necessary to support these training programs?
2. An individual who has been on a diet that eliminates dairy products complains of muscular spasms and nervousness. Why might these symptoms result from such a diet?
3. Your responsibility as a nurse includes giving intramuscular (IM) injections. (a) Why is an IM preferred over an injection directly into the circulation? (b) What muscles are best suited as sites for IM injections?

CHAPTER 8

Neural Tissue & the Central Nervous System

■ Overview

The nervous system is the control center and communication network of the body, and its overall function is the maintenance of homeostasis. The nervous system and the endocrine system acting in a complementary way regulate and coordinate the activities of the body's organ systems. The nervous system generally affects short-term control, whereas endocrine regulation is slower to develop and the general effect is long-term control.

In this chapter the introductory material begins with an overview of the nervous system and the cellular organization in neural tissue. The chapter then covers the structure and function of neurons, information processing, and the functional patterns of neural organization. Finally, the central nervous system, the brain and spinal cord, will be discussed.

The integration and interrelation of the nervous system with all the other body systems is an integral part of understanding many of the body's activities, which must be controlled and adjusted to meet changing internal and external environmental conditions.

The central nervous system (CNS) consists of the brain and the spinal cord. Both of these parts of the CNS are covered with meninges, both are bathed in cerebrospinal fluid, and both areas contain gray and white matter. Even though there are structural and functional similarities, the brain and the spinal cord show significant independent structural and functional differences.

Emphasis is placed on the importance of the spinal cord as a communication link between the brain and the peripheral nervous system (PNS), and as an integrating center that can be independently involved with somatic reflex activity.

The brain is a large, complex organ located in the cranial cavity. It is completely surrounded by cerebrospinal fluid (CSF), the cranial meninges, and the bony structures of the cranium. The development of the brain is one of the primary factors that have been used to classify us as "human." The ability to think and reason separates us from all other forms of life. The brain consists of billions of neurons organized into hundreds of neuronal pools with extensive interconnections that provide great versatility and variability. The same basic principles of neural activity and information processing that occur in the spinal cord also apply to the brain; however, because of the increased amount of neural tissue, there is an expanded versatility and complexity in response to neural stimulation and neural function. Included are exercises and test questions that focus on the major regions and structures of the brain. The concept maps of the brain will be particularly helpful in making the brain come "alive" structurally.

☐ LEVEL 1   REVIEW OF CHAPTER OBJECTIVES

1. Describe the anatomical organization and general functions of the nervous system.
2. Distinguish between neurons and neuroglia and compare their structure and functions.
3. Discuss the events that generate action potentials in the membranes of nerve cells.
4. Distinguish between continuous and saltatory nerve impulse conduction.
5. Explain the mechanism of nerve impulse transmission at the synapse.
6. Describe the process of a neural reflex.
7. Describe the three meningeal layers that surround the central nervous system.
8. Discuss the structure and functions of the spinal cord.
9. Name the major regions of the brain and describe their functions.
10. Locate the motor, sensory and association areas of the cerebral cortex and discuss their functions.

[L1]   Multiple Choice:

Place the letter corresponding to the correct answer in the space provided.

OBJ. 1 ___ 1. Sensory neurons are responsible for carrying impulses:

    a. to the CNS
    b. away from the CNS
    c. to the PNS
    d. from the CNS to the PNS

OBJ. 1 ___ 2. Interneurons, or association neurons, differ from sensory and motor neurons because of their:

    a. structural characteristics
    b. inability to generate action potentials
    c. exclusive location in the brain and spinal cord
    d. functional capabilities

OBJ. 1 ___ 3. Efferent pathways consist of axons that carry impulses:

    a. toward the CNS
    b. from the PNS to the CNS
    c. away from the CNS
    d. to the spinal cord and into the brain

OBJ. 1 ___ 4. The two major anatomical subdivisions of the nervous system are:

    a. central nervous system (CNS) and peripheral nervous system (PNS)
    b. somatic nervous system and autonomic nervous system
    c. neurons and neuroglia
    d. afferent division and efferent division

126 Chapter 8 Neural Tissue & the Central Nervous System

[OBJ. 1] ____ 5. The central nervous system (CNS) consists of:
   a. afferent and efferent divisions
   b. somatic and visceral divisions
   c. brain and spinal cord
   d. autonomic and somatic division

[OBJ. 1] ____ 6. The primary functions of the nervous system include:
   a. providing sensation of the internal and external environments
   b. integrating sensory information
   c. regulating and controlling peripheral structures and systems
   d. a, b, and c are correct

[OBJ. 2] ____ 7. The two major cell populations of neural tissue are:
   a. astrocytes and oligodendrocytes
   b. microglia and ependymal cells
   c. satellite cells and Schwann cells
   d. neurons and neuroglia

[OBJ. 2] ____ 8. The types of glial cells in the central nervous system are:
   a. astrocytes, oligodendrocytes, microglia, and ependymal cells
   b. unipolar, bipolar, multipolar cells
   c. efferent, afferent, association cells
   d. motor, sensory, interneuron cells

[OBJ. 2] ____ 9. The white matter of the CNS represents a region dominated by the presence of:
   a. astrocytes
   b. oligodendrocytes
   c. neuroglia
   d. a, b, and c are correct

[OBJ. 2] ____ 10. Neurons are responsible for:
   a. creating a three-dimensional framework for the CNS
   b. performing repairs in damaged neural tissue
   c. information transfer and processing in the nervous system
   d. controlling the interstitial environment

[OBJ. 2] ____ 11. Neurons are classified on the basis of their structure as:
   a. astrocytes, oligodendrocytes, microglia, ependymal cells
   b. efferent, afferent, association, interneurons
   c. motor, sensory, association, interneurons
   d. unipolar, bipolar, multipolar

Level -1-

Level 1 Review of Chapter Objectives 127

OBJ. 2 ___ 12. Neurons are classified on the basis of their function as:
- a. unipolar, bipolar, multipolar
- b. motor, sensory, association
- c. somatic, visceral, autonomic
- d. central, peripheral, somatic

OBJ. 3 ___ 13. Depolarization of the membrane will shift the membrane potential toward:
- a. -90 mV
- b. -85 mV
- c. -70 mV
- d. 0 mV

OBJ. 3 ___ 14. The resting membrane potential (RMP) of a typical neuron is:
- a. -85 mV
- b. -60 mV
- c. -70 mV
- d. 0 mV

OBJ. 3 ___ 15. If resting membrane potential is -70 mV and the threshold is 60 mV, a membrane potential of -62 mV will:
- a. produce an action potential
- b. depolarize the membrane to 0 mV
- c. repolarize the membrane to -80 mV
- d. not produce an action potential

OBJ. 3 ___ 16. At the site of an action potential the membrane contains:
- a. an excess of negative ions inside and an excess of negative ions outside
- b. an excess of positive ions inside and an excess of negative ions outside
- c. an equal amount of positive and negative ions on either side of the membrane
- d. an equal amount of positive ions on either side of the membrane

OBJ. 3 ___ 17. If the resting membrane potential is -70 mV, a hyperpolarized membrane is:
- a. 0 mV
- b. +30 mV
- c. -80 mV
- d. -65 mV

OBJ. 4 ___ 18. A node along the axon represents an area where there is:
- a. a layer of fat
- b. interwoven layers of myelin and protein
- c. a gap in the cell membrane
- d. an absence of myelin

128 Chapter 8 Neural Tissue & the Central Nervous System

OBJ. 4 ___ 19. At an electrical synapse, the presynaptic and postsynaptic membranes are locked together at:
   a. gap junctions
   b. synaptic vesicles
   c. myelinated axons
   d. neuromuscular junctions

OBJ. 5 ___ 20. Exocytosis and the release of acetylcholine into the synaptic cleft is triggered by:
   a. calcium ions leaving the cytoplasm
   b. calcium ions flooding into the neuron's cytoplasm
   c. reabsorption of calcium into the endoplasmic reticulum
   d. active transport of calcium into synaptic vesicles

OBJ. 5 ___ 21. The final step involved in a neural reflex is:
   a. information processing
   b. the activation of a motor neuron
   c. a response by an effector
   d. the activation of a sensory neuron

OBJ. 6 ___ 22. The goals of information processing during a neural reflex are the selection of:
   a. appropriate sensor selections and specific motor responses
   b. an appropriate motor response and the activation of specific motor neurons
   c. appropriate sensory selections and activation of specific sensory neurons
   d. appropriate motor selections and specific sensory responses

OBJ. 6 ___ 23. In the reflex arc, information processing is performed by the:
   a. activation of a sensory neuron
   b. activation of a receptor
   c. release of the neurotransmitter by the synaptic terminal
   d. motor neuron that controls peripheral effectors

OBJ. 7 ___ 24. If cerebrospinal fluid was withdrawn during a spinal tap, a needle would be inserted into the:
   a. pia mater
   b. subdural space
   c. subarachnoid space
   d. b and c are correct

OBJ. 7 ___ 25. The meninge that is firmly bound to neural tissue and deep to other meninges is the:
   a. pia mater
   b. arachnoid membrane
   c. dura mater
   d. epidural space

Level -1-

Level 1   Review of Chapter Objectives   129

OBJ. 8 ___ 26. The spinal cord is part of the:
   a. peripheral nervous system
   b. somatic nervous system
   c. autonomic nervous system
   d. central nervous system

OBJ. 8 ___ 27. The identifiable areas of the spinal cord that are based on the regions they serve include:
   a. cervical, thoracic, lumbar, sacral
   b. pia mater, dura mater, arachnoid mater
   c. axillary, radial, median, ulnar
   d. cranial, visceral, autonomic, spinal

OBJ. 8 ___ 28. The white matter of the spinal cord contains:
   a. cell bodies of neurons and glial cells
   b. somatic and visceral sensory nuclei
   c. large numbers of myelinated and unmyelinated axons
   d. sensory and motor nuclei

OBJ. 8 ___ 29. The area of the spinal cord that surrounds the central canal and is dominated by the cell bodies of neurons and glial cells is the:
   a. white matter
   b. gray matter
   c. ascending tracts
   d. descending tracts

OBJ. 8 ___ 30. The posterior gray horns of the spinal cord contain:
   a. somatic and visceral sensory nuclei
   b. somatic and visceral motor nuclei
   c. ascending and descending tracts
   d. anterior and posterior columns

OBJ. 9 ___ 31. The major region of the brain responsible for conscious thought processes, sensations, intellectual functions, memory, and complex motor patterns is the:
   a. cerebellum
   b. medulla
   c. pons
   d. cerebrum

OBJ. 9 ___ 32. The region of the brain that adjusts and smooths voluntary and involuntary motor activities on the basis of sensory information and stored memories of previous movements is the:
   a. cerebrum
   b. cerebellum
   c. medulla
   d. diencephalon

Level -1-

130   Chapter 8   Neural Tissue & the Central Nervous System

OBJ. 9 ____ 33. The brain stem consists of:
- a. diencephalon, mesencephalon (midbrain), pons, medulla oblongata
- b. cerebrum, cerebellum, medulla, pons
- c. thalamus, hypothalamus, cerebellum, medulla
- d. diencephalon, spinal cord, cerebellum, medulla

OBJ. 9 ____ 34. Mechanical protection for the brain is provided by:
- a. the bones of the skull
- b. the cranial meninges
- c. the cerebrospinal fluid
- d. a, b, and c are correct

OBJ. 9 ____ 35. The cranial meninges offer protection to the brain by:
- a. protecting the brain from extremes of temperature
- b. affording mechanical protection to the brain tissue
- c. providing a barrier against invading pathogenic organisms
- d. acting as shock absorbers that prevent contact with surrounding bones

OBJ. 9 ____ 36. The brain is protected from shocks generated during locomotion by the:
- a. bones of the cranium
- b. the cerebrospinal fluid
- c. the spinal meninges
- d. intervertebral discs of the vertebral column and the muscles and vertebrae of the neck

OBJ. 9 ____ 37. Excess cerebrospinal fluid is returned to venous circulation by:
- a. diffusion across the arachnoid villi
- b. active transport across the choroid plexus
- c. diffusion through the lateral ventricles
- d. passage through the subarachnoid space

OBJ. 10 ____ 38. The neurons in the primary sensory cortex receive somatic sensory information from:
- a. exchange fibers in the white matter
- b. touch, pressure, pain, taste, and temperature receptors
- c. visual and auditory receptors in the eyes and ears
- d. receptors in muscle spindles and Golgi tendon organs

OBJ. 10 ____ 39. The neurons of the primary motor cortex are responsible for directing:
- a. visual and auditory responses
- b. responses to taste and temperature
- c. voluntary movements
- d. involuntary movements

Level -1-

Level 1 Review of Chapter Objectives 131

OBJ. 10 ___ 40. All communication between the brain and the spinal cord involves tracts that ascend or descend through the:
- a. cerebellum
- b. diencephalon
- c. medulla
- d. thalamus

OBJ. 10 ___ 41. The thalamus contains:
- a. centers involved with emotions and hormone production
- b. relay and processing centers for sensory information
- c. centers for involuntary somatic motor responses
- d. nuclei involved with visceral motor control

OBJ. 10 ___ 42. The hypothalamus contains centers involved with:
- a. voluntary somatic motor responses
- b. somatic and visceral motor control
- c. maintenance of consciousness
- d. emotions, autonomic function, and hormone production

[L1] Completion:

Using the terms below, complete the following statements.

cholinergic	microglia	saltatory	corpus callosum
afferent	threshold	shunt	third ventricle
collaterals	adrenergic	divergence	choroid plexus
neural reflexes	receptor	nuclei	autonomic nervous system
columns	cerebral cortex	postcentral gyrus	

OBJ. 1 43. The visceral motor system that provides automatic, involuntary regulation of smooth and cardiac muscle and glandular secretions is the _____.

OBJ. 2 44. In times of infection or injury the type of neuroglia that will increase in numbers is _____.

OBJ. 2 45. The "branches" that enable a single neuron to communicate with several other cells are called _____.

OBJ. 2 46. Sensory information is brought to the CNS by means of the _____ fibers.

OBJ. 3 47. An action potential occurs only if the membrane is lowered to the level known as the _____.

OBJ. 4 48. The process that conducts impulses along an axon at a high rate of speed is called _____ conduction.

OBJ. 5 49. Chemical synapses that release the neurotransmitter acetylcholine are known as _____ synapses.

OBJ. 5 50. Chemical synapses that release the neurotransmitter norepinephrine are known as _____ synapses.

OBJ. 5 51. The spread of nerve impulses from one neuron to several neurons is called _____.

OBJ. 6 52. Automatic motor responses, triggered by specific stimuli, are called _____.

132 Chapter 8 Neural Tissue & the Central Nervous System

OBJ. 6 53. A specialized cell that monitors conditions in the body or the external environment is called a(n) _____.

OBJ. 7 54. The cell bodies of neurons in the gray matter of the spinal cord from groups called _____.

OBJ. 8 55. The white matter of the spinal cord is divided into regions called _____.

OBJ. 9 56. The layer of gray matter found on the surface of the cerebrum is the _____.

OBJ. 9 57. The diencephalic chamber is called the _____.

OBJ. 9 58. The site of cerebrospinal fluid production is the _____.

OBJ. 9 59. A bypass that drains excess cerebrospinal fluid and reduces intracranial pressure is called a(n) _____.

OBJ. 10 60. The primary sensory cortex forms the surface of the _____.

OBJ. 10 61. The major connective pathway between the two cerebral hemispheres is the _____.

[L1] Matching:

Match the terms in column "B" with the terms in column "A." Use letters for answers in the spaces provided.

	COLUMN "A"	COLUMN "B"
OBJ. 1 ___ 62.	Somatic nervous system	A. -70mV
OBJ. 1 ___ 63.	Autonomic nervous system	B. Saltatory conduction
OBJ. 2 ___ 64.	Neuroglia	C. cAMP
OBJ. 2 ___ 65.	Axons	D. Involuntary control
OBJ. 3 ___ 66.	Neuron resting membrane potential	E. Voluntary control
		F. Supporting cells
OBJ. 3 ___ 67.	Potassium ion movement	G. Continuous conduction
OBJ. 4 ___ 68.	Unmyelinated axons	H. Action potential
OBJ. 4 ___ 69.	Nodes of Ranvier	I. Simultaneous responses
OBJ. 5 ___ 70.	Second messenger	J. Repolarization
OBJ. 5 ___ 71.	Parallel processing	K. Specialized protective membranes
OBJ. 6 ___ 72.	Neural "wiring"	
OBJ. 6 ___ 73.	Peripheral effector	L. Reflex arc
OBJ. 6 ___ 74.	Somatic Reflexes	M. Controls activities of muscular system
OBJ. 7 ___ 75.	Spinal meninges	
OBJ. 7 ___ 76.	White matter	N. Ascending, descending tracts
OBJ. 8 ___ 77.	Dorsal roots	O. Muscle or gland cell
OBJ. 8 ___ 78.	Ventral roots	P. Sensory information to spinal cord
OBJ. 9 ___ 79.	Ventricles	
OBJ. 9 ___ 80.	Arachnoid	Q. Contains axons or motor neurons
OBJ. 9 ___ 81.	Choroid Plexus	R. Coordinates motor activities
OBJ. 10 ___ 82.	Cerebellum	S. CSF production
OBJ. 10 ___ 83.	Medulla oblongata	T. Cerebrospinal fluid circulation
		U. Meninge
		V. Continuous with spinal cord

Level -1-

Level 1   Review of Chapter Objectives   133

[L1] Drawing/Illustration Labeling:

OBJ. 2   **FIGURE 8.1**   Structure and Classification of Neurons

Identify each numbered structure by labeling the following figures:

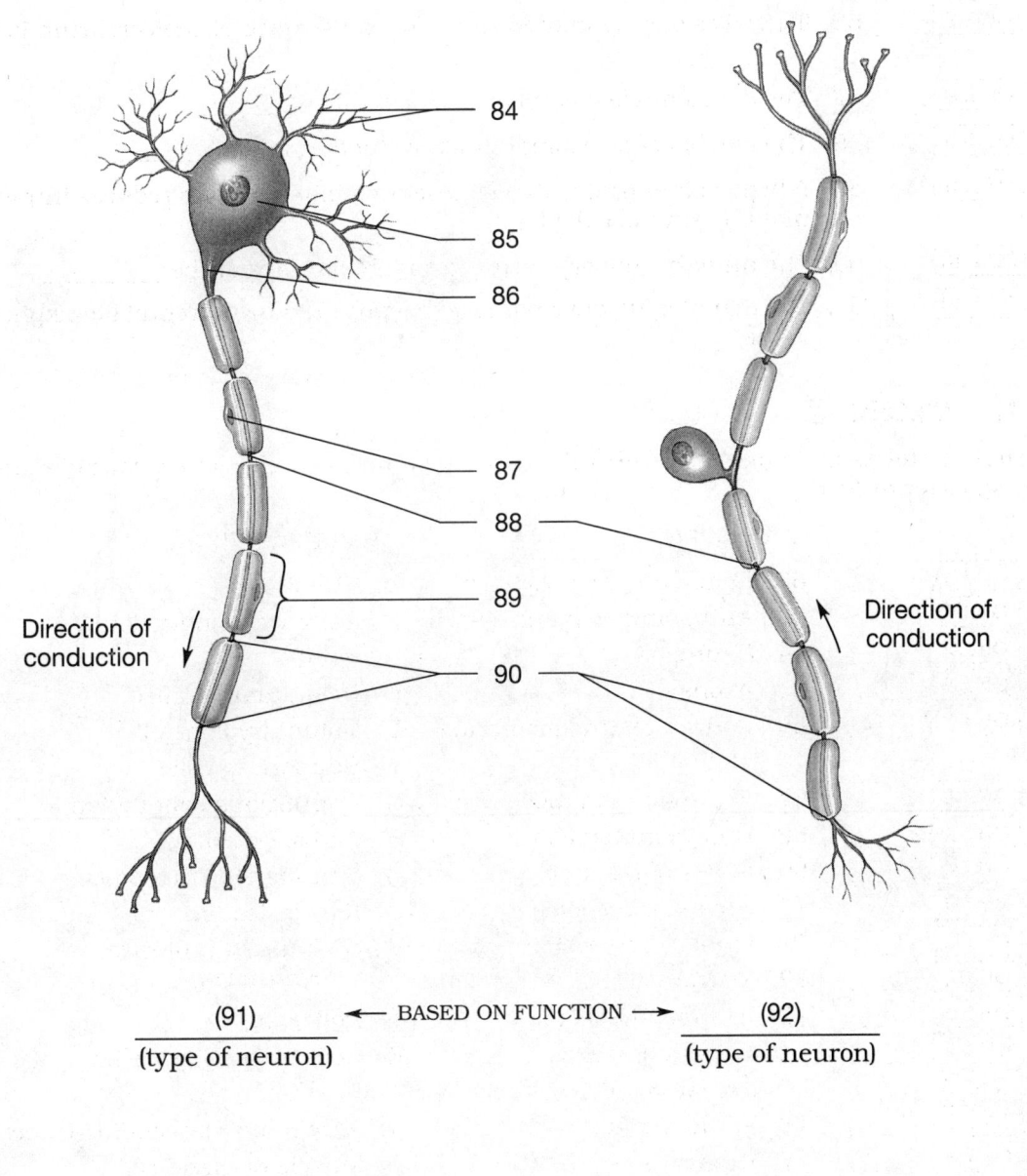

Direction of conduction

Direction of conduction

_____(91)_____ ← BASED ON FUNCTION → _____(92)_____
(type of neuron)   (type of neuron)

84 _____   87 _____   90 _____
85 _____   88 _____   91 _____
86 _____   89 _____   92 _____

134 Chapter 8 Neural Tissue & the Central Nervous System

OBJ. 2 **FIGURE 8.2** Neuron Classification (Based on Structure)

(Identify the types of neurons)

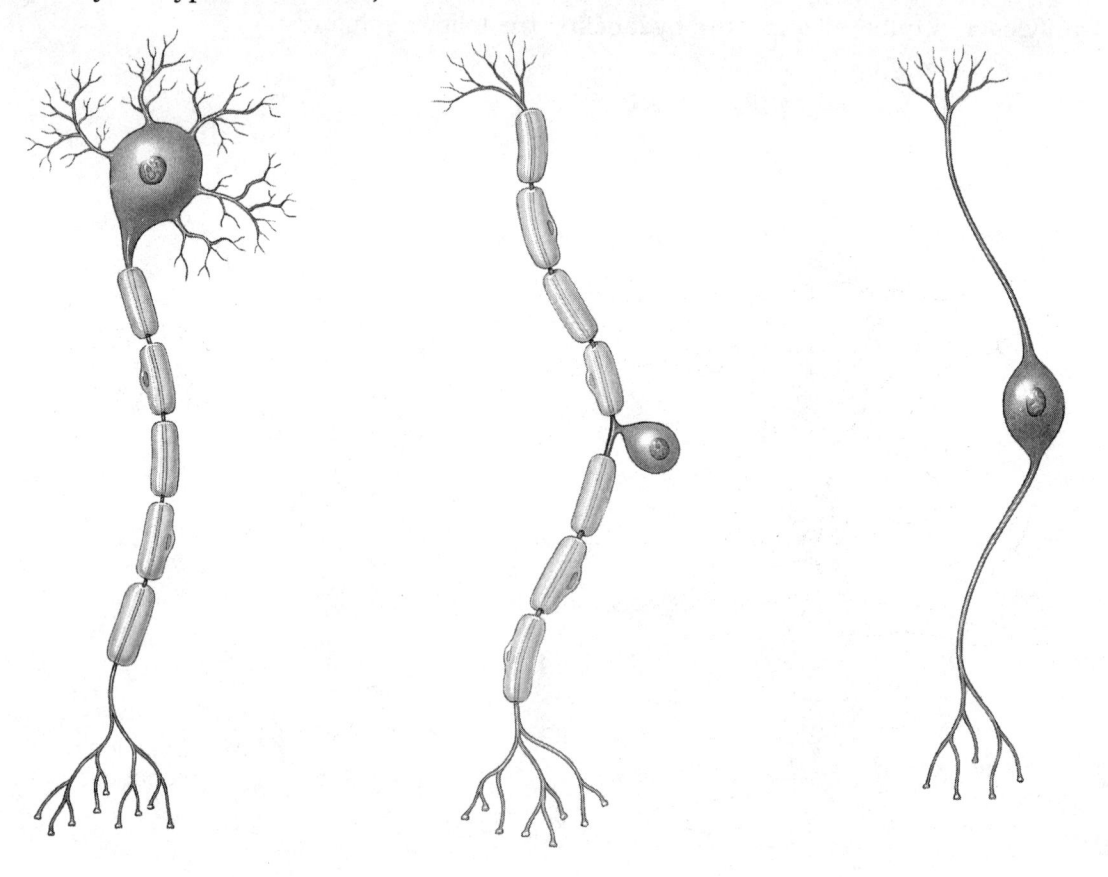

93 _____   94 _____   95 _____

Level 1 Review of Chapter Objectives 135

OBJ. 6 **FIGURE 8.3** Structure of a Reflex Arc

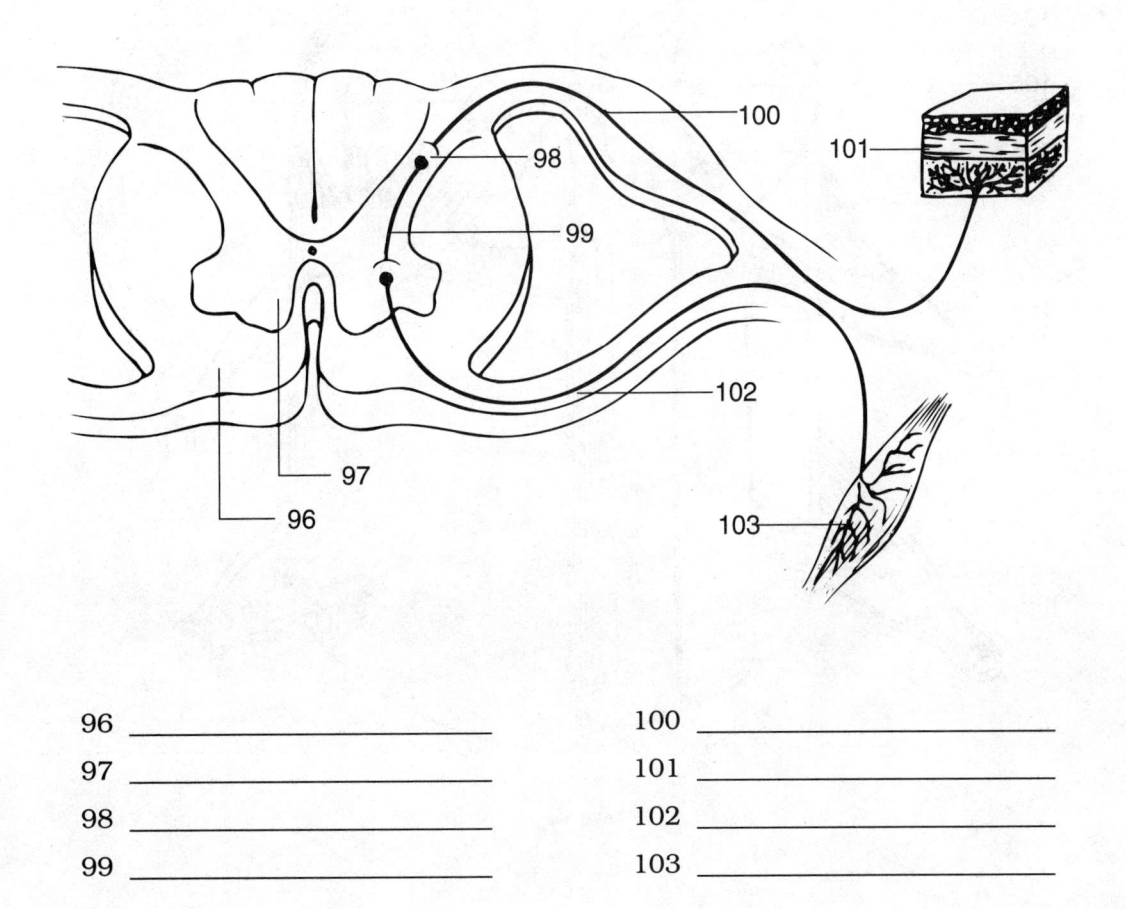

96 _____   100 _____
97 _____   101 _____
98 _____   102 _____
99 _____   103 _____

Level
-1-

136 **Chapter 8 Neural Tissue & the Central Nervous System**

OBJ. 8 **FIGURE 8.4** Organization of the Spinal Cord

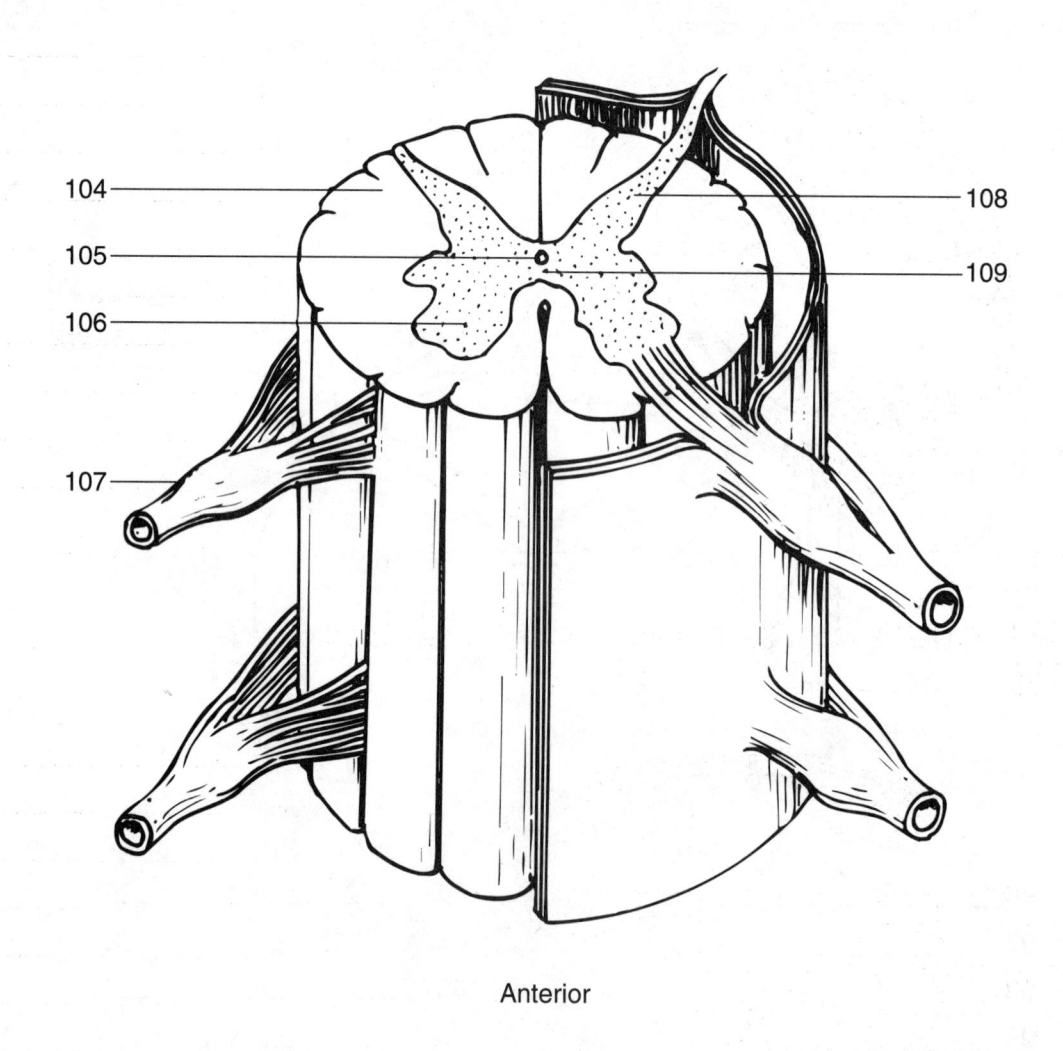

Anterior

104 _____   107 _____
105 _____   108 _____
106 _____   109 _____

Level 1 Review of Chapter Objectives 137

OBJ. 9
OBJ. 10

FIGURE 8.5 Lateral View of the Human Brain

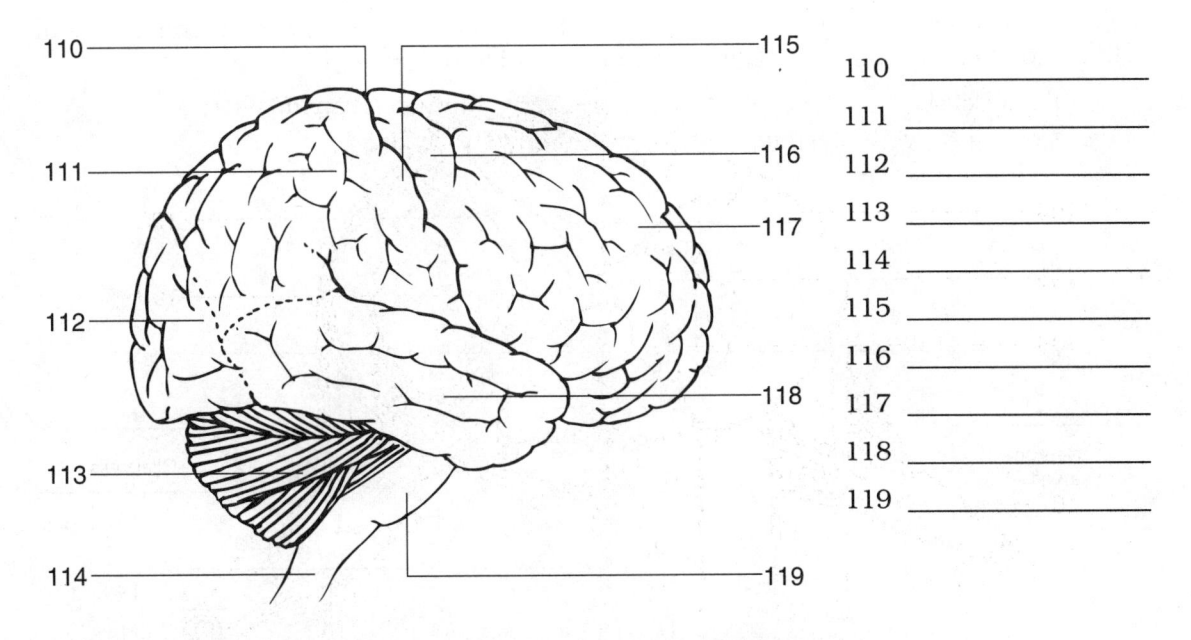

110 _____
111 _____
112 _____
113 _____
114 _____
115 _____
116 _____
117 _____
118 _____
119 _____

OBJ. 9
OBJ. 10

FIGURE 8.6 Sagittal View of the Human Brain

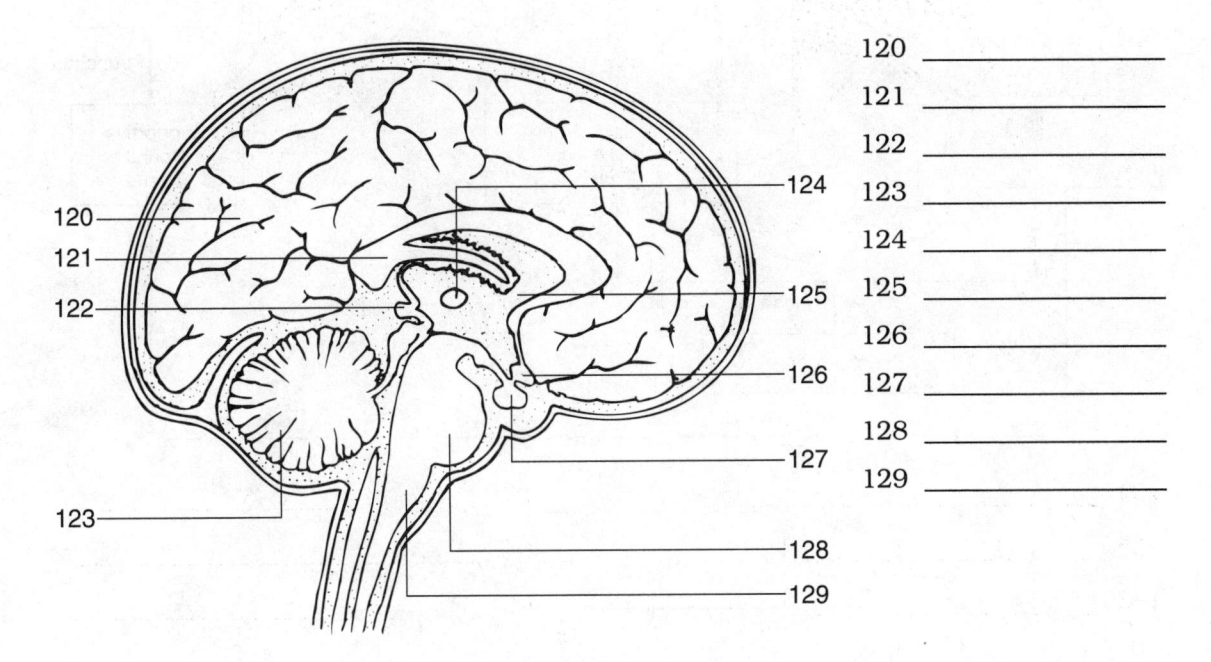

120 _____
121 _____
122 _____
123 _____
124 _____
125 _____
126 _____
127 _____
128 _____
129 _____

When you have successfully completed the exercises in L1 proceed to L2.

☐ LEVEL 2   CONCEPT SYNTHESIS

Concept Map I:

Using the following terms, fill in the numbered, blank spaces to complete the concept map. Follow the numbers that comply with the organization of the map.

- Glial Cells
- Central Nervous System
- Nerve Impulse Transmission
- Schwann Cells

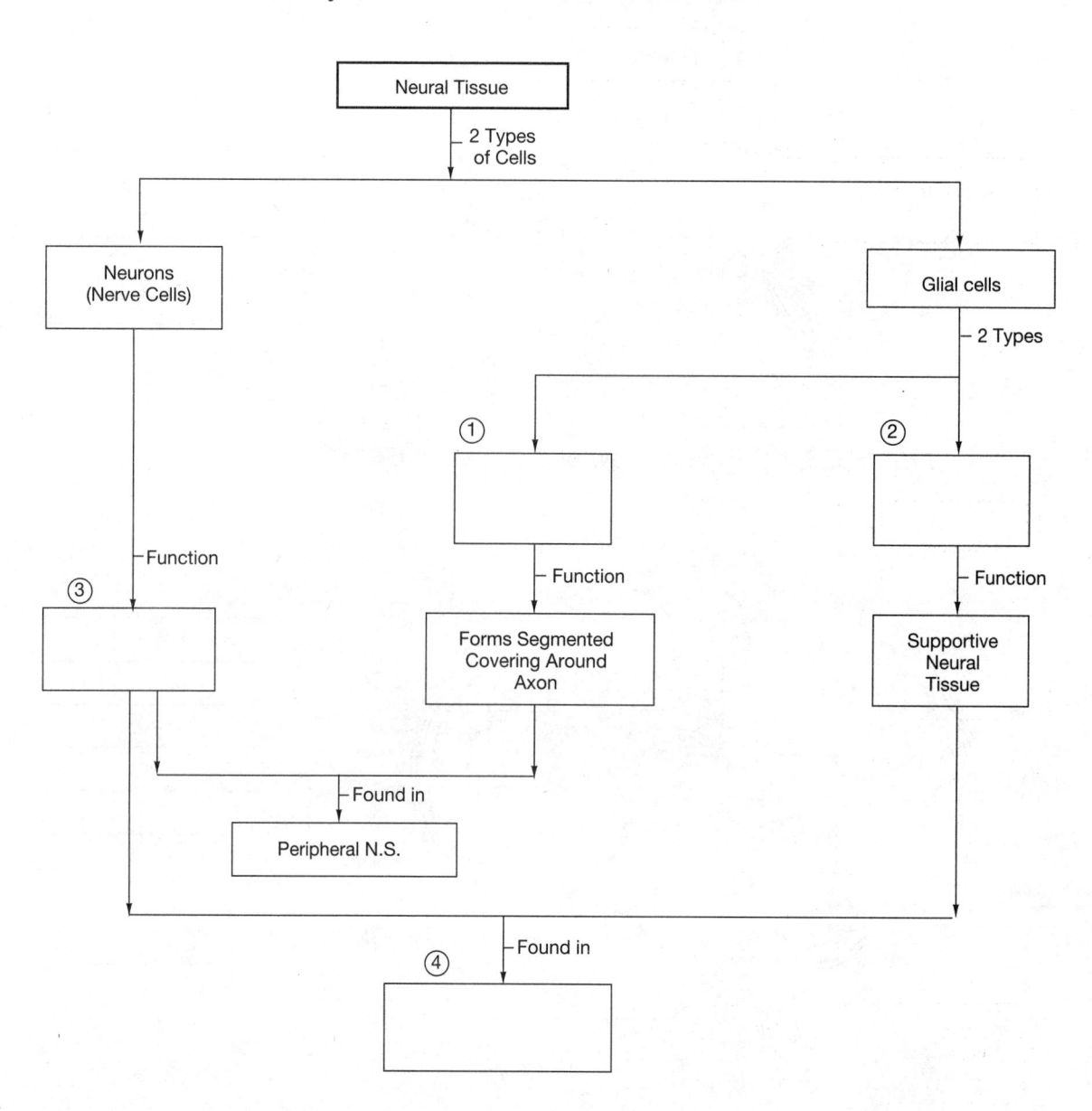

```
                    Neural Tissue
                         │
                    ┌ 2 Types
                    │ of Cells
         ┌──────────┴──────────┐
         ▼                     ▼
    Neurons                 Glial cells
  (Nerve Cells)                 │
         │                  ┌ 2 Types
         │          ┌───────┴───────┐
         │          ▼               ▼
         │         (1)             (2)
         │          │               │
      Function      │ Function      │ Function
         ▼          ▼               ▼
        (3)    Forms Segmented   Supportive
               Covering Around    Neural
                   Axon           Tissue
         │          │               │
         │       Found in           │
         │          ▼               │
         │    Peripheral N.S.       │
         │                          │
         └──────── Found in ────────┘
                    ▼
                   (4)
```

Concept Map II:

Using the terms below, fill in the numbered spaces to complete the concept maps. Follow the numbers which comply with the organization of the maps. (Follow the numbers in the circuit from CNS in upper left corner, clockwise to lower right, and return to Spinal Cord.)

- Brain
- Smooth Muscle
- Somatic Nervous System
- Peripheral Nervous System
- Afferent Division
- Motor System
- Sympathetic Nervous System

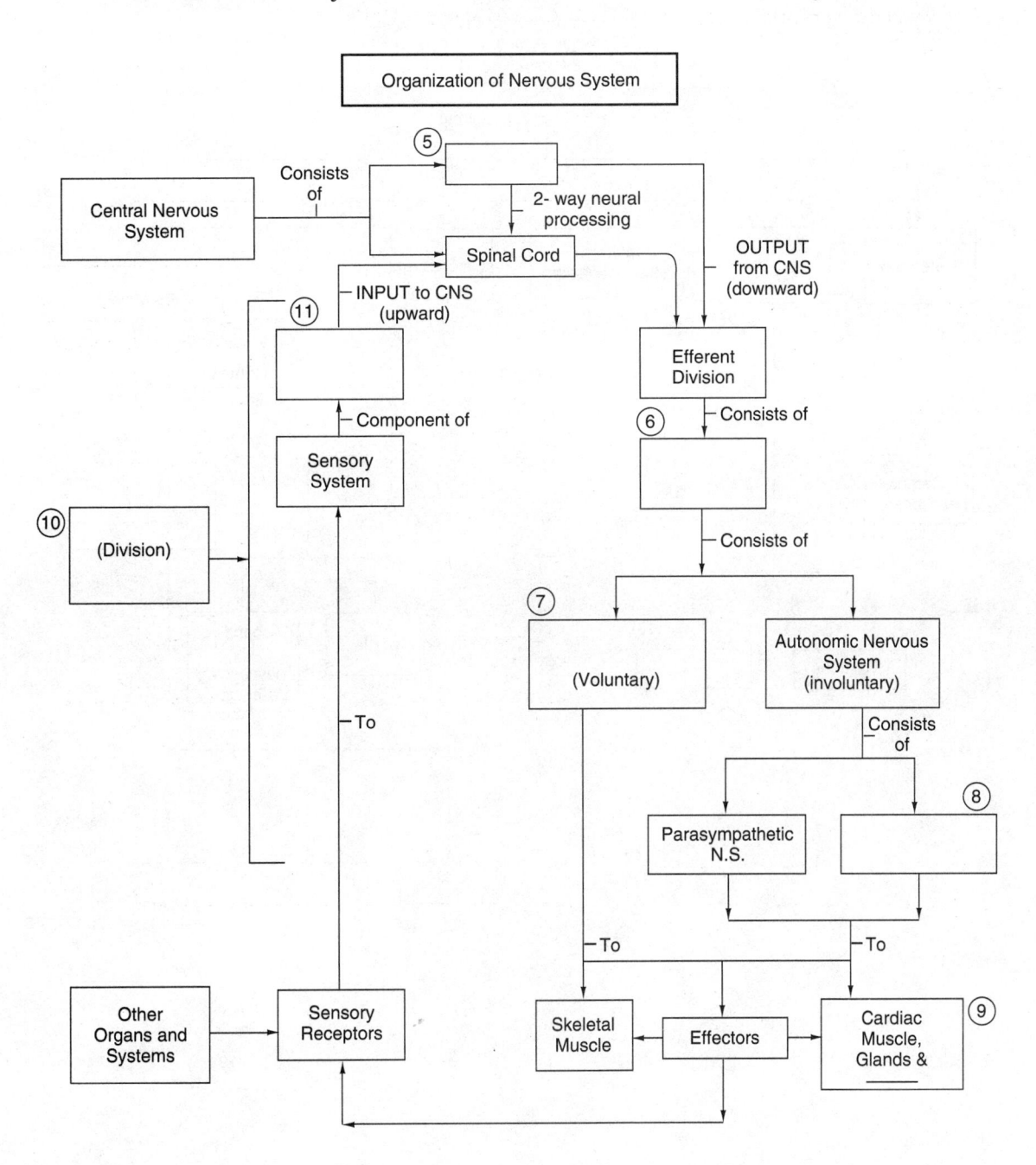

Chapter 8 Neural Tissue & the Central Nervous System

Concept Map III:

Using the terms below, fill in the numbered spaces to complete the concept map. Follow the numbers which comply with the organization of the map.

Cerebellar Hemispheres   Pons   Hypothalamus
Diencephalon   Medulla Oblongata   Ascending & Descending Tracts

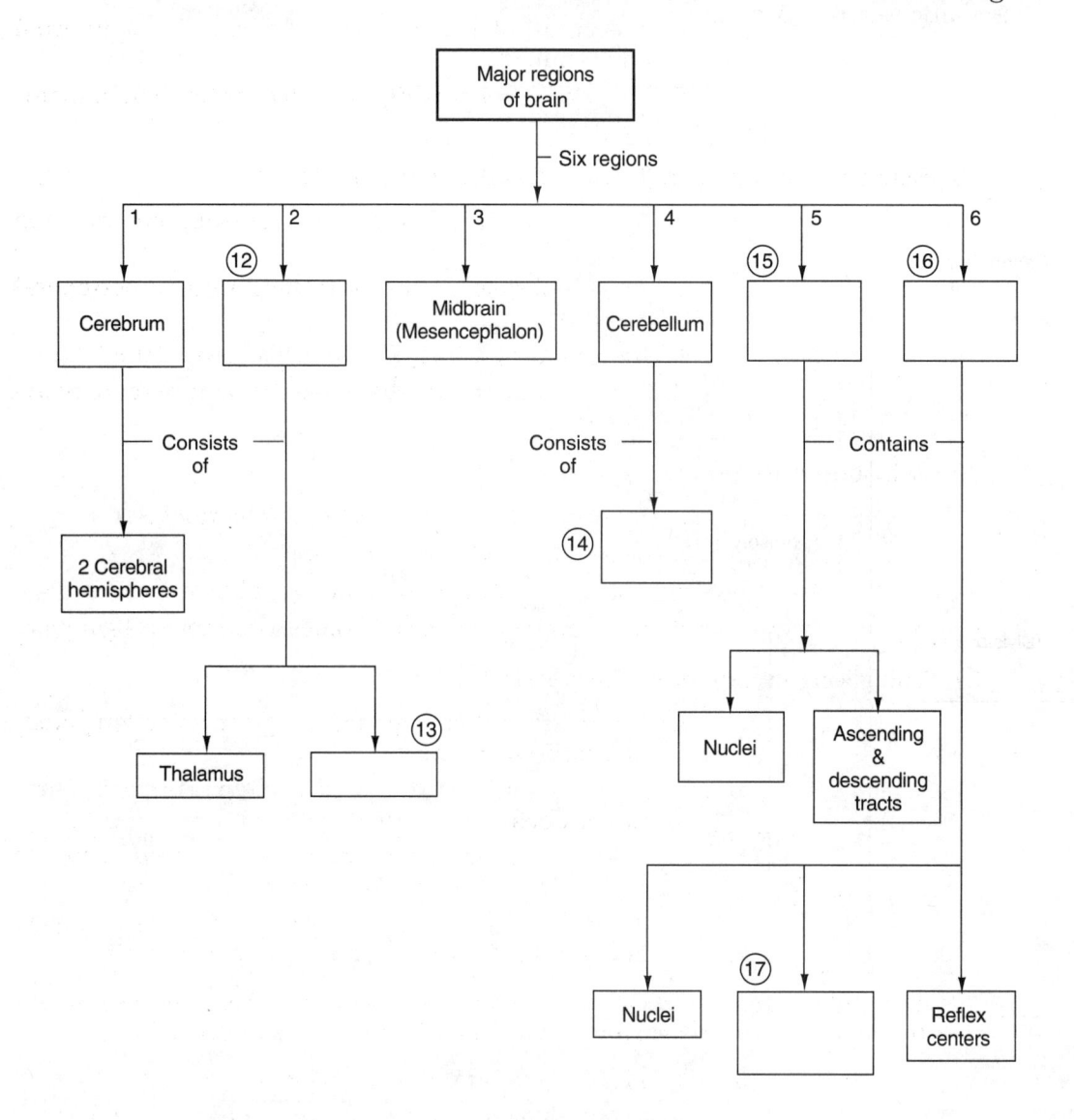

[L2] Multiple Choice:

Place the letter corresponding to the correct answer in the space provided.

_____ 18. Interneurons are responsible for:
   a. carrying instructions from the CNS to peripheral effectors
   b. delivery of information to the CNS
   c. collecting information from the external or internal environment
   d. analysis of sensory inputs and coordination of motor outputs

_____ 19. Sensory (ascending) pathways distribute information:
   a. from peripheral receptors to processing centers in the brain
   b. from processing centers in the brain to peripheral receptors
   c. from motor pathways to interneurons in the CNS
   d. the central nervous system to the peripheral nervous system

_____ 20. Schwann cells are glial cells responsible for:
   a. producing a myelin sheath peripheral axons
   b. secretion of cerebrospinal fluid
   c. phagocytic activities in the neural tissue of the PNS
   d. surrounding nerve cell bodies in peripheral ganglia

_____ 21. The all-or-nothing principle states:
   a. When a stimulus is applied it triggers an action potential in the membrane.
   b. A given stimulus either triggers a typical action potential or does not produce one at all.
   c. A hyperpolarized membrane always results in the production of an action potential.
   d. Action potentials occur in all neurons if a stimulus is applied that lowers the membrane potential.

_____ 22. The main functional difference between the autonomic nervous system and the somatic nervous system is that the activities of the ANS are:
   a. primarily voluntary controlled
   b. primarily involuntary or under "automatic" control
   c. involved with affecting skeletal muscle activity
   d. involved with carrying impulses to the CNS

_____ 23. Motor (descending) pathways begin at CNS centers concerned with motor control and end at:
   a. the cerebral cortex in the brain
   b. the cerebrum for conscious control
   c. the skeletal muscles they control
   d. reflex arcs within the spinal cord

_____ 24. The specialized membranes that provide physical stability and protection as shock absorbers are the:

    a. septal membranes
    b. spinal meninges
    c. dorsal membranes
    d. dorsal ligaments

_____ 25. Spinal nerves are classified as mixed nerves because they contain:

    a. both sensory and motor fibers
    b. both dorsal and ventral roots
    c. white matter and gray matter
    d. ascending and descending pathways

_____ 26. The three (3) meningeal layers of the spinal cord include:

    a. spinal meninges, cranial meninges, dorsal meninges
    b. dorsal meninges, ventral meninges, lateral meninges
    c. white matter, gray matter, central canal
    d. dura mater, pia mater, arachnoid mater

_____ 27. The axons in the white matter of the spinal cord that carry sensory information up toward the brain are organized into:

    a. descending tracts
    b. anterior white columns
    c. ascending tracts
    d. posterior white columns

_____ 28. Pain receptors are literally:

    a. dendrites of sensory neurons
    b. axons of motor neurons
    c. specialized sensory cells
    d. activators of motor neurons

_____ 29. The most complicated responses are produced by polysynaptic responses because:

    a. the interneurons can control several different muscle groups
    b. a delay between stimulus and response is minimized
    c. the postsynaptic motor neuron serves as the processing center
    d. there is an absence of interneurons, which minimizes delay

_____ 30. In an adult, CNS injury is suspected if:

    a. there is a plantar reflex
    b. there is an increase in synaptic pathways
    c. there is a positive Babinski reflex
    d. there is a negative Babinski reflex

Level 2   Concept Synthesis   143

_____ 31. The versatility of the brain to respond to stimuli is greater than that of the spinal cord because of:

    a. the location of the brain in the cranial vault
    b. the size of the brain and the number of myelinated neurons
    c. the fast-paced processing centers located in the brain
    d. the number of neurons and complex interconnections between the neurons

_____ 32. An individual with a damaged visual association area:

    a. is incapable of receiving somatic sensory information
    b. cannot read because he or she is blind
    c. is red-green color blind and experiences glaucoma
    d. can see letters clearly, but cannot recognize or interpret them

_____ 33. The functions of the limbic system involve:

    a. unconscious processing of visual and auditory information
    b. adjusting muscle tone and body position to prepare for a voluntary movement
    c. emotional states and related behavioral drives
    d. controlling reflex movements and processing of conscious thought

_____ 34. Hypothalamic or thalamic stimulation that depresses reticular formation activity in the brain stem results in:

    a. heightened alertness and a generalized excitement
    b. emotions of fear, rage, and pain
    c. sexual arousal and pleasure
    d. generalized lethargy or actual sleep

_____ 35. The part(s) of the diencephalon responsible for coordination of activities of the central nervous system and the endocrine system is (are) the:

    a. thalamus
    b. hypothalamus
    c. postcentral gyrus
    d. a, b, and c are correct

_____ 36. The effortless serve of a tennis player is a result of establishing:

    a. cerebral motor responses
    b. cerebellar motor patterns
    c. sensory patterns within the medulla
    d. motor patterns in the pons

_____ 37. The cardiovascular centers and the respiratory rhythmicity center are found in the:

    a. cerebrum
    b. cerebellum
    c. pons
    d. medulla oblongata

Chapter 8 Neural Tissue & the Central Nervous System

_____ 38. The large veins found between the inner and outer layers of the dura mater are called the:

   a. dural venules
   b. dural sinuses
   c. dural veins
   d. b and c are correct

_____ 39. The ventricles in the brain form hollow chambers that serve as passageways for the circulation of:

   a. blood
   b. cerebrospinal fluid
   c. interstitial fluid
   d. a and b are correct

_____ 40. The central white matter of the cerebrum is found:

   a. in the superficial layer of the neural cortex
   b. beneath the neural cortex and around the cerebral nuclei
   c. in the deep cerebral nuclei and the neural cortex
   d. in the cerebral cortex and in the cerebral nuclei

_____ 41. The series of elevated ridges that increase the surface area of the cerebral hemispheres and the number of neurons in the cortical area are called:

   a. sulci
   b. fissures
   c. gyri
   d. a, b, and c are correct

[L2] Completion:

Using the terms below, complete the following statements.

fissures	hypothalamus	hippocampus	pituitary gland
sulci	tracts	gated	interneurons
convergence	ganglia	nuclei	nerve impulse
motor nuclei	nerve plexus	reflexes	gray commissures

42. Nerve cell bodies in the PNS are clustered together in masses called _____.
43. Ion channels that open or close in response to specific stimuli are called _____.
44. An action potential traveling along an axon is called a(n) _____.
45. Axons extending from the CNS to a ganglion are called _____.
46. Axons connecting the ganglionic cells with peripyeral effectors are known as _____.
47. Several neurons synapsing on the same postsynaptic neuron are called _____.
48. Collections of nerve cell bodies in the CNS are called _____.
49. The axonal bundles that make up the white matter of the CNS are called _____.
50. The cell bodies of neurons that issue commands to peripheral effectors are called _____.
51. The area of the spinal cord where axons cross from one side of the cord to the other is the _____.
52. A complex, interwoven network of nerves is called a _____.
53. Programmed, automatic, involuntary motor responses and motor patterns are called _____.

54. The primary link betwen the nervous and endocrine system is the _____.
55. The part of the limbic system that appears to be important in learning and storage of long-term memory is the _____.
56. The shallow depressions that separate the cortical surface of the cerebral hemispheres are called _____.
57. Deep grooves separating the cortical surface of the cerebral hemispheres are called _____.
58. The component of the brain that integrates with the endocrine system is the _____.

[L2] Short Essay:

Briefly answer the following questions in the spaces provided below.

59. What are the major functions of the nervous system?

60. What are the major components of the central nervous system and the peripheral system?

61. Functionally, what is the major difference between neurons and neuroglia?

62. Using a generalized model, list and describe the steps that describe an action potential.

63. How are neurons categorized functionally and how does each group function? How are they categorized structurally?

64. What structural components make the white matter different from gray matter in the spinal cord?

65. List the five (5) steps involved in a neural reflex.

66. Why can polysynaptic reflexes produce more complicated reaponses than monosynaptic reflexes?

When you have successfully completed the exercises in L2 proceed to L3.

☐ LEVEL 3   CRITICAL THINKING/APPLICATION

Using principles and concepts learned about the nervous system, answer the following questions. Write your answers on a separate sheet of paper.

1. How does starting each day with a few cups of coffee and a cigarette affect a person's behavior and why?
2. Even though microglia are found in the CNS, why might these specialized cells be considered a part of the body's immune system?
3. What structural features make it possible to do a spinal tap without damaging the spinal cord?
4. How might damage to the following areas of the vertebral column affect the body?
   a. damage to the 4th or 5th vertebrae
   b. damage to the region C3 to C5
   c. damage to the thoracic vertebrae
   d. damage to the lumbar vertebrae
5. How does a blockage in reabsorption of cerebrospinal fluid (CSF) cause irreversible brain damage?
6. Ever since the mid-1980s an increasing number of young people have developed Parkinson's Disease. The reason has been linked to a "street drug" that had a contaminant that destroyed neurons in the substantia nigra of the mesencephalon (midbrain). What clinical explanation substantiates the relationship between this street drug and the development of Parkinson's Disease?
7. Suppose you are participating in a contest where you are blindfolded and numerous objects are placed in your hands to identify. The person in the contest who identifies the most objects while blindfolded receives a prize. What neural activities and areas in the CNS are necessary in order for you to name the objects correctly and win the prize?

CHAPTER 9

The Peripheral Nervous System and Integrated Nervous Functions

■ Overview

You probably have heard the statement that "No man is an island, no man can stand alone," implying that man is a societal creature, depending on and interacting with other people in the world in which one lives. So it is with the parts of the human nervous sytem.

The many diverse and complex physical and mental activities require that all component parts of the nervous sytem function in an integated and coordinated way if homeostasis is to be maintained within the human body.

Chapter 8 considered the structure and functions of the spinal cord and the brain. The present chapter focuses on how communication processes take place via pathways, nerve tracts and nuclei that relay sensory and motor information from the spinal cord to the higher centers in the brain. The following exercises, in part, are designed to test your understanding of patterns and principles of the brain's sensory, motor and higher-order functions.

Can you imagine what life would be like if you were responsible for coordinating the involuntary activities that occur in the cardiovascular, respiratory, digestive, excretory, and reproductive systems? Your entire life would be consumed with monitoring and giving instructions to maintain homeostasis in the body. The autonomic nervous system (ANS), a division of the peripheral nervous system, does this involuntary work in the body with meticulous efficiency.

The ANS consists of efferent motor fibers that innervate smooth and cardiac muscle as well as glands. The controlling centers of the ANS are found in the brain, whereas the nerve fibers of the ANS, which are subdivided into the sympathetic and parasympathetic fibers, belong to the peripheral nervous system. The sympathetic nervous system originates in the thoracic and lumbar regions of the spinal cord, whereas the parasympathetic nervous system originates in the brain and sacral region of the spinal cord. Both divisions terminate on the smooth muscle, cardiac muscle or glandular tissue of numerous organs.

The primary focus of the last portion of this chapter is on the structural and functional properties of the sympathetic and parasympathetic divisions of the ANS. Integration and control of autonomic functions are included to show how the ANS coordinates involuntary activities throughout the body to make homeostatic adjustments necessary for survival.

Chapter 9 The Peripheral Nervous System and Integrated Nervous Functions

☐ LEVEL 1   REVIEW OF CHAPTER OBJECTIVES

1. Identify the cranial nerves and relate each pair of cranial nerves to its principal functions.
2. Relate the distribution pattern of spinal nerves to the regions they innervate.
3. Distinguish between the motor responses produced by simple and complex reflexes.
4. Explain how higher centers control and modify reflex responses.
5. Identify the principal sensory and motor pathways.
6. Explain how we can distinguish among sensations that originate in different areas of the body.
7. Compare the autonomic nervous system with the other divisions of the nervous system.
8. Explain the functions and structures of the sympathetic and parasympathetic divisions.
9. Discuss the relationship between the sympathetic and parasympathetic divisions and explain the implications of dual innervation.
10. Summarize the effects of aging on the nervous system.

[L1]   Multiple Choice:

Place the letter corresponding to the correct answer in the space provided.

OBJ. 1   ____ 1. The special sensory cranial nerves include the:
- a. oculomotor, trochlear, and abducens
- b. spinal accessory, hypoglossal, and glossopharyngeal
- c. olfactory, optic, and vestibulocochlear
- d. vagus, trigeminal, and facial

OBJ. 1   ____ 2. Cranial nerves III, IV, VI, and XI, which provide motor control, are:
- a. trigeminal, facial, glossopharyngeal, vagus
- b. oculomotor, trochlear, abducens, spinal accessory
- c. olfactory, optic, vestibulocochlear, hypoglossal
- d. oculomotor, hypoglossal, optic, olfactory

OBJ. 1   ____ 3. The cranial nerves that carry sensory information and involuntary motor commands are:
- a. I, II, III, IV
- b. II, IV, VI, VIII
- c. V, VI, VIII, XII
- d. V, VII, IX, X

OBJ. 1   ____ 4. Cranial reflexes are reflex arcs that involve the:
- a. sensory and motor fibers of cranial nerves
- b. sensory and motor fibers of spinal nerves
- c. sensory and motor fibers of the cerebellum
- d. sensory and motor fibers in the medulla oblongata

OBJ. 2   ____ 5. The delicate connective tissue fibers that surround individual axons of spinal nerves comprise a layer called the:
- a. perineurium
- b. epineurium
- c. endoneurium
- d. commissures

Level 1 Review of Chapter Objectives 149

OBJ. 2 ____ 6. The branches of the cervical plexus innervate the muscles of the:
 a. shoulder girdle and arm
 b. pelvic girdle and leg
 c. neck and extend into the thoracic cavity to control the diaphragm
 d. back and lumbar region

OBJ. 2 ____ 7. The brachial plexus innervates the:
 a. neck and shoulder girdle
 b. shoulder girdle and arm
 c. neck and arm
 d. thorax and arm

OBJ. 3 ____ 8. When a sensory neuron synapses directly on a motor neuron, which itself serves as the processing center, the reflex is called a (an):
 a. polysynaptic reflex
 b. innate reflex
 c. monosynaptic reflex
 d. acquired reflex

OBJ. 3 ____ 9. The sensory receptors in the stretch reflex are the:
 a. muscle spindles
 b. Golgi tendon organs
 c. free nerve endings
 d. chemical receptors

OBJ. 3 ____ 10. All polysynaptic reflexes share the same basic characteristics(s), which include:
 a. they involve pools of neurons
 b. they are intersegmental in distribution
 c. they have at least one interneuron between sensory afferent and motor efferent
 d. a, b, and c are correct

OBJ. 4 ____ 11. As descending inhibitory synapses develop:
 a. the Babinski response disappears
 b. there is a positive Babinski response
 c. there will be a noticeable fanning of the toes in adults
 d. there will be a decrease in the reactivity of spinal reflexes

OBJ. 4 ____ 12. The highest level of motor control involves a series of interactions that occur:
 a. as monosynaptic reflexes that are rapid but stereotyped
 b. in centers in the brain that can modulate or build upon reflexive motor patterns
 c. in the descending pathways that increase or inhibit reflex patterns
 d. in the ascending pathways that increase or inhibit reflex patterns

OBJ. 5 ___ 13. The somatic nervous system issues somatic motor commands that direct the:

    a. activities of the autonomic nervous system
    b. contractions of smooth and cardiac muscles
    c. activities of glands and fat cells
    d. contractions of skeletal muscles

OBJ. 5 ___ 14. The autonomic nervous system issues motor commands that control:

    a. the somatic nervous system
    b. smooth and cardiac muscles, glands, and fat cells
    c. contractions of skeletal muscles
    d. voluntary activities

OBJ. 5 ___ 15. Proprioceptive data from peripheral structures, visual information from the eyes, and equilibrium-related sensations are processed and integrated in the:

    a. cerebral cortex
    b. cerebral nuclei
    c. cerebellum
    d. thalamus

OBJ. 6 ___ 16. The integrative activities performed by neurons in the cerebellar cortex and cerebellar nuclei are essential to the:

    a. involuntary regulation of posture and muscle tone
    b. involuntary regulation of autonomic functions
    c. voluntary control of smooth and cardiac muscle
    d. precise control of voluntary and involuntary movements

OBJ. 6 ___ 17. The autonomic nervous system is a subdivision of the:

    a. central nervous system
    b. somatic nervous system
    c. peripheral nervous system
    d. visceral nervous system

OBJ. 7 ___ 18. The lower motor neurons of the somatic nervous system (SNS) exert direct control over skeletal muscles. By contrast, in the ANS there is:

    a. voluntary and involuntary control of skeletal muscles
    b. always voluntary control of skeletal muscles
    c. indirect voluntary control of skeletal muscles
    d. a synapse interposed between the CNS and the peripheral effector

OBJ. 8 ___ 19. Sympathetic (preganglionic) neurons originate between:

    a. T1 and T2 of the spinal cord
    b. T1 and L2 of the spinal cord
    c. L1 and L4 of the spinal cord
    d. S2 and S4 of the spinal cord

Level 1 Review of Chapter Objectives 151

OBJ. 8 ___ 20. The important function(s) of the postganglionic fibers that enter the thoracic cavity in autonomic nerves include:
   a. accelerating the heart rate
   b. increasing the force of cardiac contractions
   c. dilating the respiratory passageways
   d. a, b, and c are correct

OBJ. 8 ___ 21. Preganglionic neurons in the parasympathetic division of the ANS originate in the:
   a. peripheral ganglia adjacent to the target organ
   b. thoracolumbar area of the spinal cord
   c. walls of the target organ
   d. brain stem and sacral segments of the spinal cord

OBJ. 8 ___ 22. Since second-order neurons in the parasympathetic division are all located in the same ganglion, the effects of parasympathetic stimulation are:
   a. more diversified and less localized than those of the sympathetic division.
   b. less diversified but less localized than those of the sympathetic division
   c. more specific and localized than those of the sympathetic division
   d. more diversified and more localized than those of the sympathetic division

OBJ. 8 ___ 23. The parasympathetic division of the ANS includes visceral motor nuclei associated with cranial nerves:
   a. I, II, III, IV
   b. III, VII, IX, X
   c. IV, V, VI, VIII
   d. V, VI, VIII, XII

OBJ. 8 ___ 24. At their synapses with ganglionic neurons, all ganglionic neurons in the sympathetic division release:
   a. epinephrine
   b. norepinephrine
   c. acetylcholine
   d. a, b, and c are correct

OBJ. 8 ___ 25. At neuroeffector junctions, typical sympathetic postganglionic fibers release:
   a. epinephrine
   b. norepinephrine
   c. acetylcholine
   d. dopamine

OBJ. 8 ___ 26. At synapses and neuroeffector junctions, all preganglionic and postganglionic fibers in the parasympathetic division release:
   a. epinephrine
   b. norepinephrine
   c. acetylcholine
   d. a, b, and c are correct

152 Chapter 9 The Peripheral Nervous System and Integrated Nervous Functions

OBJ. 8   ___ 27. The sympathetic division can change tissue and organ activities by:
  a. releasing norepinephrine at peripheral synapses
  b. distribution of norepinephrine by the bloodstream
  c. distribution of epinephrine by the bloodstream
  d. a, b, and c are correct

OBJ. 8   ___ 28. Cholinergic postganglionic sympathetic fibers which innervate the sweat glands of the skin and the blood vessels of the skeletal muscles are stimulated during exercise to:
  a. constrict the blood vessels and inhibit sweat gland secretion
  b. keep the body cool and provide oxygen and nutrients to active skeletal muscles
  c. increase the smooth muscle activity in the digestive tract for better digestion
  d. decrease the body temperature and decrease the pH in the blood

OBJ. 9   ___ 29. When vital organs receive dual innervation, the result is usually:
  a. a stimulatory effect within the organ
  b. an inhibitory effect within the organ
  c. sympathetic-parasympathetic opposition
  d. sympathetic-parasympathetic inhibitory effect

OBJ. 9   ___ 30. Autonomic tone exists in the heart because:
  a. ACh (acetylcholine) released by the parasympathetic division decreases the heart rate, and norepinephrine (NE) released by the sympathetic division accelerates the heart rate
  b. ACh released by the parasympathetic division accelerates the heart rate, and NE released by the sympathetic division decreases the heart rate
  c. NE released by the parasympathetic division accelerates the heart rate, and ACh released by the sympathetic division decreases the heart rate
  d. NE released by the sympathetic division and ACh released by the parasympathetic division accelerate the heart rate

OBJ. 9   ___ 31. In the absence of stimuli, autonomic tone is important to autonomic motor neurons because:
  a. it can increase their activity on demand
  b. it can decrease their activity to avoid overstimulation
  c. it shows a resting level of spontaneous activity
  d. its activity is determined by the degree to which they are stimulated

OBJ. 9   ___ 32. The lowest level of integration in the ANS consists of:
  a. centers in the medulla that control visceral functions
  b. regulatory centers in the posterior and lateral hypothalamus
  c. regulatory centers in the midbrain that control the viscera
  d. lower motor neurons that participate in cranial and spinal visceral reflexes function

Level 1 Review of Chapter Objectives 153

OBJ. 10 ___ 33. A reduction in brain size and weight associated with aging results primarily from:
- a. a decrease in blood flow to the brain
- b. a change in the synaptic organization of the brain
- c. a decrease in the volume of the cerebral cortex
- d. a, b, and c are correct

OBJ. 10 ___ 34. Abnormal intracellular and extracellular deposits in CNS neurons associated with the aging process include:
- a. lipofuscin
- b. amyloid
- c. neurofibrillary tangles
- d. a, b, and c are correct

[L1] Completion:

Using the terms below, complete the following statements.

hypoglossal	spinal accessory	flexor reflex	"fight or flight"
cranial reflexes	epineurium	somatic reflexes	involuntary
Babinski sign	sensation	pyramidal system	opposing
cerebral nuclei	Parkinson's disease	Alzheimer's disease	"rest or repose"
cerebellum	visceral reflexes	acetylcholine	autonomic tone
limbic	synapse		

OBJ. 1 35. The cranial nerve that controls the tongue muscle is N XII, the _____.

OBJ. 1 36. The cranial nerve that directs voluntary motor control of the large superficial muscles of the back is the _____.

OBJ. 2 37. The outermost layer of a spinal nerve is called the _____.

OBJ. 3 38. Reflexes processed in the brain are called _____.

OBJ. 3 39. Reflexes that control activities of the muscular system are called _____.

OBJ. 3 40. The withdrawal reflex affecting the muscles of a limb is a(n) _____.

OBJ. 4 41. Stroking an infant's foot on the side of the sole produces a fanning of the toes known as the _____.

OBJ. 5 42. The information that arrives in the form of an action potential in a sensory fiber is called a _____.

OBJ. 5 43. Voluntary control of skeletal muscles is provided by the _____.

OBJ. 6 44. The processing centers whose functions blur the distinction between the "conscious" and "unconscious" motor control are the _____.

OBJ. 6 45. Motor patterns associated with learned movement patterns are controlled by the _____.

OBJ. 7 46. The points at which information is transmitted from one excitable cell to another is the _____.

OBJ. 7 47. The motor neurons of the somatic nervous system exert voluntary control over skeletal muscles, while in the ANS the control of smooth and cardiac muscles is _____.

OBJ. 8 48. Because the sympathetic division of the ANS stimulates tissue metabolism and increases alertness during times of emergency, it is called the _____.

154 Chapter 9 The Peripheral Nervous System and Integrated Nervous Functions

OBJ. 8 — 49. Because the parasympathetic division of the ANS conserves energy and promotes sedentary activity, it is known as the _____.

OBJ. 8 — 50. At their synaptic terminals, cholinergic autonomic fibers release _____.

OBJ. 9 — 51. Sympathetic-parasympathetic innervation in an organ produces action that is described as _____.

OBJ. 9 — 52. The release of small amounts of acetylcholine and norepinephrine on a continuous basis in an organ innervated by sympathetic and parasympathetic fibers is referred to as _____.

OBJ. 9 — 53. The simplest functional units in the ANS are _____.

OBJ. 9 — 54. The system (area) of the brain that would most likely exert an influence on autonomic control if an emotional condition is present is the _____ system.

OBJ. 10 — 55. Inadequate dopamine production causes the motor problems of _____.

OBJ. 10 — 56. A progressive disorder characterized by the loss of higher brain functions is _____.

[L1] Matching:

Match the terms in column "B" with the terms in column "A". Use letters for answers in the spaces provided.

	COLUMN "A"	COLUMN "B"
OBJ. 1	57. C.N. X	A. Spinal nerves C5-T1
OBJ. 1	58. C.N. II	B. Voluntary motor control
OBJ. 2	59. Cervical plexus	C. Golgi tendon organ
OBJ. 2	60. Brachial plexus	D. Pupillary dilation
OBJ. 3	61. Stretch reflex	E. Monosynaptic reflex
OBJ. 3	62. Tendon reflex	F. Dilates blood vessels
OBJ. 4	63. Descending pathways	G. Constricts blood vessels
OBJ. 5	64. Pyramidal system	H. Postcentral gyrus
OBJ. 6	65. Cortical sensations	I. Optic
OBJ. 7	66. Thoracolumbar axons and ganglia	J. Motor
OBJ. 7	67. Craniosacral axons and ganglia	K. Vagus
OBJ. 8	68. Acetylcholine	L. Spinal nerves C1-C5
OBJ. 8	69. Norepinephrine	M. Alzheimer's
OBJ. 9	70. Sympathetic-parasympathetic opposition	N. Defecation and urination
		O. Autonomic tone
OBJ. 9	71. Parasympathetic reflex	P. Sympathetic division
OBJ. 9	72. Sympathetic reflex	Q. Parasympathetic divison
OBJ. 10	73. Plaques	

Level -1-

Level 1 Review of Chapter Objectives 155

[L1] Drawing/Illustration Labeling:

OBJ. 5   **FIGURE 9.1** Preganglionic and Postganglionic Cell Bodies of Sympathetic Neurons

Using the terms below, identify and label the numbered structures of the sympathetic system.

inferior mesenteric ganglion   postganglionic neuron   celiac ganglion
preganglionic axon   superior mesenteric ganglion L2
collateral ganglia   sympathetic chain ganglion   T1
preganglionic cell body in
   gray matter of spinal cord

74 _____   78 _____   81 _____

75 _____   79 _____   82 _____

76 _____   80 _____   83 _____

77 _____

When you have successfully completed the exercises in L1 proceed to L2.

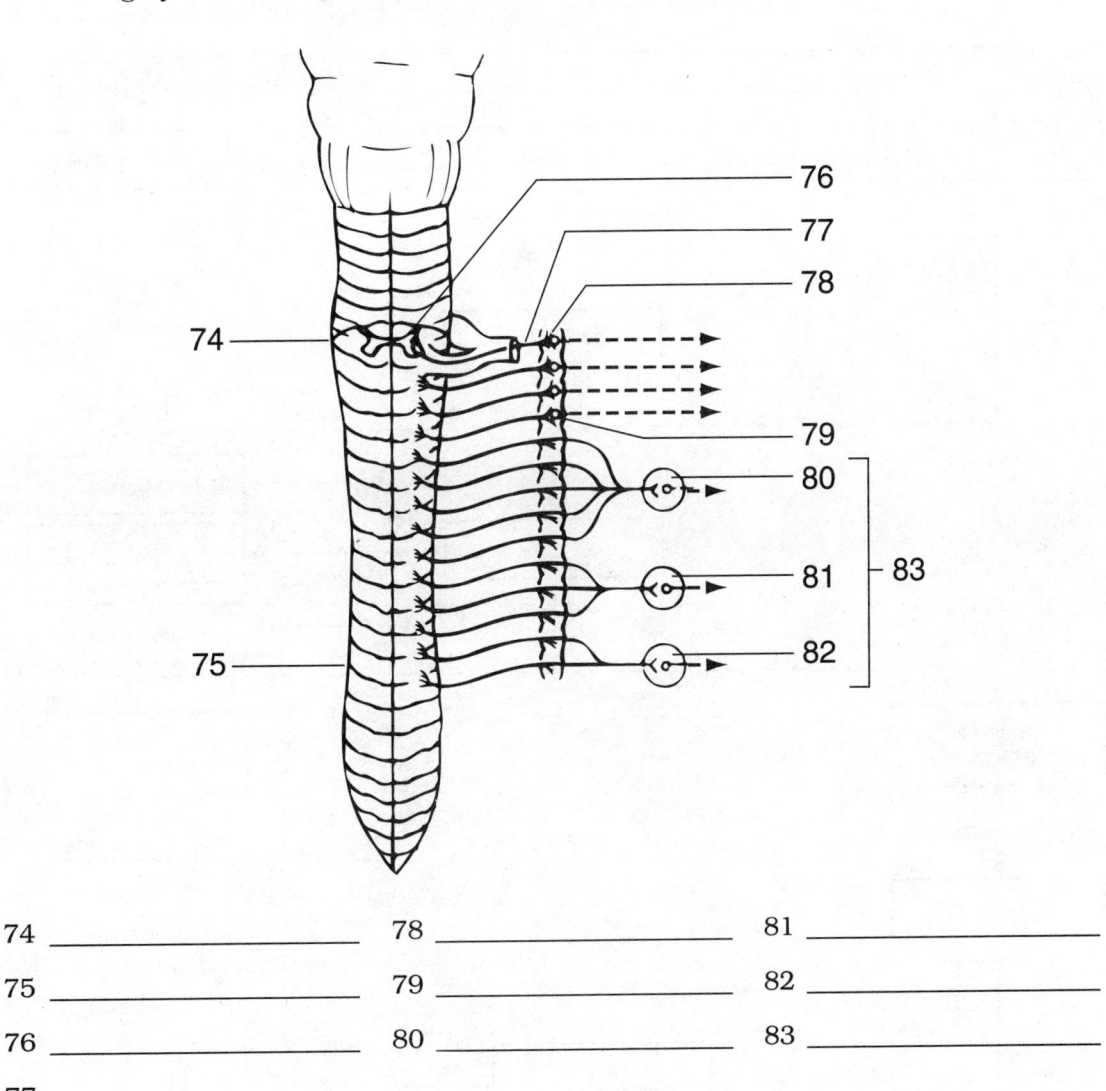

Chapter 9 The Peripheral Nervous System and Integrated Nervous Functions

LEVEL 2 CONCEPT SYNTHESIS

Concept Map I:

Using the following terms, fill in the numbered, blank spaces to complete the concept map. Follow the numbers that comply with the organization of the map.

- Ganglia outside CNS
- Smooth muscle
- Motor neurons
- Postganglionic
- Sympathetic

Concept map structure:

- Autonomic N.S. (organization) → Involuntary Nervous System
- Functional division:
  - (1) _____ → Serves same organ ← Parasympathetic
  - Serves same organ — Has → Opposing effects
- Consists of (2) _____
  - To → Heart, (3) _____, Internal glands
  - Two chains in:
    - Brain or spinal cord — Contains → Neurons — Called → Preganglionic → Axons synapse with → (5) _____
    - (4) _____ — Contains → Neurons — Called → (5) _____ — Axon extends to → Organ it serves

Body Trek

Using the terms below, fill in the blanks to complete the trek through the spinal cord on an ascending nerve tract.

cerebral cortex	synapse	pons	dorsal root ganglion
receptor	medulla oblongata	posterior horn	thalamus
midbrain	diencephalon	pyramidal	

Robo is activated and programmed to trek along an ascending tract in the spinal cord while "carrying" an impulse that is a result of a stimulus applied to the left hand of a subject. The robot is injected into the spinal canal and immediately begins the trek by proceeding to the posterior horn of the spinal cord.

The stimulus is applied at a (6) _____ area on the palm on the left hand of the subject. The impulse is transmitted on a sensory neuron into the (7) _____ and relayed into the (8) _____ of the spinal cord. Robo "picks up" the impulse at the synapse in the posterior horn. The impulse is "carried" from the left side of the spinal cord to the right side across the gray commissure. Continuing on this postsynaptic pathway Robo carries the impulse "uphill" as it ascends through the entrance to the brain, the (9) _____, then on into the (10) _____ and into the (11) _____, finally arriving in the (12) _____. Here the robot pushes the impulse into the (13) _____, an important relay "station" to higher brain regions. After a brief pause at a chemical (14) _____, Robo proceeds farther "uphill" on a neuron to the (15) _____ where the determination is made that the stimulus caused PAIN! (Ouch!) Robo is anxious to get out of the "pain area" because the "pain" interferes with its electronic abilities to operate normally. With its extended ultramicro-arm it grasps onto a neuron and travels "downhill" until it can complete its trek on another neuron, this time of the (16) _____ system into the spinal cord where it proceeds to the spinal canal for its exit during the next spinal tap.

[L2] Multiple Choice:

Place the letter corresponding to the correct answer in the space provided.

_____ 17. In the thalamus, data arriving over the integrated, sorted, and projected to the:
   a. cerebellum
   b. spinal cord
   c. primary sensory cortex
   d. a and c are correct

_____ 18. If a sensation arrives at the wrong part of the sensory cortex we will:
   a. experience pain in the posterior column of the white matter of the spinal cord
   b. reach an improper conclusion about the source of the stimulus
   c. be incapable of experiencing pain or pressure
   d. lose all capability of receiving and sending information

_____ 19. If the central cortex were damaged a person would be able to detect light touch but would be unable to:
   a. determine its source
   b. determine the magnitude of the stimulus
   c. determine the amount of pressure
   d. a, b, and c are correct

Chapter 9 The Peripheral Nervous System and Integrated Nervous Functions

_____ 20. Voluntary and involuntary somatic motor commands issued by the brain reach peripheral targets by traveling over the:
- a. sensory and motor fibers
- b. pyramidal system
- c. ganglionic and preganglionic fibers
- d. ascending tracts

_____ 21. An individual whose primary motor cortex has been destroyed retains the ability to walk and maintain balance but the movements:
- a. are restricted and result in partial paralysis
- b. are under involuntary control and are poorly executed
- c. are characteristic involuntary motor commands
- d. lack precision and are awkward and poorly controlled

_____ 22. When someone touches a hot stove, the rapid, automatic preprogrammed response that preserves homeostasis is provided by the:
- a. cerebellum
- b. primary sensory cortex
- c. spinal reflex
- d. a, b, and c are correct

_____ 23. At the highest level of processing, the complex, variable, and voluntary motor patterns are dictated by the:
- a. cerebral cortex
- b. frontal lobe
- c. cerebellum
- d. diencephalon

_____ 24. Hemispheric specialization does not mean that the two hemispheres are independent but that:
- a. there is a genetic basis for the distribution of functions
- b. the left hemisphere is categorized in left-handed individuals
- c. 90 percent of the population have an enlarged right hemisphere at birth
- d. specific centers have evolved to process information gathered by the system as a whole

_____ 25. The axon of a ganglionic neuron is called a postganglionic fiber because:
- a. it carries impulses away from the ganglion
- b. it carries impulses to the target organ
- c. it carries impulses toward the ganglion
- d. a, b, and c are correct

_____ 26. The effect(s) produced by sympathetic postganglionic fibers in spinal nerves include(s):
- a. stimulation of secretion by sweat glands
- b. acceleration of blood flow to skeletal muscles
- c. dilation of the pupils and focusing of the eyes
- d. a, b, and c are correct

27. The major structural difference between sympathetic pre- and postganglionic fibers is that:
   a. preganglionic fibers are short and postganglionic fibers are long
   b. preganglionic fibers are long and postganglionic fibers are short
   c. preganglionic fibers are close to target organs and postganglionic fibers are close to the spinal cord
   d. preganglionic fibers innervate target organs while postganglionic fibers originate from cranial nerves

28. The effects of parasympathetic stimulation are usually:
   a. brief in duration and restricted to specific organs and sites
   b. long in duration and diverse in distribution
   c. brief in duration and diverse in distribution
   d. long in duration and restricted to specific organs and sites

29. The functions of the parasympathetic division center on:
   a. accelerating the heart rate and the force of contraction
   b. dilation of the respiratory passageways
   c. relaxation, food processing, and energy absorption
   d. a, b, and c are correct

30. During a crisis, the event necessary for the individual to cope with stressful and potentially dangerous situations is called:
   a. the effector response
   b. sympathetic activation
   c. parasympathetic activation
   d. a, b, and c are correct

31. Parasympathetic preganglionic fibers of the vagus nerve entering the thoracic cavity join the:
   a. cardiac plexus
   b. pulmonary plexus
   c. hypogastric plexus
   d. a and b are correct

32. Sensory nerves deliver information to the CNS along:
   a. spinal nerves
   b. cranial nerves
   c. autonomic nerves that innervate peripheral effectors
   d. a, b, and c are correct

[L2] Completion:

Using the terms below, complete the following statements.

- hypothalamus
- splanchnic
- cerebral nuclei
- postganglionic
- dopamine
- dyslexia
- norepinephrine
- arousal
- electroencephalogram

33. The fibers that innervate peripheral organs are called _____ fibers.
34. Adrenergic postganglionic sympathetic terminals release the neurotransmitter _____.
35. In the dorsal wall of the abdominal cavity, preganglionic fibers that innervate the collateral ganglia form the _____ nerves.
36. Sympathetic activation is controlled by sympathetic centers in the _____.
37. Motor patterns associated with walking and body positioning are controlled by _____.
38. One of the most common methods involved in monitoring the electrical activity of the brain is the _____.
39. A disorder affecting the compehension and use of words is referred to as _____.
40. One of the functions of the reticular formation is _____.
41. Parkinson's disease is associated with inadequate production of the neurotransmitter _____.

[L2] Short Essay:

Briefly answer the following questions in the spaces provided below.

42. What are the primary functions of the cerebellum?

43. List the anatomical changes in the nervous system that are commonly associated with aging.

44. Why is the sympathetic division of the ANS called the "fight or flight" system? Why is the parasympathetic division of the ANS called the "rest and repose" system?

45. What are the major components of the sympathetic division of the ANS?

46. What are the major components of the parasympathetic division of the ANS?

47. What effect does dual innervation have on automatic control throughout the body?

When you have successfully completed the exercises in L2 proceed to L3.

☐ LEVEL 3   CRITICAL THINKING/APPLICATION

Using the principles and concepts learned about the peripheral nervous system and integrated neural functions, answer the following questions. Write your answers on a separate sheet of paper.

1. A friend of yours complains of pain radiating down through the left arm. After having an EKG it was discovered that there were signs of a mild heart attack. Why would the pain occur in the arm instead of the cardiac area?
2. An individual whose primary motor cortex has been destroyed retains the ability to walk, maintain balance, and perform other voluntary and involuntary movement. Even though the movements lack precision and may be awkward and poorly controlled, why is the ability to walk and maintain balance possible?
3. Your parents have agreed to let your grandmother live in their home because recently she has exhibited some "abnormal" behaviors usually associated with Alzheimer's disease. What behaviors would you look for to confirm the possibility of Alzheimer's?
4. You have probably heard stories about "superhuman" feats that have been performed during times of crisis. What autonomic mechanisms are involved in producing a sudden, intensive physical activity that, under ordinary circumstances, would be impossible?
5. Recent surveys show that 30 to 35 percent of the American adult population is involved in some type of exercise program. What contributions does sympathetic activation make to help the body adjust to the changes that occur during exercise and still maintain homeostasis?

CHAPTER 10

Sensory Function

■ Overview

Do we really see with our eyes, hear with our ears, smell with our nose, and taste with our tongue? Ask the ordinary layperson and the answer will probably be yes. Ask the student of anatomy and physiology and the most likely response will be "not really." Our awareness of the world within and around us is aroused by sensory receptors that react to stimuli within the body or to stimuli in the environment outside the body. The previous chapters on the nervous system described the mechanisms by which the body perceives stimuli as neural events and not necessarily as environmental realities.

Sensory receptors receive stimuli and neurons transmit action potentials to the CNS where the sensations are processed, resulting in motor responses that serve to maintain homeostasis.

Chapter 10 considers the general senses of temperature, pain, touch, pressure, vibration, and proprioception and the special senses of smell, taste, balance, hearing, and vision. The activities in this chapter will reinforce your understanding of the structure and function of general sensory receptors and specialized receptor cells that are structurally more complex than those of the general senses.

☐ LEVEL 1   REVIEW OF CHAPTER OBJECTIVES

1. Distinguish between the general and special senses.
2. Identify the receptors for the general senses and describe how they function.
3. Describe the receptors and processes involved in the sense of smell.
4. Describe the receptors and processes involved in the sense of taste.
5. Identify the parts of the eye and their functions.
6. Explain how we are able to see objects and distinguish colors.
7. Discuss how the central nervous system processes information related to vision.
8. Discuss the receptors and processes involved in the sense of equilibrium.
9. Describe the parts of the ear and their roles in the process of hearing.

Level 1   Review of Chapter Objectives   163

[L1]   Multiple Choice:

Place the letter corresponding to the correct answer in the space provided.

OBJ. 1   ____   1. The term "general senses" refers to the sensations of:
   a. smell, taste, balance, hearing, and vision
   b. pain, smell, pressure, balance, and vision
   c. temperature, pain, touch, pressure, vibration, and proprioception
   d. touch, taste, balance, vibration, and hearing

OBJ. 1   ____   2. The "special senses" refer to:
   a. balance, taste, smell, hearing, and vision
   b. temperature, pain, taste, touch, and hearing
   c. touch, pressure, vibration, and proprioception
   d. proprioception, smell, touch, and taste

OBJ. 1   ____   3. We cannot hear high-frequency sounds that dolphins respond to nor detect scents that excite bloodhounds because:
   a. our CNS is incapable of interpreting these stimuli
   b. our receptors have characteristic ranges of sensitivity
   c. these stimuli cause abnormal receptor function
   d. the stimuli produce inappropriate stimulation with no basis of fact

OBJ. 1   ____   4. Which of the following describes free nerve endings?
   a. are dendrites of neurons
   b. are sensory in function
   c. are sensitive to a variety of stimuli
   d. a, b, and c are correct

OBJ. 2   ____   5. The receptors for the general senses are the:
   a. axons of the sensory neurons
   b. dendrites of sensory neurons
   c. cell bodies of the sensory neurons
   d. a, b, and c are correct

OBJ. 2   ____   6. The three classes of mechanoreceptors are:
   a. heavy pressure, light pressure, and pain
   b. fine touch, crude touch, and pressure receptors
   c. tactile, baroreceptors, proprioceptors
   d. slow-adapting, fast-adapting, and central adapting receptors

OBJ. 2   ____   7. Pain receptors are also known as:
   a. baroreceptors
   b. osmoreceptors
   c. nociceptors
   d. salviceptors

164 Chapter 10 Sensory Function

OBJ. 2 ___ 8. Baroreceptors:
a. consist of free nerve endings
b. monitor changes in pressure
c. may be found in the walls of the respiratory, digestive or urinary tracts
d. a, b, and c are correct

OBJ. 3 ___ 9. The first step in olfactory reception occurs on the surface of the:
a. olfactory cilia
b. columnar cells
c. basal cells
d. olfactory glands

OBJ. 3 ___ 10. The CNS interprets smell on the basis of the particular pattern of:
a. cortical arrangement
b. neuronal replacement
c. receptor activity
d. sensory impressions

OBJ. 4 ___ 11. The four (4) primary taste sensations are:
a. sour, bitter, salty, and sweet
b. bitter, stringent, wet, and saline
c. sour, bitter, sweet, and composite
d. cold, sweet, sour, and composite

OBJ. 4 ___ 12. Taste buds are monitored by cranial nerves:
a. VII, IX, X
b. IV, V, VI
c. I, II, III
d. VIII, XI, XII

OBJ. 5 ___ 13. The extrinsic muscle of the eye responsible for rotating the eye medially is the:
a. inferior rectus
b. medial rectus
c. superior rectus
d. superior oblique

OBJ. 5 ___ 14. The extrinsic muscle of the eye responsible for rolling the eye is the:
a. superior rectus
b. superior oblique
c. inferior oblique
d. inferior rectus

OBJ. 5 ___ 15. The fibrous tunic, the outermost layer covering the eye, consists of the:
a. iris and choroid
b. pupil and ciliary body
c. sclera and cornea
d. lacrimal sac and orbital fat

Level 1

OBJ. 5 ___ 16. The vascular tunic consists of three distinct structures that include:
   a. sclera, cornea, iris
   b. choroid, pupil, lacrimal sac
   c. retina, cornea, iris
   d. iris, ciliary body, choroid

OBJ. 5 ___ 17. The function of the vitreous body in the eye is to:
   a. provide a fluid cushion for protection of the eye
   b. serve as a route for nutrient and waste transport
   c. stabilize the shape of the eye and give physical support to the retina
   d. serve as a medium for cleansing the inner eye

OBJ. 5 ___ 18. The primary function of the lens of the eye is to:
   a. absorb light after it passes through the retina
   b. biochemically interact with the photoreceptors of the retina
   c. focus the visual image on retinal receptors
   d. integrate visual information for the retina

OBJ. 5 ___ 19. When looking directly at an object, its image falls upon the portion of the retina called the:
   a. fovea centralis
   b. choroid layer
   c. sclera
   d. focal point

OBJ. 6 ___ 20. When photons of all wavelengths stimulate both rods and cones, the eye perceives:
   a. "black" objects
   b. all the colors of the visible light spectrum
   c. either "red" or "blue" light
   d. "white" light

OBJ. 7 ___ 21. Axons converge on the optic disc, penetrate the wall of the eye, and proceed toward the:
   a. retina at the posterior part of the eye
   b. diencephalon as the optic nerve (N II)
   c. retinal processing areas below the choroid coat
   d. cerebral cortex area of the parietal lobes

OBJ. 7 ___ 22. The sensation of vision arises from the integration of information arriving at the:
   a. lateral left side of the midbrain
   b. visual cortex of the cerebrum
   c. lateral right side of the midbrain
   d. reflex centers in the brain stem

166   Chapter 10   Sensory Function

OBJ. 8 ____ 23. The senses of equilibrium and hearing are provided by receptors in the:
      a. external ear
      b. middle ear
      c. inner ear
      d. b and c are correct

OBJ. 8 ____ 24. Ascending auditory sensations synapse in the thalamus and then are delivered by fibers to the:
      a. auditory cortex of the parietal lobe
      b. auditory cortex of the temporal lobe
      c. auditory cortex of the occipital lobe
      d. auditory cortex of the frontal lobe

OBJ. 9 ____ 25. The bony labyrinth of the iner ear is subdivided into the:
      a. auditory meatus, auditory canal, ceruminous glands
      b. saccule, utricle, vestibule
      c. vestibule, semicircular canals, and the cochlea
      d. ampulla, crista, cupula

OBJ. 9 ____ 26. The dividing line between the external ear and the middle ear is the:
      a. pharyngotympanic tube
      b. tympanic membrane
      c. sacculus
      d. utriculus

OBJ. 9 ____ 27. The auditory ossicles of the middle ear include the:
      a. sacculus, utriculus, ampulla
      b. vestibule, cochlea, organ of Corti
      c. malleus, stapes, incus
      d. otoliths, maculae, otoconia

OBJ. 9 ____ 28. The structure in the cochlea of the inner ear that provides information to the CNS is the:
      a. scala tympani
      b. organ of Corti
      c. tectorial membrane
      d. basilar membrane

OBJ. 9 ____ 29. The receptors that provide the sensation of hearing are located in the:
      a. vestibule
      b. ampulla
      c. tympanic membrane
      d. cochlea

Level -1-

[L1] Completion:

Using the terms below, complete the following statements.

rods	endolymph	occipital
sensitivity	mechanoreceptors	somatosensory cortex
cerebral cortex	sclera	(postcentral gyrus)
saccule, utricle	bipolar	pupil
thermoreceptors	otoliths	round window
cones	taste buds	

OBJ. 1   30. The ultimate destination of sensations from the general senses is the _____.

OBJ. 1   31. The information provided by receptors of the special senses is distributed to specific areas of the _____.

OBJ. 1   32. The reason we cannot hear extreme high frequency sounds is that our receptors have characteristic ranges of _____.

OBJ. 2   33. The receptors that respond to extremes of temperature are called _____.

OBJ. 2   34. Receptors that are sensitive to stimuli that distort their cell membranes are _____.

OBJ. 3   35. Structurally, olfactory receptors are _____ neurons.

OBJ. 4   36. Gustatory receptors are clustered in individual _____.

OBJ. 5   37. Most of the ocular surface of the eye is covered by the _____.

OBJ. 5   38. The opening surrounded by the iris is called the _____.

OBJ. 5   39. The photoreceptors that enable us to see in dimly lit rooms, at twilight, or in pale moonlight are the _____.

OBJ. 6   40. The photoreceptors that account for the perception of color are the _____.

OBJ. 7   41. Visual information is integrated in the cortical area of the _____ lobe.

OBJ. 8   42. The receptors in the inner ear that provide sensations of gravity and linear acceleration are located in the _____ and the _____.

OBJ. 8   43. Macula contain sensory receptors which respond to the movement of _____ when the head is tilted.

OBJ. 9   44. The chambers and canals in the inner ear contain a fluid called _____.

OBJ. 9   45. The thin membranous partition that separates the perilymph of the cochlear chambers from the air spaces of the middle ear is the _____.

Chapter 10 Sensory Function

[L1] Matching:

Match the terms in column "B" with the terms in column "A." Use letters for answers in the spaces provided.

	COLUMN "A"	COLUMN "B"
OBJ. 1	____ 46. Nose, ear, eye	A. Ganglion cells
OBJ. 1	____ 47. Somatosensory cortex	B. Smell
OBJ. 2	____ 48. Nociceptors	C. Equilibrium
OBJ. 2	____ 49. Chemoreceptors	D. Ear wax
OBJ. 3	____ 50. Olfaction	E. Sensation of pain
OBJ. 4	____ 51. Gustation	F. Aqueous humor
OBJ. 5	____ 52. Anterior cavity	G. Visual pigment
OBJ. 5	____ 53. Lacrimal glands	H. Tears
OBJ. 5	____ 54. Sharp vision	I. Response to specific molecules
OBJ. 6	____ 55. Rhodopsin	J. Fovea centralis
OBJ. 7	____ 56. Component of Optic Nerve	K. Sense organs
OBJ. 8	____ 57. Utricle, saccule	L. Inner ear
OBJ. 9	____ 58. Ceruminous glands	M. Taste
OBJ. 9	____ 59. Membranous labyrinth	N. General senses

[L1] Drawing/Illustration Labeling:

Identify each numbered structure by labeling the following figures:

OBJ. 5   **FIGURE 10.1**   Sectional Anatomy of the Eye

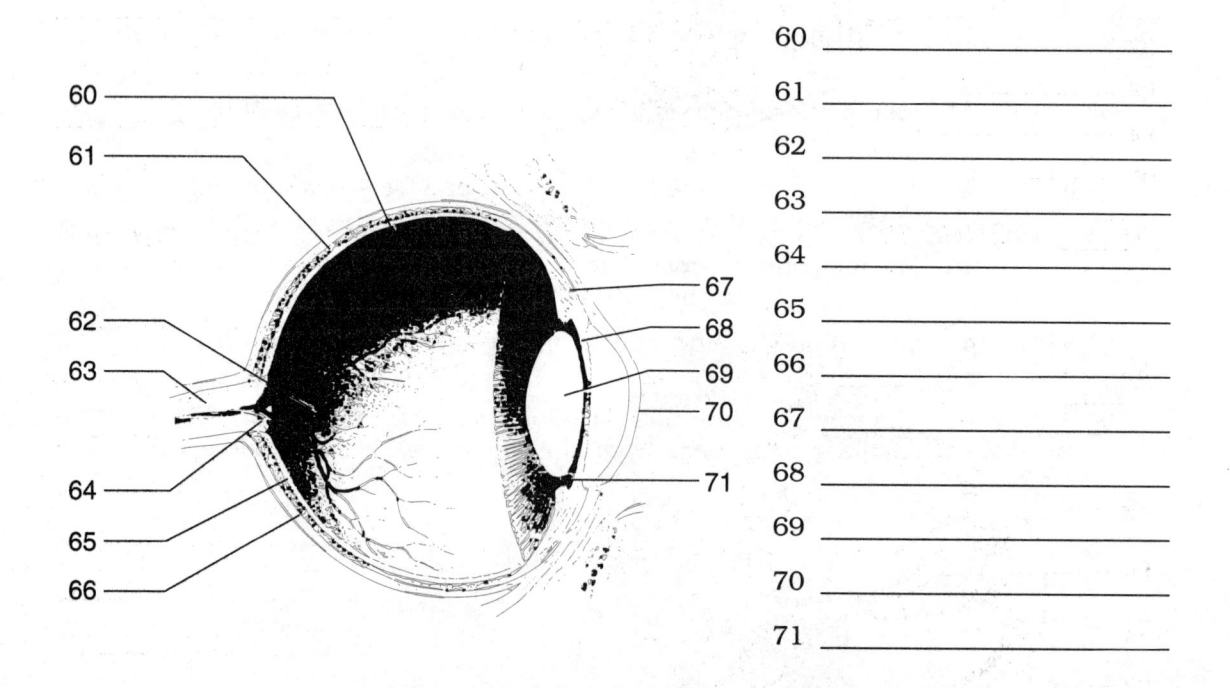

60 _____
61 _____
62 _____
63 _____
64 _____
65 _____
66 _____
67 _____
68 _____
69 _____
70 _____
71 _____

Level 1   Review of Chapter Objectives   169

[OBJ. 9]   *FIGURE 10.2*   Anatomy of the Ear: External, Middle and Inner Ears

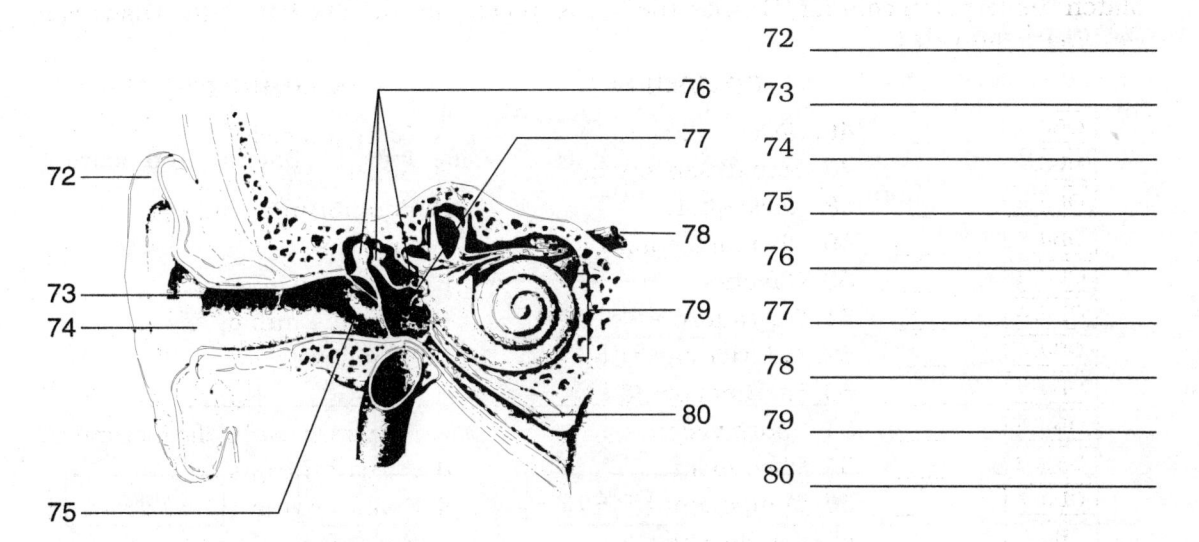

72 _____
73 _____
74 _____
75 _____
76 _____
77 _____
78 _____
79 _____
80 _____

[OBJ. 9]   *FIGURE 10.3*   Anatomy of the Ear: Bony Labyrinth

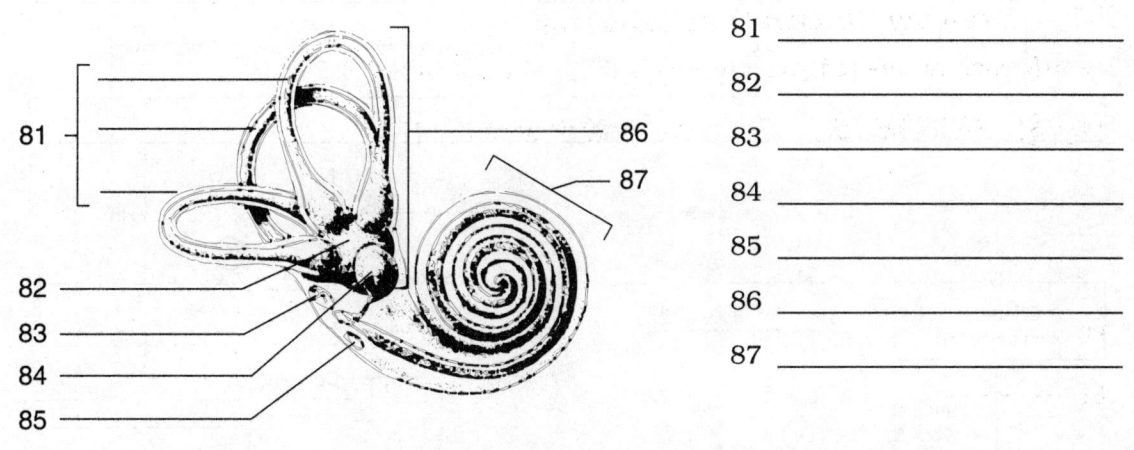

81 _____
82 _____
83 _____
84 _____
85 _____
86 _____
87 _____

[OBJ. 9]   *FIGURE 10.4*   Gross Anatomy of the Cochlea: Details Visible in Section

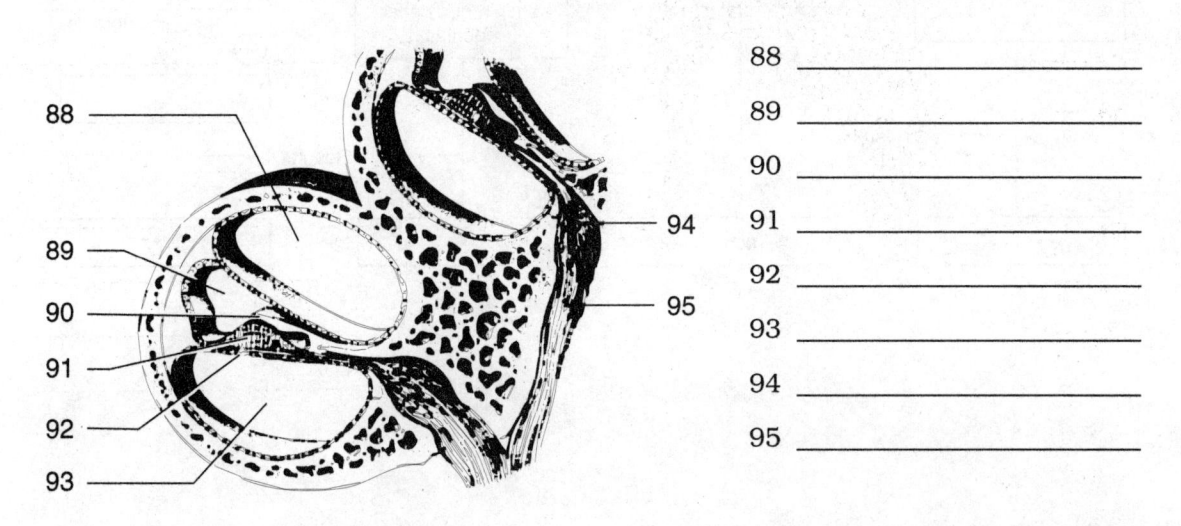

88 _____
89 _____
90 _____
91 _____
92 _____
93 _____
94 _____
95 _____

When you have successfully completed the exercises in L1 proceed to L2.

Level -1-

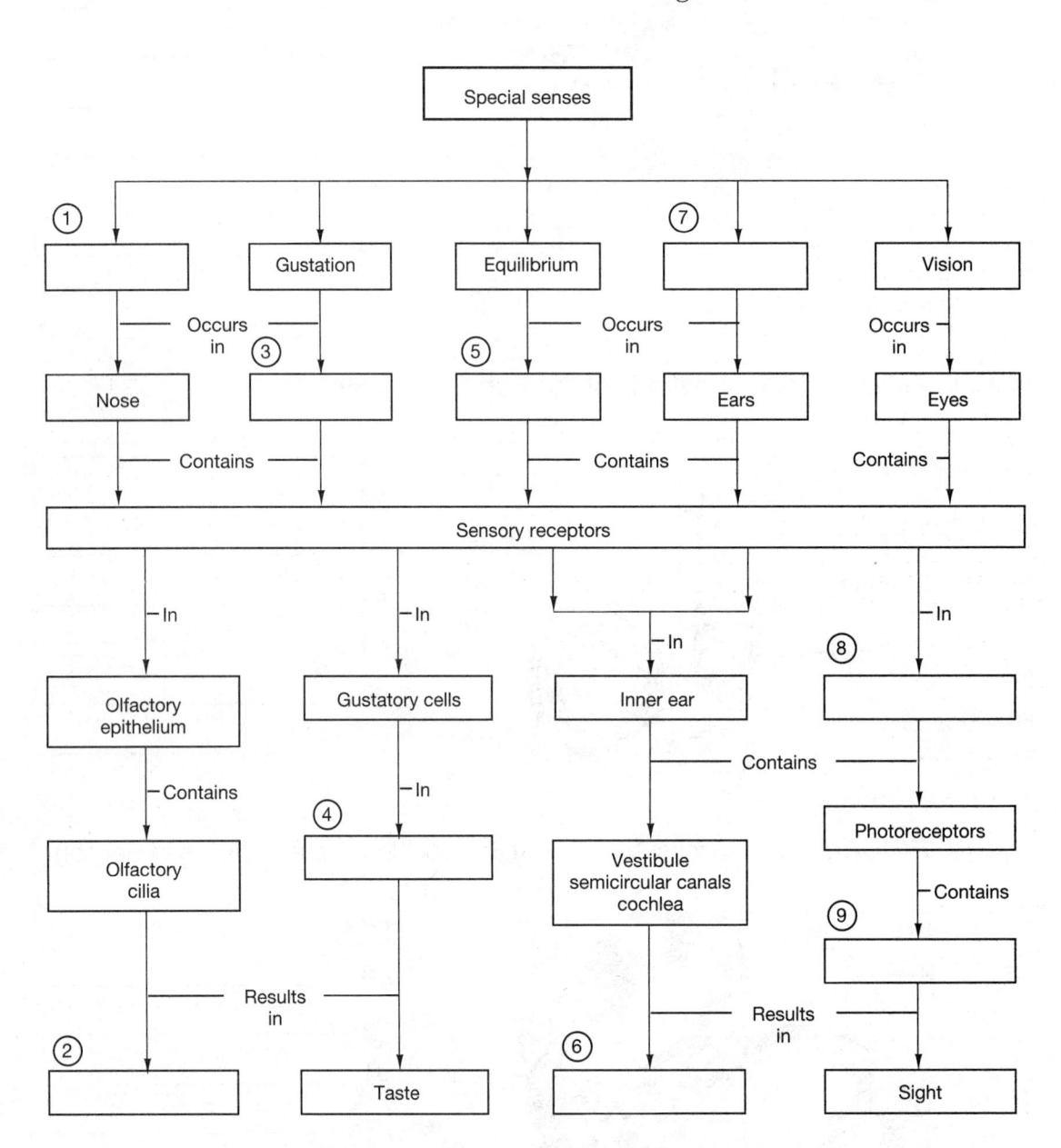

☐ LEVEL 2 CONCEPT SYNTHESIS

Concept Map I:

Using the following terms, fill in the numbered, blank spaces to complete the concept map. Follow the numbers that comply with the organization of the map.

Retina   Hearing   Rods and cones   Olfaction   Balance and hearing
Smell   Ears   Taste buds   Tongue

Body Trek:

Using the terms below, fill in the blanks to complete the trek through the outer, middle, and inner ear.

pharyngotympanic	oval window	hairs atop the hair cell
endolymph	scala vestibule	scala tympani
incus	organ of Corti	round window
pinna	cochlear	middle ear
tympanic membrane	malleus	external ear
ceruminous	nasopharynx	ossicles
tectorial	basilar membrane	external auditory meatus
stapes		

Robo's programming for this trek involves following sound waves through the outer and middle ear until the sound (mechanical) waves are converted into nerve (electrical) in the inner ear.

Robo's trek begins as sound waves are funnelled by the (10) _____ into the (11) _____, the entrance to the external auditory canal. The robot's progress is slowed in this area because of the presence of a "waxy" material secreted by (12) _____ glands along the canal. All of a sudden Robo is thrust against the (13) _____, or eardrum, causing a tremendous vibration that pushes the robot from the (14) _____ into the (15) _____, or tympanic cavity. This compartment is an air-filled space containing three bones, the auditory (16) _____. One of the bones looks like a "hammer," the (17) _____, while another one looks like an "anvil," the (18) _____, and the third has an appearance like a "stirrup," or (19) _____. Robo's trek is momentarily halted because of an opening that leads into an elongated channel, the (20) _____ tube, which allows for communication between the tympanic cavity and the (21) _____. After trekking around the opening Robo is "waved" through an ovoid "pane-like" covering, the (22) _____, which is waving back and forth and creating vibrations that set up pressure waves in a clear fluid, the (23) _____ of the bony labyrinth in the inner ear. The robot is propelled by the pressure waves as they are propagated through the perilymph of the (24) _____ and (25) _____. These pressure waves distort the (26) _____ on their way to the (27) _____ of the tympanic duct. As Robo treks into the duct, it senses a distorted membrane forcing hair cells of the (28) _____ toward or away from the (29) _____ membrane. This movement moves Robo along, and leads to displacement of (30) _____ and stimulation of sensory neurons of the (31) _____ nerve.

Mission Control orders Robo to use the programmed route by picking up a pressure wave as it "rolls" back toward the entrance to the vestibular duct. Robo's handlers are happy to retrieve their robot, which is covered with wax and needs recharging because of a run-down battery.

[Level 2]   Multiple Choice:

Place the letter corresponding to the correct answer in the space provided.

_____ 32. Our knowledge of the environment is limited to those characteristics that stimulate our:

    a. eyes and ears
    b. peripheral receptors
    c. nose and tongue
    d. central nervous system

_____ 33. The system that helps to focus attention and either heightens or reduces awareness of arriving sensations is the:

    a. reticular activating system in the midbrain
    b. limbic system in the cerebrum
    c. endocrine system
    d. autonomic nervous system

_____ 34. The receptors that provide information which plays a major role in regulating cardiac function and adjusting blood flow to vital tissues are:

    a. mechanoreceptors
    b. baroreceptors
    c. tactile receptors
    d. a, b, and c are correct

_____ 35. The position of joints, the tension in tendons and ligaments, and the state of muscular contractions are monitored by:

    a. proprioceptors
    b. baroreceptors
    c. mechanoreceptors
    d. tactile receptors

_____ 36. When a neuron responds to an excitatory or inhibitory neurotransmitter, it functions as a:

    a. mechanoreceptor
    b. tactile receptor
    c. chemoreceptor
    d. proprioceptor

_____ 37. The chemoreceptive neurons that monitor the oxygen concentration of the arterial blood are found within the:

    a. carotid and aortic sinus
    b. supporting and stem cells
    c. papillae
    d. carotid and aortic bodies

_____ 38. There are no known structural differences between warm and cold thermoreceptors because they are all:

    a. mechanically regulated ion channels
    b. affected by excitatory or inhibitory neurotransmitters
    c. free nerve endings
    d. affected by the extremes of temperature

_____ 39. The only known example of neuronal replacement in the human adult is the:

    a. olfactory receptor population
    b. gustatory receptor population
    c. optic receptor population
    d. vestibuloreceptor population

_____ 40. During the focusing process, when light travels from the air into the relatively dense cornea:

    a. the sclera assumes an obvious color
    b. the light path is bent
    c. pupillary reflexes are triggered
    d. reflexive adjustments occur in both pupils

Level 2

_____ 41. Exposure to bright light produces a:
   a. rapid reflexive increase in pupillary diameter
   b. slow reflexive increase in pupillary diameter
   c. very slow reflexive decrease in pupillary diameter
   d. rapid reflexive decrease in pupillary diameter

_____ 42. The color of the eye is determined by:
   a. light reflecting through the cornea onto the retina
   b. the thickness of the iris and the number and distribution of pigment cells
   c. the reflection of light from the aqueous humor
   d. the number and distribution of pigment cells in the lens

_____ 43. After an intense exposure to light, a "ghost" image remains on the retina and a photoreceptor cannot respond to stimulation until:
   a. the rate of neurotransmitter release declines at the receptor membrane
   b. the receptor membrane channels close
   c. its supply of rhodopsin has been ceompletely broken down
   d. its rhodopsin molecules have been regenerated

_____ 44. The reason everything appears to be black and white when we enter dimly lighted surroundings is:
   a. both rods and cones are stimulated
   b. only cones are stimulated
   c. only rods are stimulated
   d. only the blue cones are stimulated

_____ 45. When one or more classes of cones are nonfunctional, the result is:
   a. a blind spot occurs
   b. color blindness
   c. image inversion
   d. the appearance of "ghost" images

_____ 46. The most detailed information about the visual image is provided by the:
   a. cones
   b. rods
   c. optic disc
   d. rods and cones together

_____ 47. The region of the retina called the "blind spot" is an area that structurally comprises the:
   a. choroid coat
   b. suprachiasmatic nucleus
   c. optic disc
   d. visual cortex

[L2] Completion:

Using the terms below, complete the following statements.

retina	accommodation	referred pain	pupil
hyperopia	adaptation	cataract	sensory receptor
myopia	aqueous humor	ampulla	

48. A specialized cell that monitors conditions in the body or the external environment is a _____.
49. A reduction in sensitivity in the presence of a constant stimulus is _____.
50. Pain sensations from visceral organs that are often perceived as originating in more superficial regions innervated by the same spinal nerves are known as _____.
51. Sensory receptors in the semicircular canals in the inner ear are located in the _____.
52. When the muscles of the iris contract, they change the diameter of the central opening referred to as the _____.
53. The posterior chamber of the eye contains a fluid called _____.
54. The visual receptors and associated neurons in the eye are contained in the _____.
55. When the lens of the eye loses its transparency, the abnormal lens is known as a _____.
56. When the lens of the eye becomes rounder to focus on the image of a nearby object on the retina, the mechanism is called _____.
57. If a person sees objects at close range under normal conditions, the individual is said to be "nearsighted," a condition formally termed _____.
58. If a person sees distant objects more clearly under normal conditions, the individual is said to be "farsighted," a condition formally termed _____.

[L2] Short Essay:

Briefly answer the following questions in the spaces provided below.

59. What sensations are included as "general senses?"

60. What sensations are included as "special senses?"

61. What four (4) kinds of "general sense" receptors are found throughout the body and to what kind(s) of stimuli do they respond?

62. What is the functional difference between a baroreceptor and a proprioceptor?

63. What sensations are provided by the saccule and utricle in the vestibule of the inner ear?

64. When referring to the eye, what is the purpose of accommodation and how does it work?

When you have successfully completed the exercises in L2 proceed to L3.

☐ LEVEL 3   CRITICAL THINKING/APPLICATION

Using principles and concepts learned about sensory functions, answer the following questions. Write your answers on a separate sheet of paper.

1. Grandmother and Granddad are all "decked out" for a night of dining and dancing. Grandma has doused herself with her finest perfume and Grandpa has soaked his face with aftershave. The pleasant scents are overbearing to others; however, the old folks can barely smell the aromas. Why?
2. Suppose you were small enough to wander around in the middle ear. What features in this region would make you think that you might be in a blacksmith's shop or perhaps a shop involved with equestrian enterprises?
3. A bright flash of light temporarily blinds normal, well-nourished eyes. As a result, a "ghost" image remains on the retina. Why?

CHAPTER 11

The Endocrine System

■ Overview

The nervous system and the endocrine system are the metabolic control systems in the body. Together they monitor and adjust the physiological activities throughout the body to maintain homeostasis. The effects of nervous system regulation are usually rapid and short term, whereas the effects of endocrine regulation are ongoing and long term.

Endocrine cells are glandular secretory cells that release chemicals, called hormones, into the bloodstream for distribution to target tissues throughout the body. The influence of these chemical "messengers" results in facilitating processes that include growth and development, sexual maturation and reproduction, and the maintenance of homeostasis within other systems.

Chapter 11 consists of exercises that will test your knowledge of the endocrine organs and their functions. The integrative and complementary activities of the nervous and endocrine systems are presented to show the coordinated effort necessary to regulate adequately physiological activities in the body.

☐ LEVEL 1   REVIEW OF CHAPTER OBJECTIVES

1. Compare the endocrine and nervous systems.
2. Compare the major chemical classes of hormones.
3. Explain the general mechanisms of hormonal action.
4. Describe how endocrine organs are controlled.
5. Describe the location, hormones, and functions of the following endocrine glands and tissues: pituitary, thyroid, parathyroids, thymus, adrenals, kidneys, heart, pancreas, testes, ovaries, and pineal gland.
6. Explain how hormones interact to produce coordinated physiological responses.
7. Identify the hormones that are especially important to normal growth and discuss their roles.
8. Explain how the endocrine system responds to stress.
9. Discuss the results of abnormal hormone production.
10. Discuss the functional relationships between the endocrine system and other body systems.

[L1] Multiple Choice:

Place the letter corresponding to the correct answer in the space provided.

OBJ. 1 ____ 1. Response patterns in the endocrine system are particularly effective in:
   a. regulating ongoing metabolic processes
   b. rapid short-term specific responses
   c. the release of chemical neurotransmitters
   d. a, b, and c are correct

OBJ. 1 ____ 2. An example of a functional similarity between the nervous system and the endocrine system is:
   a. both systems secrete hormones into the bloodstream
   b. the cells of the endocrine and nervous systems are functionally the same
   c. compounds used as hormones by the endocrine system and may also function as neurotransmitters inside the CNS
   d. both produce very specific responses to environmental stimuli

OBJ. 1 ____ 3. Neurons communicate with one another and with effectors by:
   a. releasing chemicals into the bloodstream
   b. interacting with a hormone and a receptor complex
   c. receptor binding at the cell membrane
   d. releasing chemical neurotransmitters

OBJ. 1 ____ 4. The release of hormones by endocrine cells alters the:
   a. rate at which chemical neurotransmitters are released
   b. metabolic activities of many tissues and organs simultaneously
   c. very specific responses to environmental stimuli
   d. anatomical boundary between the nervous and endocrine systems

OBJ. 2 ____ 5. The protein hormone prolactin is involved with the:
   a. synthesis of melanin
   b. production of milk
   c. production of testosterone
   d. labor contractions and milk ejection

OBJ. 2 ____ 6. The amino acid derivative hormone epinephrine is responsible for:
   a. increased cardiac activity
   b. glycogen breakdown
   c. release of lipids by adipose tissue
   d. a, b, and c are correct

Chapter 11 The Endocrine System

OBJ. 3 ___ 7. The most notable effect of ADH produced in the posterior pituitary is to:
  a. increase the amount of water lost at the kidneys
  b. decrease the amount of water lost at the kidneys
  c. stimulate the contraction of uterine muscles
  d. increase or decrease calcium ion concentrations in body fluids

OBJ. 3 ___ 8. Hormones alter cellular operations by changing the:
  a. cell membrane permeability properties
  b. identities, activities, quantities, or properties of important enzymes
  c. arrangement of the molecular complex of the cell membrane
  d. rate at which hormones affect the target organ cells

OBJ. 3 ___ 9. Peptide hormones affect target organ cells by:
  a. binding to receptors in the cytoplasm
  b. binding to target receptors in the nucleus
  c. enzymatic reactions that occur in the ribosomes
  d. second messengers released when receptor binding occurs at the membrane surface

OBJ. 3 ___ 10. Steroid hormones affect target organ cells by:
  a. targeting receptors in peripheral tissues
  b. releasing second messengers at cell membrane receptors
  c. binding to receptors in the cell membrane
  d. binding to target receptors in the nucleus

OBJ. 4 ___ 11. Endocrine cells responding directly to changes in the composition of the extracellular fluid is an example of:
  a. a neural reflex
  b. a reflex arc
  c. an endocrine reflex
  d. a hypothalamic control mechanism

OBJ. 4 ___ 12. The hypothalamus is a major coordinating and control center because:
  a. it contains autonomic centers and acts as an endocrine organ
  b. it initiates endocrine and neural reflexes
  c. it stimulates appropriate responses by peripheral target cells
  d. it stimulates responses to restore homeostasis

OBJ. 5 ___ 13. The protein hormone FSH in the male is responsible for:
  a. maturation of germinative cells in the gonads
  b. production of interstitial cells in the male
  c. sperm formation and testosterone secretion
  d. the male doesn't secrete FSH

Level -1-

Level 1   Review of Chapter Objectives   179

OBJ. 5   ___ 14. The inability to tolerate stress due to underproduction of glucocorticoids results in a syndrome called:
    a. Cushing's disease
    b. Addison's disease
    c. myxedema
    d. eunuchoidism

OBJ. 5   ___ 15. The posterior pituitary secretes:
    a. growth hormone and prolactin
    b. oxytocin and antidiuretic hormone
    c. thyroid stimulating and adrenocorticotrophic hormone
    d. melanocyte-stimulating and luteinizing hormone

OBJ. 5   ___ 16. The gonadotropic hormones secreted by the anterior pituitary are:
    a. TSH, ACTH, ADH
    b. PRL, GH, MSH
    c. FSH, LH
    d. ADH, MSH, FSH

OBJ. 5   ___ 17. The hormone produced by the pineal gland is:
    a. melanocyte-stimulating hormone
    b. pinealtonin
    c. oxytocin
    d. melatonin

OBJ. 6   ___ 18. When a cell receives instructions from two different hormones at the same time the results may be:
    a. antagonistic
    b. synergistic
    c. integrative
    d. a, b, and c are correct

OBJ. 7   ___ 19. The hormones that are of primary importance to normal growth include:
    a. TSH, ACTH, insulin, parathormone, and LH
    b. prolactin, insulin, growth hormone, ADH, and MSH
    c. growth hormone, prolactin, thymosin, androgens, and insulin
    d. growth hormone, thyroid hormones, insulin, parathormone, and gonadal hormones

OBJ. 7   ___ 20. The reason insulin is important to normal growth is that it promotes:
    a. changes in skeletal proportions and calcium deposition in the body
    b. passage of glucose and amino acids across cell membranes
    c. muscular development via protein synthesis
    d. a, b, and c are correct

180 Chapter 11 The Endocrine System

OBJ. 8   ___ 21. Despite the variety of potential stresses, the human body responds to each one:

   a. in a variety of ways to make the adjustments necessary for homeostasis
   b. with the same basic pattern of hormonal and physiological adjustments
   c. by suppressing the stress using psychological conditioning
   d. by reducing the stress via relaxation exercises

OBJ. 9   ___ 22. The overproduction syndrome aldosteronism results in;

   a. high blood potassium concentrations
   b. low blood volume
   c. dependence on lipids for energy
   d. increased body weight due to water retention

OBJ. 10   ___ 23. Which of the following hormones has an anti-inflammatory effect?

   a. atrial natriuretic hormone
   b. glucocorticoids
   c. mineralocorticoids
   d. b and c are correct

[L1] Completion:

Using the terms below, complete the following statements.

gigantism	cytoplasm	neurotransmitters
exhaustive	general adaptation syndrome	parathyroids
diabetes mellitus	reflex	adrenal gland
testosterone	hypothalamus	thymus
amino acid derivatives	sex hormones	

OBJ. 1   24. Many compounds used as hormones by the endocrine system also function inside the CNS as _____.

OBJ. 2   25. An example of a gland in the body that functions as a neural tissue and an endocrine tissue is the _____.

OBJ. 2   26. Epinephrine and norepinephrine are structurally similar and belong to a class of compounds sometimes called _____.

OBJ. 3   27. The hormone that stimulates the production of enzymes and proteins in skeletal muscle fibers, causing an increase in muscle size and strength is _____.

OBJ. 4   28. The control of calcium ion concentrations by parathormone or calcitonin is an example of an endocrine _____.

OBJ. 4   29. The most complex endocrine responses are directed by the _____.

OBJ. 5   30. The glands that are primarily responsible for increasing calcium ion concentrations in body fluids are the _____.

OBJ. 5   31. The gland that affects maturation and functional competence of the immune system is the _____.

OBJ. 6   32. Steroid hormones bind to receptors in the _____.

OBJ. 7   33. Oversecretion of the growth hormone (GH) leads to a disorder called _____.

Level -1-

OBJ. 8   34. The collapse of vital systems due to stress represents the _____ phase of the GAS syndrome.

OBJ. 8   35. Patterns of hormonal and physiological adjustments to stress constitute the _____.

OBJ. 9   36. The underproduction syndrome in insulin results in the condition called _____.

OBJ. 10   37. The hormones which stimulate sebaceous gland activity and growth of body hair at puberty are the _____.

[L1] Matching:

Match the terms in column "B" with the terms in column "A." Use letters for answers in the spaces provided.

	COLUMN "A"	COLUMN "B"
OBJ. 1 ___ 38.	Neurotransmitters	A. Amino acid derivative
OBJ. 1 ___ 39.	Release of hormones	B. Calcitonin
OBJ. 1 ___ 40.	Endocrine cells	C. Pituitary
OBJ. 1 ___ 41.	Neural cells	D. Nervous system
OBJ. 2 ___ 42.	Thyroid stimulating hormone	E. Stimulates RBC production
OBJ. 2 ___ 43.	Epinephrine	F. Overproduction of thyroid hormone
OBJ. 3 ___ 44.	Erythropoietin	G. Endocrine system
OBJ. 3 ___ 45.	Glucagon	H. Dwarfism
OBJ. 4 ___ 46.	"Master Gland"	I. Produces releasing-inhibiting hormones
OBJ. 4 ___ 47.	Hypothalamus	
OBJ. 5 ___ 48.	Thyroid C cells	J. Peptide hormone
OBJ. 5 ___ 49.	Adrenal medulla	K. Release of chemicals
OBJ. 6 ___ 50.	Enzyme activator or inhibitor	L. Kidneys
		M. Action potentials
OBJ. 6 ___ 51.	Hormone	N. Underproduction of thyroid hormone
OBJ. 7 ___ 52.	Undersecretion of GH	
OBJ. 8 ___ 53.	Alarm phase of GAS	O. Regulates blood glucose concentration
OBJ. 9 ___ 54.	Cretinism	
OBJ. 9 ___ 55.	Graves' disease	P. Second messenger
OBJ. 10 ___ 56.	Site of production of renin	Q. Immediate response to crisis
		R. Secretion of epinephrine
		S. First messenger

182 **Chapter 11 The Endocrine System**

[L1] Drawing/Illustration Labeling:

Identify each numbered structure by labeling the following figures:

OBJ. 2 ***FIGURE 11.1*** Structural Classification of Hormones

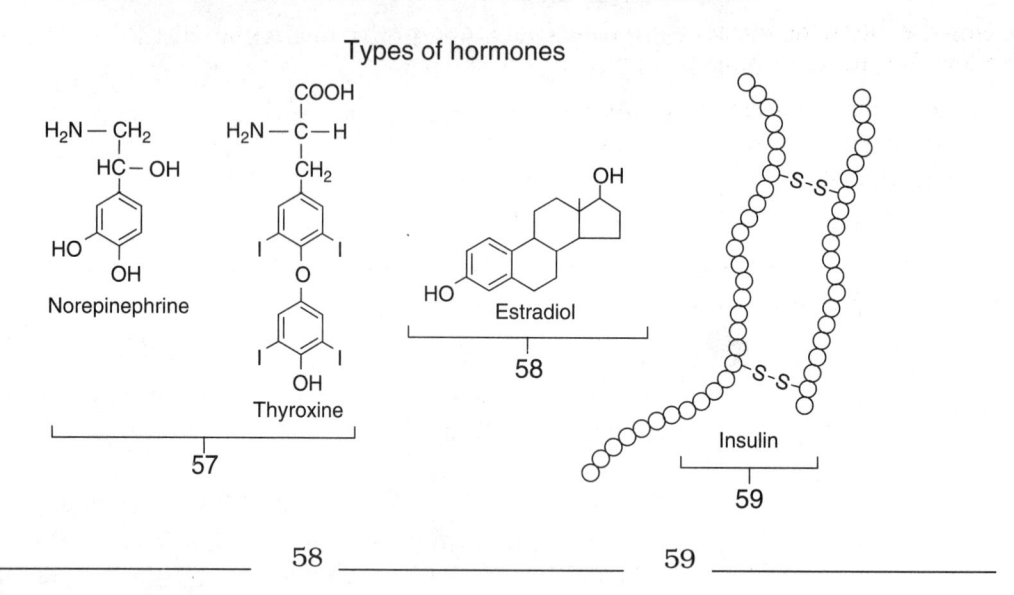

Types of hormones

Norepinephrine

Thyroxine

57

Estradiol

58

Insulin

59

57 _____   58 _____   59 _____

OBJ. 5 ***FIGURE 11.2*** The Endocrine System

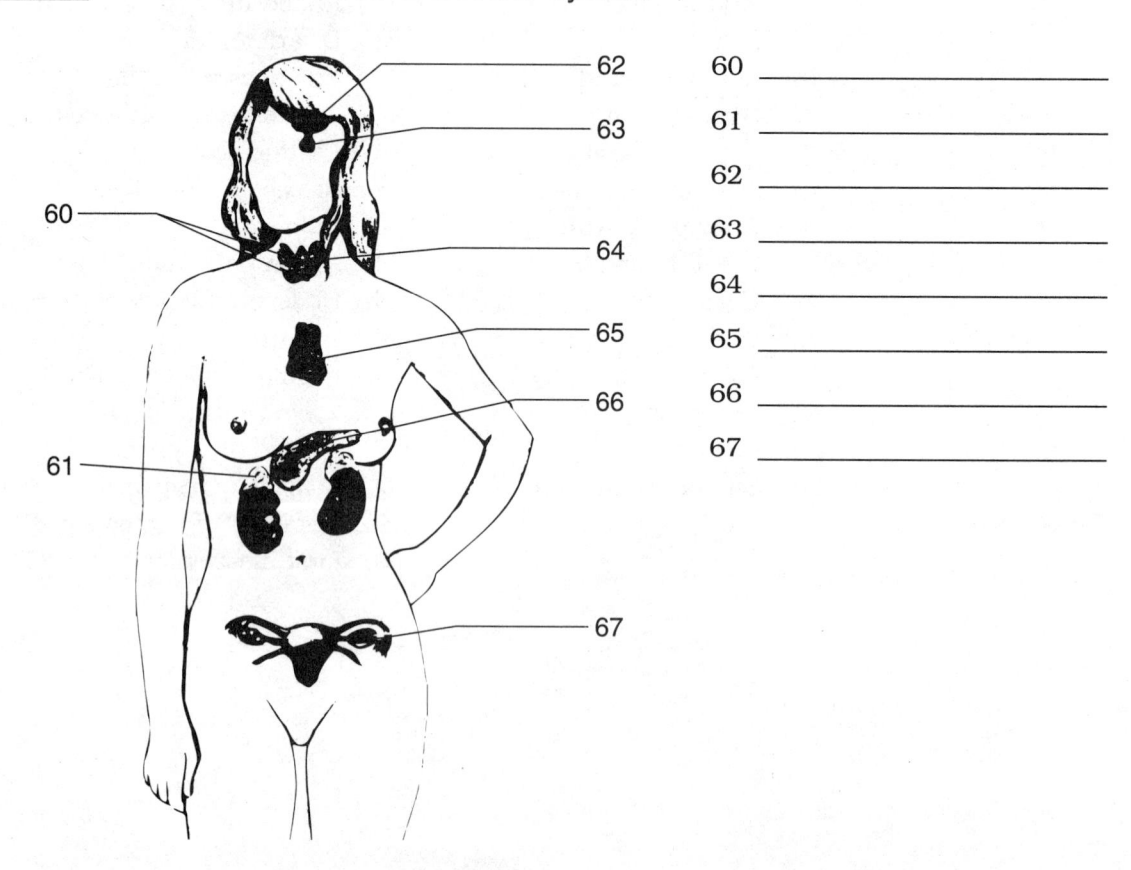

60 _____
61 _____
62 _____
63 _____
64 _____
65 _____
66 _____
67 _____

Level -1- **When you have successfully completed the exercises in L1 proceed to L2.**

☐ LEVEL 2   CONCEPT SYNTHESIS

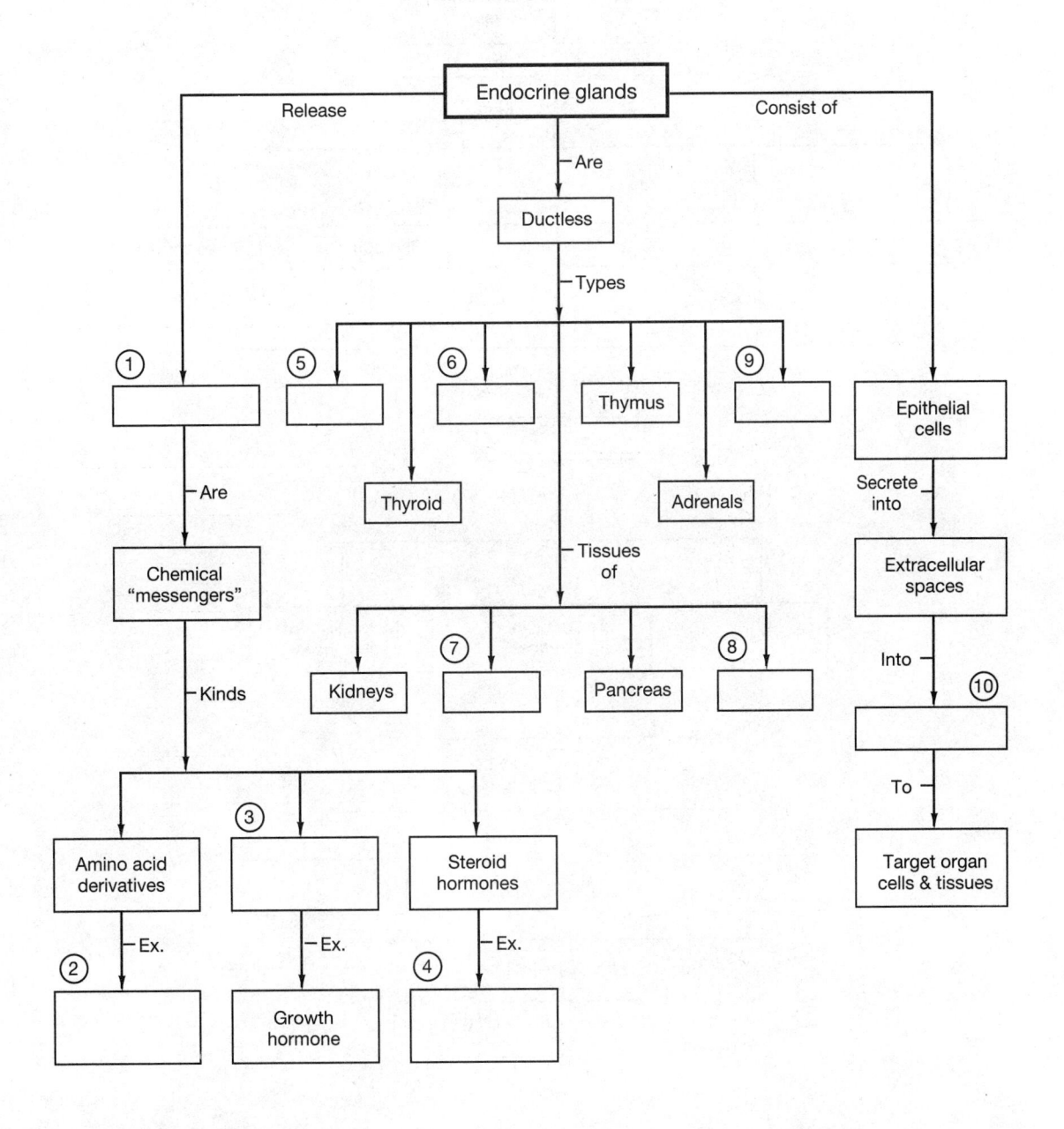

Concept Map I:

Using the following terms, fill in the numbered, blank spaces to complete the concept map. Follow the numbers that comply with the organization of the map.

- Male/female gonads
- Hormones
- Parathyroids
- Epinephrine
- Bloodstream
- Peptide hormones
- Pineal
- Testosterone
- Pituitary
- Heart

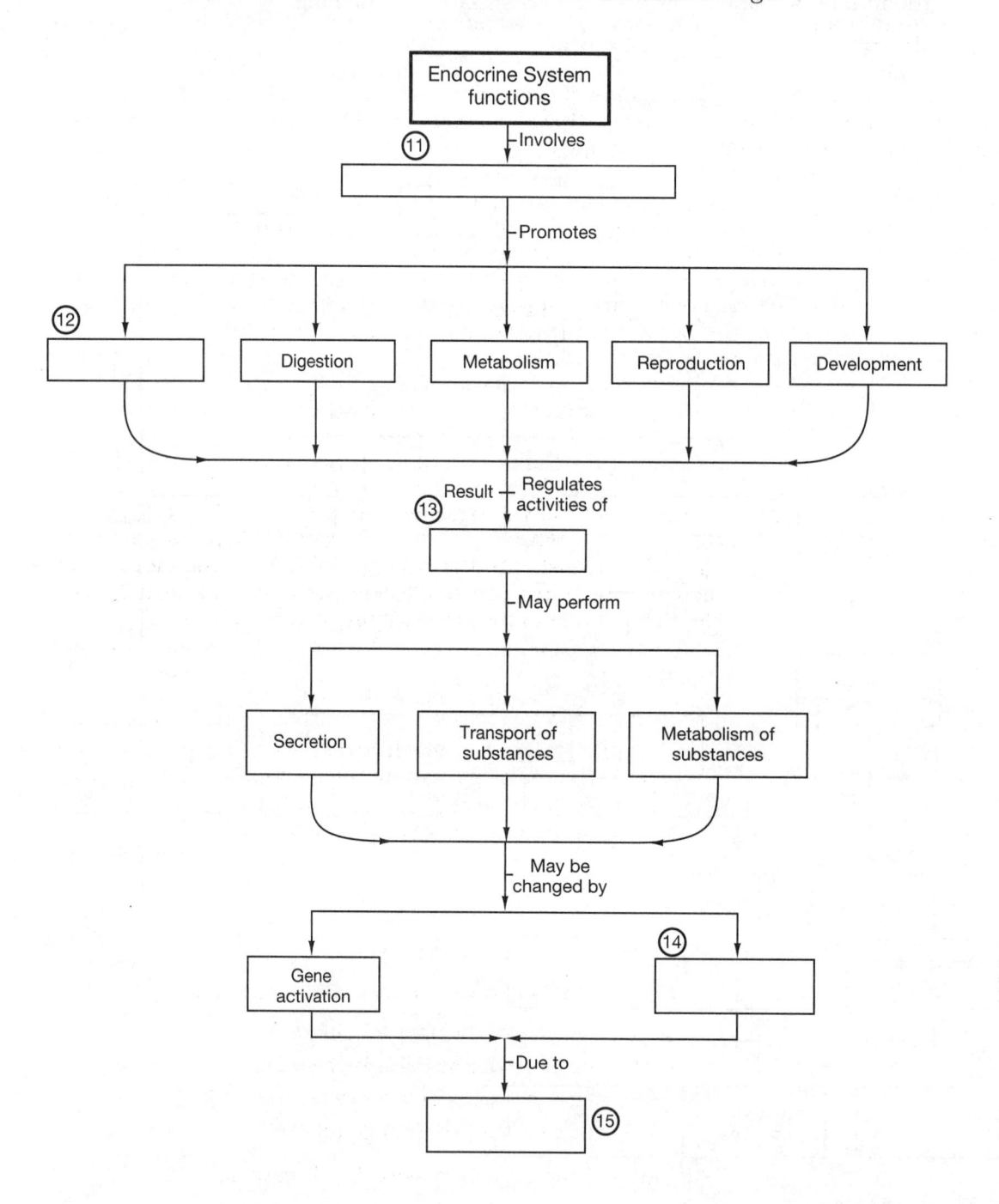

Chapter 11 The Endocrine System

Concept Map II:

Using the following terms, fill in the numbered, blank spaces to complete the concept map. Follow the numbers that comply with the organization of the map.

Homeostasis   Target cells   Hormones
Cellular communication   Formation of second messenger

11. Hormones
12. Cellular communication
13. Target cells
14. Formation of second messenger
15. Homeostasis

Level 2 Concept Synthesis

Body Trek:

Using the terms below, fill in the blanks to complete a trek through the endocrine system

progesterone	erythropoietin	adrenal	sella turcica
kidneys	heart	estrogen	ovaries
thymus	pituitary	testosterone	insulin
infundibulum	melatonin	pineal	pancreas
testes	parathyroid	RBCs	thyroid

The body trek to "visit" the glands of the endocrine system will be taken by using an imaginary pathway through the body. Specific directions will be used to locate and identify the glands comprising the endocrine system.

The trek begins in the roof of the thalamus where the (16) _____ gland synthesizes the hormone (17) _____. Continuing in an anterior-inferior direction, the trek down the stalk of the hypothalamus, called the (18) _____, leads to the base of the brain, the location of the (19) _____ gland, which is housed in a bony encasement, the (20) _____. This pea-sized "master" gland secretes approximately nine tropic hormones that exert their effects on target organs, tissues, and cells throughout the body. Trekking southward in the body, the next "landmarks" are located in the neck region. Situated on the anterior surface of the trachea is the (21) _____ gland with four small (22) _____ glands embedded in its posterior surface. Just below and posterior to the sternum is the (23) _____, a gland that is primarily concerned with the functional competence of the immune system.

Moving slightly downward and away from the midline of the thorax, the production of atrial natriuretic hormone is taking place in the tissues of the (24)_____. Trekking inferiorly and moving to a position behind the stomach, the (25) _____ can be seen secreting glucagon and (26) _____ which are used to control blood glucose levels. Leaving the stomach region and progressing to the superior borders of the kidneys, the (27) _____ glands, which secrete hormones that affect the kidneys and most cells throughout the body, are identified. While in the area, the much larger (28) _____ are sighted. Their endocrine tissues release (29) _____ which stimulates the production of (30) _____ by the bone marrow.

The imaginary trek within a female ends with a visit to the (31) _____, located near the lateral wall of the pelvic cavity. Here, the hormone (32) _____, which supports follicle maturation, and the hormone (33) _____, which prepares the uterus for implantation, are released. The trek ends in the male by a visit to the scrotal sac, the location of the (34) _____, which release the hormone (35) _____, the hormone that supports functional maturation of sperm and promotes development of male characteristics in the body.

[L2] Multiple choice:

Place the letter corresponding to the correct answer in the space provided.

_____ 36. Corticosteroids are hormones that are produced and secreted by the:

    a. medulla of the adrenal glands
    b. cortex of the cerebral hemispheres
    c. sensory cortex of the cerebrum
    d. cortex of the adrenal glands

_____ 37. The adrenal medulla produces and releases the hormones:

    a. mineralocorticoids and gluco corticoids
    b. epinephrine and norepinephrine
    c. androgens and estrogens
    d. aldosterone and cortisone

_____ 38. The endocrine functions of the kidney and the heart include the production and secretion of the hormones:

    a. renin and angiotensinogen
    b. insulin and glucagon
    c. erythropoietin and atrial natriuretic peptide
    d. epinephrine and norepinephrine

_____ 39. The endocrine tissues of the reproductive system of the female produce:

    a. estrogens, inhibin, and progesterone
    b. androgens, estrogens, and glucocorticoids
    c. FSH and LH
    d. a and c are correct

_____ 40. The overall effect of the hormones secreted by the thyroid gland is:

    a. to increase calcium ion concentrations in body fluids
    b. maturation and functional competence of the immune system
    c. increase cellular rates of metabolism and oxygen consumption
    d. increased reabsorption of sodium ions and water from urine

_____ 41. The parathyroid glands secrete hormones that:

    a. afffect the circulating concentration of calcium ions
    b. affect the functional competence of the immune system
    c. affect blood pressure and other cardiac activity
    d. affect the release of amino acids from skeletal muscles

_____ 42. One of the major effects of ANP produced by the heart is that it:

    a. assists in the production of red blood cells
    b. constricts peripheral blood vessels
    c. promotes water retention at the kidneys
    d. a and c are correct

_____ 43. Glucagon and insulin secreted by the islets of Langerhans regulate:

    a. blood calcium levels
    b. blood glucose concentrations
    c. protein synthesis in muscle cells
    d. blood glucose utilization by the brain

_____ 44. Testosterone produced in the interstitial cells of the testes is responsible for:

    a. promoting the production of functional sperm
    b. determining male secondary sexual characteristics
    c. affecting metabolic operations throughout the body
    d. a, b, and c are correct

_____ 45. The estrogens produced in follicle cells surrounding the eggs in the ovary are responsible for:

    a. supporting the maturation of eggs and stimulating the growth of the uterine lining
    b. preparing the uterus for the arrival of the developing embryo
    c. accelerating the movement of the fertilized egg along the oviduct
    d. enlargement of the mammary glands

_____ 46. The binding of a peptide hormone to its receptor starts a biochemical chain of events that changes the pattern of:

    a. enzymatic activity within the cell
    b. calcium ion release or entry into the cell
    c. diffusion through the lipid portion of the cell membrane
    d. an RNA transcription in the nucleus

_____ 47. Aldosterone targets kidney cells and causes the:

    a. loss of sodium ions and water, increasing fluid losses in the urine
    b. retention of sodium ions and water, reducing fluid losses in the urine
    c. production and release of angiotensin II by the kidneys
    d. secretion of the enzyme renin by the kidneys

_____ 48. The most dramatic functional change that occurs in the endocrine system due to aging is:

    a. a decrease in blood and tissue concentrations of ADH and TSH
    b. an overall decrease in circulating hormone levels
    c. a decline in the concentration of reproductive hormones
    d. a, b, and c are correct

_____ 49. The two basic categories of endocrine disorders are:

    a. abnormal hormone production or abnormal cellular sensitivity
    b. the underproduction and overproduction syndrome
    c. muscular weakness and the inability to tolerate stress
    d. a and b are correct

[L2] Completion:

Using the terms below, complete the following statements.

    portal   cyclic-AMP   nucleus   aldosterone
    hypothalamus   glucocorticoids   epinephrine   target cells

50. The interface between the neural and endocrine systems is the _____.
51. The peripheral cells that are modified by the activities of a hormone are referred to as _____.
52. Thyroid hormones target receptors in the _____.

53. Many hormones produce their effects by increasing intracellular concentrations of _____.
54. Blood vessels that link two capillary networks are called _____ vessels.
55. The principal mineralocorticoid produced by the human adrenal cortex is _____.
56. The dominant hormone of the alarm phase of the general adaptation syndrome is _____.
57. The dominant hormones of the resistance phase of the GAS are _____.

[L2] Short Essay:

Briefly answer the following questions in the spaces provided below.

58. What mechanisms does the hypothalamus use to regulate the activities of the nervous and endocrine systems?

59. What hypothalamic control mechanisms are used to effect endocrine activity in the anterior pituitary?

60. How does the calorigenic effect of thyroid hormones help us to adapt to cold temperatures?

61. How does the kidney hormone erythropoietin cause an increase in blood pressure?

62. What are the possible results when a cell receives instructions from two different hormones at the same time?

When you have successfully completed the exercises in L2 proceed to L3.

☐ LEVEL 3   CRITICAL THINKING/APPLICATION

Using principles and concepts learned about the endocrine system, answer the following questions. Write your answers on a separate sheet of paper.

1. Negative feedback is an important mechanism for maintaining homeostasis in the body. Using the criteria below, create a model that shows how negative feedback regulates hormone production.

    Criteria:

    Gland X secretes hormone 1.

    Gland Y secretes hormone 2.

    Organ Z contains gland Y.

2. (a) As a diagnostic clinician, what endocrine malfunctions and conditions would you associate with the following symptoms in patients A, B, and C?

    Patient A: Marked increase in daily fluid intake, 12-15 liters of urine per day, glycosuria (the presence of glucose in the urine), lethargic.

    Patient B: Blood pressure 100/60 mm Hg, pulse 50 beats/min, abnormal weight gain, dry skin and hair, always tired, body temperature 95 degrees F, feelings of weakness.

    Patient C: Blood pressure 160/100 mm Hg, glucose 130 mg %, muscle weakness, poor wound healing, thin arms, legs, and skin, and red cheeks.

    (b) What glands are associated with each disorder?

3. An anatomy and physiology peer of yours makes a claim stating that the hypothalamus is exclusively a part of the CNS. What arguments would you make to substantiate that the hypothalamus is an interface between the nervous system and the endocrine system?

4. Topical steroid creams are used effectively to control irritating allergic responses or superficial rashes. Why are they ineffective and dangerous to use in the treatment of open wounds?

5. If you have participated in athletic competitions, you have probably heard the statement, "I could feel the adrenalin flowing." Why does this feeling occur and how is it manifested in athletic performance?

CHAPTER 12

Blood

■ Overview

Fact: Every cell of the body needs a continuous supply of water, nutrients, energy, and oxygen.

Ten and one-half pints of blood, making up 7 percent of the body's total weight, circulate constantly through the body of the average adult, bringing to each cell the oxygen, nutrients, and chemical substances necessary for its proper functioning, and, at the same time, removing waste products. This life-sustaining fluid, along with the heart and a network of blood vessels, comprises the cardiovascular system, which, acting in concert with other systems, plays an important role in the maintenance of homeostasis. This specialized fluid connective tissue consists of two basic parts: the formed elements and cell fragments, and the fluid plasma in which they are carried.

Functions of the blood, including transportation, regulation, protection, and coagulation, serve to maintain the integrity of cells in the human body.

Chapter 12 provides an opportunity for you to identify and study the components of blood and review the functional roles the components play in order for cellular needs to be met throughout the body. Blood types, hemostasis, hemopoiesis (hematopoiesis), and blood abnormalities are also considered.

☐ LEVEL 1   REVIEW OF CHAPTER OBJECTIVES

1. Describe the important components and major functions of blood.
2. Discuss the composition and functions of plasma.
3. Describe the origin and production of the formed elements in blood.
4. Discuss the characteristics and functions of red blood cells.
5. Explain what determines a person's blood type and why blood types are important.
6. Categorize the various white blood cells on the basis of their structure and functions.
7. Describe the mechanisms that control blood loss after an injury.

[L1] Multiple Choice:

Place the letter corresponding to the correct answer in the space provided.

OBJ. 1 ____ 1. The formed elements of the blood consist of:
   a. antibodies, metalloproteins, and lipoproteins
   b. red and white blood cells, and platelets
   c. albumins, globulins, and fibrinogen
   d. electrolytes, nutrients, and organic wastes

OBJ. 1 ____ 2. Loose connective tissue and cartilage contain a network of insoluble fibers, whereas plasma, a fluid connective tissue, contains:
   a. dissolved proteins
   b. a network of collagen and elastic fibers
   c. elastic fibers only
   d. collagen fibers only

OBJ. 1 ____ 3. Blood transports dissolved gases, bringing oxygen from the lungs to the tissues and carrying:
   a. carbon dioxide from the lungs to the tissues
   b. carbon dioxide from one peripheral cell to another
   c. carbon dioxide from the interstitial fluid to the cell
   d. carbon dioxide from the tissues to the lungs

OBJ. 1 ____ 4. The "patrol agents" in the blood that defend the body against toxins and pathogens are:
   a. hormones and enzymes
   b. albumins and globulins
   c. white blood cells and antibodies
   d. red blood cells and platelets

OBJ. 1 ____ 5. Blood temperature is roughly ____ degrees C, and the blood pH averages ____.
   a. 0 degrees C; 6.8
   b. 32 degrees C; 7.0
   c. 38 degrees C; 7.4
   d. 98 degrees C; 7.8

OBJ. 2 ____ 6. Which one of the following statements is correct?
   a. Plasma contributes approximately 92 percent of the volume of whole blood, and H_2O accounts for 55 percent of the plasma volume.
   b. Plasma contributes approximately 55 percent of the volume of whole blood, and H_2O accounts for 92 percent of the plasma volume.
   c. H_2O accounts for 99 percent of the volume of the plasma, and plasma contributes approximately 45 percent of the volume of whole blood.
   d. H_2O accounts for 45 percent of the volume of the plasma, and plasma contributes approximately 99 percent of the volume of whole blood.

OBJ. 2 ____ 7. The three primary classes of plasma proteins are:
   a. antibodies, metalloproteins, lipoproteins
   b. serum, fibrin, fibrinogen
   c. albumins, globulins, fibrinogen
   d. heme, iron, globin

OBJ. 2 ____ 8. In addition to water and proteins, the plasma consists of:
   a. erythrocytes, leukocytes, and platelets
   b. electrolytes, nutrients, and organic wastes
   c. albumins, globulins, and fibrinogen
   d. a, b, and c are correct

OBJ. 3 ____ 9. Formed elements in the blood are produced through the process of:
   a. hemolysis
   b. hemopoiesis
   c. diapedesis
   d. erythrocytosis

OBJ. 3 ____ 10. The stem cells that produce all of the blood cells are called:
   a. erythroblasts
   b. rouleaux
   c. hemocytoblasts
   d. plasma cells

OBJ. 4 ____ 11. Circulating mature RBCs lack:
   a. mitochondria
   b. ribosomes
   c. nuclei
   d. a, b, and c are correct

OBJ. 4 ____ 12. The primary function of a mature red blood cell is:
   a. transport of respiratory gases
   b. delivery of enzymes to target tissues
   c. defense against toxins and pathogens
   d. a, b, and c are correct

OBJ. 4 ____ 13. The part of the hemoglobin molecule that directly interacts with oxygen is:
   a. globin
   b. the tertiary protein structure
   c. the iron ion
   d. the sodium ion

OBJ. 4 ____ 14. Iron is necessary in the diet because it is involved with:
   a. the prevention of sickle cell anemia
   b. hemoglobin production
   c. prevention of hemolysis
   d. a, b, and c are correct

Level 1 Review of Chapter Objectives   193

OBJ. 4 ___ 15. During RBC recycling each heme unit is stripped of its iron and converted to:
  a. biliverdin
  b. urobilin
  c. transferrin
  d. ferritin

OBJ. 4 ___ 16. The primary site of erythropoiesis in the adult is the:
  a. bone marrow
  b. kidney
  c. liver
  d. a and c are correct

OBJ. 4 ___ 17. Erythropoietin appears in the plasma when peripheral tissues, especially the kidneys, are exposed to:
  a. extremes of temperature
  b. high urine volumes
  c. excessive amounts of radiation
  d. low oxygen concentrations

OBJ. 5 ___ 18. Agglutinogens are contained (on, in) the _____, while the agglutinins are found (on, in) the _____.
  a. plasma; cell membrane of RBC
  b. nucleus of the RBC; mitochondria
  c. cell membrane of RBC; plasma
  d. mitochondria; nucleus of the RBC

OBJ. 5 ___ 19. If you have type A blood, your plasma holds circulating _____ that will attack _____ erythrocytes.
  a. anti-B agglutinins; Type B
  b. anti-A agglutinins; Type A
  c. anti-A agglutinogens; Type A
  d. anti-A agglutinins; Type B

OBJ. 5 ___ 20. A person with type O blood contains:
  a. anti-A and anti-B agglutinins
  b. anti-O agglutinins
  c. anti-A and anti-B agglutinogens
  d. type O blood lacks agglutinins

OBJ. 6 ___ 21. The two types of agranular leukocytes found in the blood are:
  a. neutrophils, eosinophils
  b. leukocytes, lymphocytes
  c. monocytes, lymphocytes
  d. neutrophils, monocytes

OBJ. 6 ___ 22. Based on their staining characteristics, the types of granular leukocytes found in the blood are:
  a. lymphocytes, monocytes, erythrocytes
  b. neutrophils, monocytes, lymphocytes
  c. eosinophils, basophils, lymphocytes
  d. neutrophils, eosinophils, basophils

[OBJ. 7] ___ 23. Megakaryocytes are specialized cells of the bone marrow responsible for:

    a. specific immune responses
    b. engulfing invading bacteria
    c. formation of platelets
    d. production of scar tissue in an injured area

[OBJ. 7] ___ 24. Basophils are specialized in that they:

    a. contain microphages that engulf invading bacteria
    b. contain histamine that exaggerates the inflammation response at the injury site
    c. are enthusiastic phagocytes, often attempting to engulf items as large or larger than themselves
    d. produce and secrete antibodies that attack cells or proteins in distant portions of the body

[OBJ. 7] ___ 25. The process of hemostasis includes five (5) phases. The correct order of the phases as they occur after injury is as follows:

    a. vascular, coagulation, platelet, clot retraction, clot destruction
    b. coagulation, vascular, platelet, clot destruction, clot retraction
    c. platelet, vascular, coagulation, clot retraction, clot destruction
    d. vascular, platelet, coagulation, clot retraction, clot destruction

[OBJ. 7] ___ 26. The extrinsic pathway involved in blood clotting involves the release of:

    a. platelet factors and platelet thromboplastin
    b. Ca^{++}, thrombin and fibrinogen
    c. tissue factors and tissue thromboplastin
    d. prothrombin and fibrinogen

[OBJ. 7] ___ 27. The "common pathway" in blood clotting involves the following events in sequential order as follows:

    a. tissue factors → Ca^{++} → plasminogen → plasmin
    b. prothrombin → thrombin → fibrinogen → fibrin
    c. platelet factors → Ca^{++} → fibrinogen → fibrin
    d. vascular → platelet → coagulation → destruction

Level 1 Review of Chapter Objectives 195

[L1] Completion:

Using the terms below, complete the following statements.

vascular	platelets	hemopoiesis	hematocrit
venepuncture	lymphocytes	formed elements	plasma
vitamin B12	fixed macrophages	agglutinins	serum
lymphopoiesis	viscosity		

OBJ. 1 28. The ground substance of the blood is the _____.

OBJ. 1 29. The blood cells and cell fragments suspended in the ground substance are referred to as _____

OBJ. 1 30. The most common clinical procedure for collecting blood for blood tests is the _____.

OBJ. 2 31. Interactions between the dissolved proteins and the surrounding water molecules determine the blood's _____.

OBJ. 2 32. When the clotting proteins are removed from the plasma, the remaining fluid is the _____.

OBJ. 3 33. The process of blood cell formation is called _____.

OBJ. 4 34. For erythropoiesis to proceed normally, the myeloid tissues must receive adequate amounts of amino acids, iron, and _____.

OBJ. 4 35. The blood test used to determine the percentage of formed elements in whole blood is the _____.

OBJ. 5 36. Immunoglobulins in plasma that react with antigens on the surfaces of foreign red blood cells when donor and recipient differ in blood type are called _____.

OBJ. 6 37. T cells and B cells are representative cell populations of WBCs identified as _____.

OBJ. 6 38. Immobile monocytes found in many connective tissues are called _____.

OBJ. 6 39. The production of lymphocytes from stem cells is called _____.

OBJ. 7 40. After a clot has formed, the clot shrinks due to the action of filaments contained in _____.

OBJ. 7 41. The first phase of homeostasis involves a period of local vasoconstriction called the _____ phase.

[L1] Matching:

Match the terms in column "B" with the terms in column "A." Use letters for answers in the spaces provided.

	COLUMN "A"	COLUMN "B"
OBJ. 1 42.	Whole blood	A. Hematocytoblasts
OBJ. 1 43.	pH regulation	B. Macrophage
OBJ. 2 44.	Antibodies	C. Buffer in blood
OBJ. 3 45.	Myeloid tissue	D. Agglutination
OBJ. 3 46.	Stem cells	E. Specific immunity
OBJ. 4 47.	Erythropoietin	F. Bone marrow
OBJ. 5 48.	Cross-reaction	G. Immunoglobulins
OBJ. 6 49.	Lymphocytes	H. Plasma and formed elements
OBJ. 6 50.	Monocyte	I. Hormone
OBJ. 7 51.	Platelets	J. Cell fragments

196 Chapter 12 Blood

[L1] Drawing/Illustration Labeling:

Identify each numbered structure by labeling the following figures:

OBJ. 4   **FIGURE 12.1**

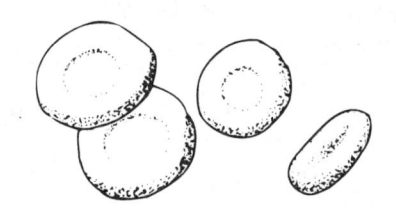

52 _____

OBJ. 6   **FIGURE 12.2**   Agranular Leukocytes

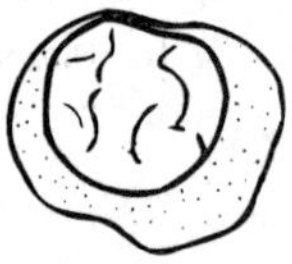

53 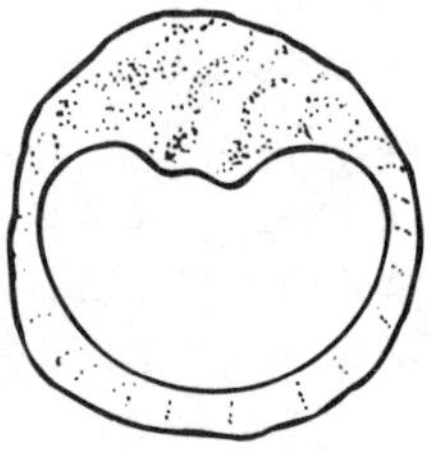 _____   54 _____

OBJ. 6   **FIGURE 12.3**   Granular Leukocytes

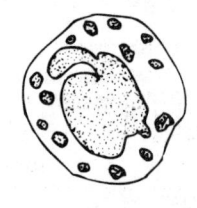

55 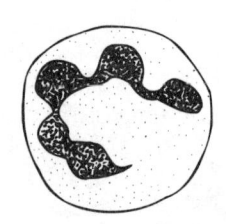 _____   56 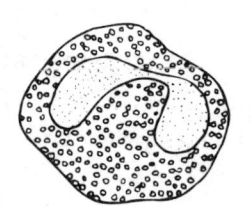 _____   57 _____

Level -1-   **When you have successfully completed the exercises in L1 proceed to L2.**

LEVEL 2 CONCEPT SYNTHESIS

Concept Map I:

Using the following terms, fill in the numbered, blank spaces to complete the concept map. Follow the numbers that comply with the organization of the map.

- Solutes
- Plasma
- Gamma
- Neutrophils
- Leukocytes
- Albumins
- Monocytes

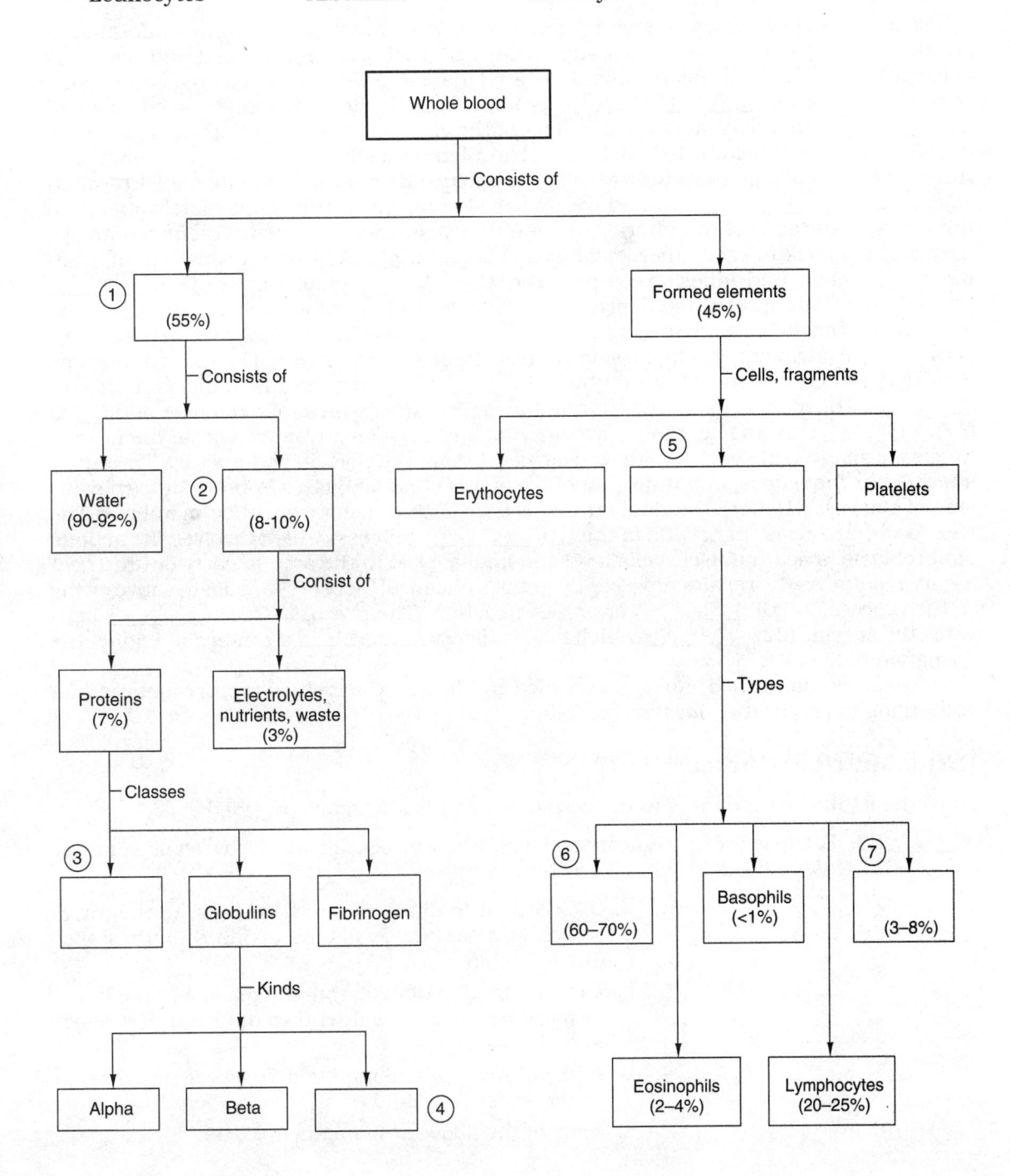

Body Trek:

Using the terms below, fill in the blanks to complete a trek into the blood vessel lining of a superficial vein.

plasminogen	coagulation	platelet	fibrinogen
vascular	fibrin	clot	clot retraction
endothelium	thrombocytes	platelet plug	fibrinolysis
RBCs	vascular spasm	plasmin	

Robo's programmed assignment for this trek is to monitor and collect information related to the clotting process in a superficial vein that has been incised and damaged because of an injury. The micro-robot is located just inside the damaged area of the blood vessel lining, the (8) _____. There is an immediate "feeling" of being crushed owing to a (9) _____ that decreases the diameter of the vessel at the site of the injury. Not only is Robo in danger of being crushed, but the turbulent and sticky "atmospheric" conditions threaten the robot's sensory devices. The turbulence increases as fragments with rough edges, the (10) _____, flow into the damaged area, where they immediately adhere to the exposed surfaces of the interior lining of the vessel wall. As more fragments arrive, they begin to stick to each other, forming a (11) _____. The vessel constriction, fragment aggregation, and adhesion comprise the (12) _____ phase and the (13) _____ phase of the clotting response. Thirty seconds to several minutes later, the damaged site is a mecca of chemical activity as the (14) _____ phase begins. Robo's "chemical sensors" are relaying messages to mission control about a series of complex, sequential steps involving the conversion of circulating (15) _____ into the insoluble protein (16) _____. The robot is maneuvered from the immediate area to make room for additional (17) _____ and fragments that are arriving and becoming trapped within the fibrous tangle, forming a (18) _____ that seals off the damaged portion of the vessel. The injury site still has torn edges, initiating a robotic response that facilitates Robo's exit to the outside of the vessel, where the final stages of the clotting response will be monitored. The trek to the outside is "tight" due to the (19) _____ process, which involves the actions of fibroblasts, smooth muscle cells, and endothelial cells in the area to carry out the necessary repairs. As the repairs proceed, the robot's chemical "sensors" are again active owing to the process of (20) _____, or clot destruction. The precursor (21) _____ activates the enzyme (22) _____ which begins digesting the fibrin strands and ending the formation of the clot.

Mission accomplished, Robo is returned to Mission Control for reprogramming and recharging in preparation for its next trek.

[L2] Multiple Choice:

Place the letter corresponding to the correct answer in the space provided.

_____ 23. Because the concentration of dissolved gases is different between plasma and tissue fluid:

  a. O_2 will tend to diffuse from the plasma to the interstitial fluid, and CO_2 will tend to diffuse in the opposite direction

  b. CO_2 will tend to diffuse from the plasma to the interstitial fluid, and O_2 will tend to diffuse in the opposite direction

  c. both O_2 and CO_2 will tend to diffuse from the plasma to the interstitial fluid

  d. none of the above statements are true

_____ 24. If blood comprises 7 percent of the body weight in kilograms, how many liters of blood would there be in an individual who weighs 85 kg?

        a. 5.25
        b. 5.95
        c. 6.25
        d. 6.95

_____ 25. The reason liver disorders can alter the composition and functional properties of the blood is because:

        a. the liver synthesizes immunoglobulins and protein hormones
        b. the proteins synthesized by the liver are filtered out of the blood by the kidneys
        c. the liver is the primary source of plasma proteins
        d. the liver serves as a filter for plasma proteins and pathogens

_____ 26. On the average, one microliter of blood contains _____ erythrocytes.

        a. 260 million
        b. 10^{13}
        c. 5.2 million
        d. 25 million

_____ 27. In a mature RBC, energy is obtained exclusively by anaerobic respiration, i.e., the breakdown of glucose in the cytoplasm.

        a. true
        b. false

_____ 28. If agglutinogen "B" meets with agglutinin "anti-A", the result would be:

        a. a cross-reaction
        b. no agglutination would occur
        c. the patient would be comatose
        d. the patient would die

_____ 29. The blood cells that may originate in the thymus, spleen and lymph nodes as well as in bone marrow are the:

        a. erythrocytes
        b. lymphocytes
        c. leukocytes
        d. monocytes

_____ 30. Rh-negative blood indicates:

        a. the presence of the Rh agglutinogen
        b. the presence of agglutinogen A
        c. the absence of the Rh agglutinogen
        d. the absence of agglutinogen B

200   Chapter 12   Blood

_____ 31. In hemolytic disease of the newborn:
   a. the newborn's agglutinins cross the placental barrier and cause the newborn's RBCs to degenerate
   b. the mother's agglutinins cross the placental barrier and destroy fetal red blood cells
   c. the mother's agglutinogens destroy her own RBCs, causing deoxygenation of the newborn
   d. all of the above occur

_____ 32. Circulating leukocytes represent a small fraction of the total population, since most WBCs are found in peripheral tissue.
   a. true
   b. false

_____ 33. A typical microliter of blood contains _____ leukocytes.
   a. 1,000-2,000
   b. 3,000-5,000
   c. 6,000-9,000
   d. 10,000-12,000

_____ 34. Platelets are unique formed elements of the blood because they:
   a. initiate the immune response and destroy bacteria
   b. are cytoplasmic enzyme packets rather than individual cells
   c. can reproduce because they contain a nucleus
   d. none of the above apply to platelets

_____ 35. The major effect of a vitamin K deficiency in the body is that it leads to:
   a. a breakdown of the common pathway, inactivating the clotting system
   b. the body becomes insensitive to situations that would necessitate the clotting mechanism
   c. an overactive clotting system, which might necessitate thinning of the blood
   d. all of the above are correct

[L2]   Completion:

Using the terms below, complete the following statements.

| leukopenia | hemolysis | differential | leukocytosis |
| fibrin | fractionated | lipoproteins | |

36. When the components of whole blood are separated, they are said to be _____.
37. The insoluble fibers that provide the basic framework for a blood clot are called _____.
38. Globulins involved in lipid transport are called _____.
39. The rupturing of red blood cells is called _____.
40. An inadequate number of white blood cells is called _____.
41. Excessive numbers of white blood cells refers to a condition called _____.
42. A blood cell count that determines the numbers and kinds of leukocytes is called a _____ white blood cell count.

[L2] Short Essay:

Briefly answer the following questions in the spaces provided below.

43. List the primary functions of blood.

44. What are the major components of the plasma?

45. List and describe the three (3) kinds of granular leukocytes and the two (2) kinds of agranular WBCs.

46. What are the primary functions of platelets?

47. List the events in the clotting response and summarize the results of each occurrence.

48. What is the difference between an embolus and a thrombus?

When you have successfully completed the exercises in L2 proceed to L3.

☐ LEVEL 3   CRITICAL THINKING/APPLICATION

Using principles and concepts learned about the blood, answer the following questions. Write your answers on a separate sheet of paper.

1. A man weighs 154 pounds and his hematocrit is 45 percent. The weight of blood is approximately 7 percent of his total body weight.
    a. What is his total blood volume in liters?
    b. What is his total cell volume in liters?
    c. What is his total plasma volume in liters?
    d. What percent of his blood constitutes the plasma volume?
    e. What percent of his blood comprises the formed elements?
       Note: 1 kilogram = 2.2 pounds

2. Considering the following condition, what effect would each have on an individual's hematocrit (percentage of erythrocytes to the total blood volume)?
    a. an increase in viscosity of the blood
    b. an increased dehydration in the body
    c. a decrease in the number of RBCs
    d. a decrease in the diameter of a blood vessel

3. A person with type B blood has been involved in an accident and excessive bleeding necessitates a blood transfusion. Due to an error by a careless laboratory technician, the person is given type A blood. Explain what will happen.

4. Your doctor has recommended that you take a vitamin supplement of your choice. You look for a supplement that lists all the vitamins; however, you cannot find one that has vitamin K.
    a. Why?
    b. What are some dietary sources of vitamin K?
    c. What is the function of vitamin K in the body?

CHAPTER 13

The Heart

■ Overview

The heart is one of nature's most efficient and durable pumps. Throughout life, it beats 60 to 80 times per minute, supplying oxygen and other essential nutrients to every cell in the body and removing waste for elimination from the lungs or the kidneys. Every day approximately 2,100 gallons of blood is pumped through a vast network of about 60,000 miles of blood vessels. The "double pump" design of this muscular organ facilitates the continuous flow of blood through a closed system that consists of a pulmonary circuit to the lungs and a systemic circuit serving all other regions of the body. A system of valves in the heart maintains the "one-way" direction of blood flow through the heart. Nutrient and oxygen supplies are delivered to the heart's tissues by coronary arteries that encircle the heart like a crown. Normal cardiac rhythm is maintained by the heart's electrical system, centered primarily in a group of specialized pacemaker cells located in a sinus node in the right atrium.

Chapter 13 examines the structural features of the heart, cardiac physiology, cardiac dynamics, and the heart and the cardiovascular system.

❑ LEVEL 1   REVIEW OF CHAPTER OBJECTIVES

1. Describe the location and general features of the heart.
2. Trace the flow of blood through the heart, identifying the major blood vessels, chambers, and heart valves.
3. Identify the layers of the heart wall.
4. Describe the differences in the action potential and twitch contractions of skeletal muscle fibers and cardiac muscle cells.
5. Describe the components of and functions of the conducting system of the heart.
6. Explain the events of the cardiac cycle and relate the heart sounds to specific events in this cycle.
7. Define stroke volume and cardiac output and describe the factors that influence these values.

[L1] Multiple Choice:

Place the letter corresponding to the correct answer in the space provided.

OBJ. 1 ____ 1. The "double pump" function of the heart includes the right side, which serves as the _____ circuit pump, while the left side serves as the _____ pump.

    a. systemic; pulmonary
    b. pulmonary; hepatic portal
    c. hepatic portal; cardiac
    d. pulmonary; systemic

OBJ. 1 ____ 2. The visceral pericardium, or epicardium, covers the:

    a. inner surface of the heart
    b. outer surface of the heart
    c. vessels in the mediastinum
    d. endothelial lining of the heart

OBJ. 2 ____ 3. Atrioventricular valves prevent backflow of blood into the _____; semilunar valves prevent backflow into the _____.

    a. atria; ventricles
    b. lungs; systemic circulation
    c. ventricles; atria
    d. capillaries; lungs

OBJ. 2 ____ 4. Blood flows from the left atrium into the left ventricle through the _____ valve.

    a. tricuspid
    b. L. atrioventricular
    c. mitral
    d. b and c are correct

OBJ. 2 ____ 5. When deoxygenated blood leaves the right ventricle through a semilunar valve, it is forced into the:

    a. pulmonary veins
    b. aortic arch
    c. pulmonary arteries
    d. lung capillaries

OBJ. 2 ____ 6. Blood from systemic circulation is returned to the right atrium by the superior and:

    a. inferior vena cava
    b. pulmonary veins
    c. pulmonary arteries
    d. brachiocephalic veins

OBJ. 2 ____ 7. Oxygenated blood from the systemic arteries flows into:

    a. peripheral tissue capillaries
    b. systemic veins
    c. the right atrium
    d. the left atrium

Level 1   Review of Chapter Objectives   205

OBJ. 2   ___ 8. The lung capillaries receive deoxygenated blood from the:
   a. pulmonary veins
   b. pulmonary arteries
   c. aorta
   d. superior and inferior vena cava

OBJ. 3   ___ 9. One of the important differences between skeletal muscle tissue and cardiac muscle tissue is that cardiac muscle tissue is:
   a. striated voluntary muscle
   b. multinucleated
   c. comprised of unusually large cells
   d. striated involuntary muscle

OBJ. 3   ___ 10. Cardiac muscle tissue:
   a. will not contract unless stimulated by nerves
   b. does not require nerve activity to stimulate a contraction
   c. is under voluntary control
   d. a, b, and c are correct

OBJ. 3   ___ 11. Blood from coronary circulation is returned to the right atrium of the heart via:
   a. anastomoses
   b. the circumflex branch
   c. coronary sinus
   d. the anterior interventricular branch

OBJ. 3   ___ 12. The correct sequential path of a normal action potential in the heart is:
   a. SA node → AV bundle → AV node → Purkinje fibers
   b. AV node → SA node → AV bundle → bundle of His
   c. SA node → AV node → bundle of His → bundle branches → Purkinje fibers
   d. SA node → AV node → bundle branches → AV bundle → Purkinje fibers

OBJ. 5   ___ 13. The sinoatrial node acts as the pacemaker of the heart because these cells are:
   a. located in the wall of the left atrium
   b. the only cells in the heart that can conduct an impulse
   c. the only cells in the heart innervated by the autonomic nervous system
   d. the ones that depolarize and reach threshold first

OBJ. 5   ___ 14. After the AV node is depolarized and the impulse spreads through the atria, there is a slight delay before the impulse spreads to the ventricles. The reason for this delay is to allow:
   a. the atria to finish contracting
   b. the ventricles to repolarize
   c. a greater venous return
   d. nothing; there is no reason for the delay

15. The P wave of a normal electrocardiogram indicates:
    a. atrial repolarization
    b. atrial depolarization
    c. ventricular repolarization
    d. ventricular depolarization

16. The QRS complex of the EKG appears as the:
    a. atria depolarize
    b. atria repolarize
    c. ventricles repolarize
    d. ventricles depolarize

17. EKGs are useful in detecting and diagnosing abnormal patterns of cardiac activity called:
    a. myocardial infarctions
    b. cardiac arrhythmias
    c. autorhythmicity
    d. a, b, and c are correct

18. The "lubb-dubb" sounds of the heart have practical clinical value because they provide information concerning:
    a. the strength of ventricular contraction
    b. the strength of the pulse
    c. the efficiency of heart valves
    d. the relative time the heart spends in systole and diastole

19. When a chamber of the heart fills with blood and prepares for the start of the next cardiac cycle the heart is in:
    a. systole
    b. ventricular ejection
    c. diastole
    d. contraction

20. The amount of blood ejected by the left ventricle per minute is the:
    a. stroke volume
    b. cardiac output
    c. diastolic volume
    d. systolic volume

21. The amount of blood pumped out of each ventricle during a single beat is the:
    a. stroke volume
    b. cardiac volume
    c. cardiac output
    d. systolic volume

Level 1 Review of Chapter Objectives 207

OBJ. 7   ___ 22. Starling's law of the heart states:
- a. stroke volume is equal to cardiac output
- b. venous return is inversely proportional to cardiac output
- c. cardiac output is equal to venous return
- d. a, b, and c are correct

OBJ. 7   ___ 23. The factor that prevents tetanization of cardiac muscle is:
- a. the cardiac muscle fibers are specialized for contraction
- b. the refractory period of cardiac muscle is relatively brief
- c. the action potential of the muscle triggers a single contraction
- d. the muscle cell completes its contraction before the membrane can respond to an additional stimulus

OBJ. 7   ___ 24. The cardioacceleratory center in the medulla is responsible for the activation of:
- a. baroreceptors
- b. parasympathetic neurons
- c. sympathetic neurons
- d. chemoreceptors

[L1] Completion:

Using the terms below, complete the following statements.

repolarization	atria	pulmonary	autonomic nervous system
chemoreceptors	electrocardiogram	carbon dioxide	fibrous skeleton
pulmonary veins	automaticity	pericardium	myocardium

OBJ. 1   25. The chambers in the heart with thin walls that are highly distensible are the _____.

OBJ. 1   26. The internal connective tissue framework of the heart is called the _____.

OBJ. 1   27. The serous membrane lining the pericardial cavity is called the _____.

OBJ. 2   28. The right side of the heart contains blood with an abundance of the gas _____.

OBJ. 2   29. Oxygenated blood is returned to the left atrium via the _____.

OBJ. 2   30. The only arteries in the body that carry deoxygenated blood are the _____ arteries.

OBJ. 3   31. The muscular wall of the heart which forms both atria and ventricles is the _____.

OBJ. 4   32. The process following depolarization of heart cells is termed _____.

OBJ. 5   33. The action of cardiac muscle tissue contracting on its own in the absence of neural stimulation is called _____.

OBJ. 6   34. The recording and evaluating of electrical events that occur in the heart constitutes a(n) _____.

OBJ. 7   35. Blood CO_2, pH, and O_2 levels are monitored by _____.

OBJ. 7   36. The most important control of heart rate is the effect of the _____.

208 Chapter 13 The Heart

[L1] Matching:

Match the terms in column "B" with the terms in column "A." Use letters for answers in the spaces provided.

		COLUMN "A"	COLUMN "B"
OBJ. 1	___ 37.	Serous membrane	A. Blood to systemic arteries
OBJ. 2	___ 38.	Aorta	B. Increasing heart rate
OBJ. 3	___ 39.	Anastomoses	C. Semilunar valve closes
OBJ. 4	___ 40.	"T" wave	D. Monitor blood pressure
OBJ. 5	___ 41.	Cardiac pacemaker	E. SA node
OBJ. 5	___ 42.	Bundle of His	F. Pericardium
OBJ. 6	___ 43.	"Lubb" sound	G. AV conducting fibers
OBJ. 6	___ 44.	"Dubb" sound	H. AV valves close; semilunar valves open
OBJ. 7	___ 45.	Baroreceptors	I. Interconnections between blood vessels
OBJ. 7	___ 46.	Epinephrine	J. Ventricular repolarization

[L1] Drawing/Illustration Labeling:

Identify each numbered structure by labeling the following figure:

OBJ. 1   **FIGURE 13.1**   Anatomy of the Heart (Ventral View)

47. _____
48. _____
49. _____
50. _____
51. _____
52. _____
53. _____
54. _____
55. _____
56. _____
57. _____
58. _____
59. _____
60. _____
61. _____
62. _____
63. _____
64. _____
65. _____
66. _____

Level -1- **When you have successfully completed the exercises in L1 proceed to L2.**

☐ LEVEL 2 CONCEPT SYNTHESIS

Concept Map I/Body Trek:

Using the terms below, fill in the blanks to complete a trek through the heart and peripheral vessels.

aortic semilunar valve	pulmonary veins	right ventricle
tricuspid valve	systemic arteries	right atrium
aorta	superior vena cava	L. common carotid
inferior vena cava	left ventricle	bicuspid valve
pulmonary semilunar valve	systemic veins	left atrium
pulmonary arteries		

Robo's instructions: On this trek you will use the "heart map" to follow a drop of blood as it goes through the heart and peripheral blood vessels. Identify each structure at the sequential, numbered locations 1 through 16.

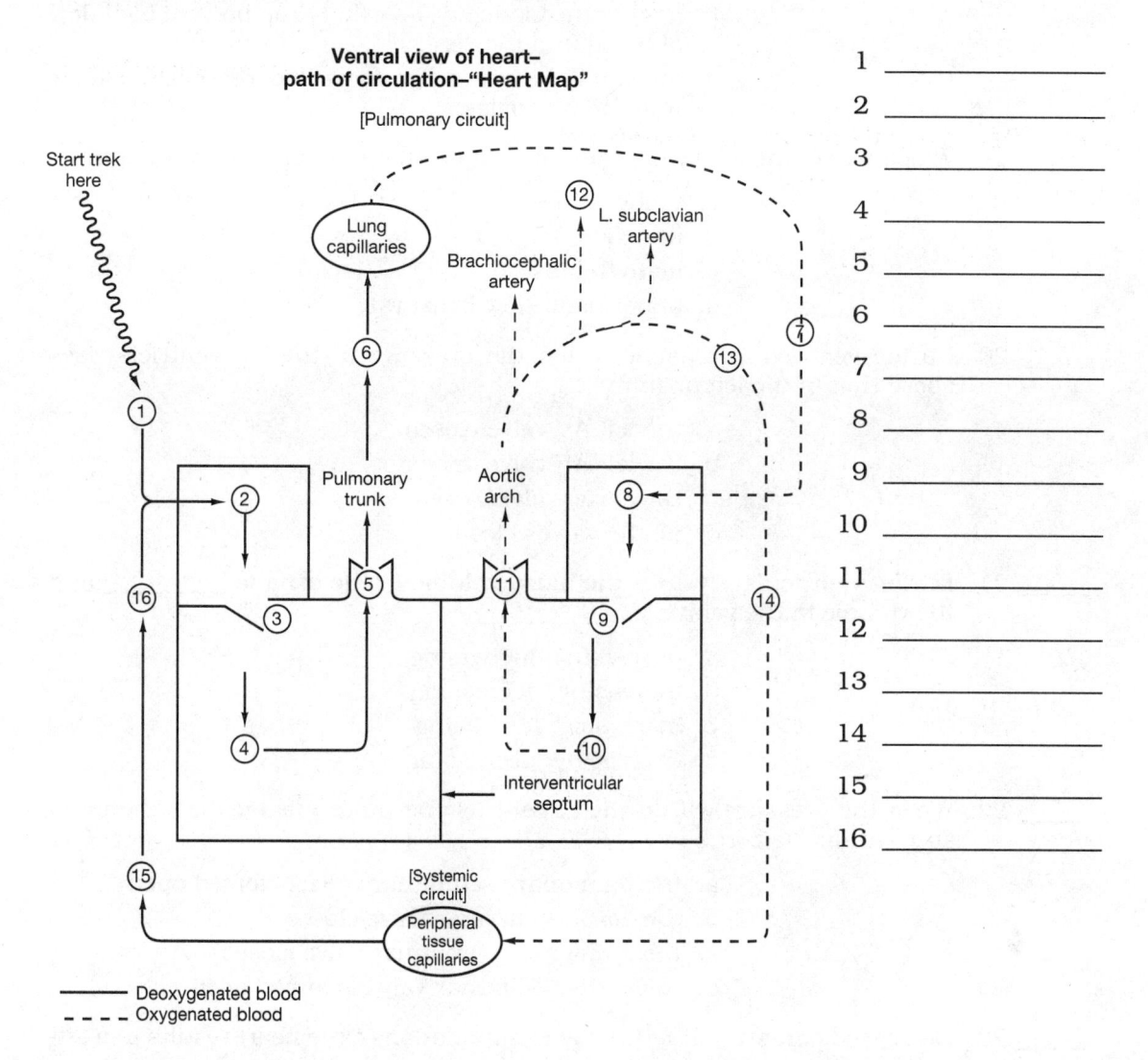

1. _____
2. _____
3. _____
4. _____
5. _____
6. _____
7. _____
8. _____
9. _____
10. _____
11. _____
12. _____
13. _____
14. _____
15. _____
16. _____

210 Chapter 13 The Heart

[L2] Multiple Choice:

Place the letter corresponding to the correct answer in the space provided.

_____ 17. Assuming anatomic position, the best way to describe the specific location of the heart in the body is:

　　a. within the mediastinum of the thorax
　　b. in the region of the fifth intercostal space
　　c. just behind the lungs
　　d. in the center of the chest

_____ 18. The function of the chordae tendinae is to:

　　a. anchor the semilunar valve flaps and prevent backward flow of blood into the ventricles
　　b. anchor the AV valve flaps and prevent backflow of blood into the atria
　　c. anchor the bicuspid valve flaps and prevent backflow of blood into the ventricle
　　d. anchor the aortic valve flaps and prevent backflow into the ventricles

_____ 19. Which one of the following would not show up on an electrocardiogram?

　　a. tachycardia
　　b. murmurs
　　c. arrhythmias
　　d. abnormally slow heart rate

_____ 20. During ventricular diastole, when the pressure in the left ventricle rises above that in the left atrium:

　　a. the left AV valve closes
　　b. the left AV valve opens
　　c. the aortic valve closes
　　d. all the valves close

_____ 21. During ventricular systole, the blood volume in the atria is _____ and the volume in the ventricle is _____.

　　a. decreasing; increasing
　　b. increasing; decreasing
　　c. increasing; increasing
　　d. decreasing; decreasing

_____ 22. When the pressure within the L. ventricle becomes greater than the pressure within the aorta:

　　a. the pulmonary semilunar valve is forced open
　　b. the aortic semilunar valve closes
　　c. the pulmonary semilunar valve closes
　　d. the aortic semilunar valve is forced open

_____ 23. Decreased parasympathetic (vagus) stimulation to the heart results in a situation known as:

　　a. bradycardia
　　b. tachycardia
　　c. fibrillation
　　d. tetany

Level 2

_____ 24. Serious arrhythmias that reduce the pumping efficiency of the heart may indicate:
- a. damage to the myocardium
- b. injury to the SA and AV nodes
- c. underlying heart disease
- d. a, b, and c are correct

_____ 25. During exercise the most important control mechanism to increase cardiac output is:
- a. increased body temperature
- b. increased end-systolic volume
- c. increased sympathetic activity to the ventricles
- d. increased epinephrine from the adrenal medulla

_____ 26. Which of the following does not control the movement of blood through the heart?
- a. opening and closing of the valves
- b. contraction of the myocardium
- c. size of the atria and ventricles
- d. relaxation of the myocardium

_____ 27. Valvular malfunction in the heart:
- a. causes an increase in the amount of blood pumped out of each ventricle
- b. interferes with ventricular contraction
- c. increases the cardiac output
- d. interferes with movement of blood through the heart

_____ 28. One of the major results of congestive heart failure is:
- a. the heart, veins, and capillaries are excessively restricted
- b. an abnormal increase in blood volume and interstitial fluid
- c. the valves in the heart cease to function
- d. the heart begins to contract spastically

[L2] Completion:

Using the terms below, complete the following statements.

| angina pectoris | endocardium | cardiac reserve |
| systemic | nodal | diuretics |

29. An improperly functioning bicuspid (mitral) valve would affect _____ circulation.
30. The inner surface of the heart that is continuous with the endothelium of the attached blood vessels is the _____.
31. The spontaneous depolarization in the heart takes place in specialized _____ cells.
32. The difference between resting and maximum cardiac output is the _____.
33. The most common treatment for congestive heart failure is to administer _____.
34. Temporary heart insufficiency and ischemia causing severe chest pain is referred to as _____.

212 Chapter 13 The Heart

[L2] Short Essay:

Briefly answer the following questions in the spaces provided below.

35. If the end-systolic volume (ESV) is 60 ml and the end-diastolic volume (EDV) is 140 ml, what is the stroke volume (SV)?

36. If the cardiac output (CO) is 5 liter/min, and the heart rate (HR) is 100 beats/min, what is the stroke volume (SV)?

37. What three (3) distinct layers comprise the tissues of the heart wall? Describe each.

38. Beginning with the SA node, trace the pathway of an action potential through the conducting network of the heart. (Use arrows to indicate direction.)

When you hve successfully completed the exercises in L2 proceed to L3.

☐ LEVEL 3   CRITICAL THINKING/APPLICATION

Using principles and concepts learned about the heart, answer the following questions. Write your answers on a separate sheet of paper.

1. Unlike the situation in skeletal muscle, cardiac muscle contraction is an active process, but relaxation is entirely passive. Why?

2. After a vigorous tennis match, Ted complained of chest pains. He was advised to see his doctor, who immediately ordered an ECG. An evaluation of the ECG showed a slight irregular wave pattern. The physician ordered a PET scan, which showed an obstruction due to an embolus (clot) in a branch of a coronary artery. What is the relationship between chest pains and the possibility of a heart attack?

3. If the oxygen debt in skeletal muscle tissue is not paid back, the muscle loses its ability to contract efficiently owing to the presence of lactic acid and a decrease in the O_2 supply to the muscle. Why is the inability to develop a significant oxygen debt consistent with the function of the heart?

4. Your anatomy and physiology instructor is lecturing on the importance of coronary circulation to the overall functional efficiency of the heart. Part of this efficiency is due to the presence of arterial anastomoses. What are arterial anastomoses and why are they important in coronary circulation?

CHAPTER 14

Blood Vessels and Circulation

■ Overview

Blood vessels form a closed system of ducts that transport blood and allow exchange of gases, nutrients, and wastes between the blood and the body cells. The general plan of the cardiovascular system includes the heart, arteries that carry blood away from the heart, capillaries that allow exchange of substances between blood and the cells, and veins that carry blood back to the heart. The pulmonary circuit carries deoxygenated blood from the right side of the heart to the lung capillaries where the blood is oxygenated. The systemic circuit carries the oxygenated blood from the left side of the heart to the systemic capillaries in all parts of the body. The cyclic nature of the system results in deoxygenated blood returning to the right atrium to continue the cycle of circulation.

Blood vessels in the muscles, the skin, the cerebral circulation, and the hepatic portal circulation are specifically adapted to serve the functions of organs and tissues in these important special areas of cardiovascular activity.

Chapter 14 describes the structure and functions of the blood vessels, the dynamics of the circulatory process, cardiovascular regulation, and patterns of cardiovascular response.

☐ LEVEL 1   REVIEW OF CHAPTER OBJECTIVES

1. Distinguish among the types of blood vessels on the basis of their structure and function.
2. Explain the mechanisms that regulate blood flow through arteries, capillaries, and veins.
3. Discuss the mechanisms and various pressures involved in the movement of fluids between capillaries and interstitial spaces.
4. Describe the factors that influence blood pressure and how blood pressure is regulated.
5. Describe how central and local control mechanisms interact to regulate blood flow and pressure in tissues.
6. Explain how the activities of the cardiac, vasomotor, and respiratory centers are coordinated to control the blood flow through the tissues.
7. Explain how the circulatory system responds to the demands of exercise and hemorrhaging.
8. Identify the major arteries and veins and the areas they serve.
9. Describe the age-related changes that occur in the cardiovascular system.

[L1] Multiple Choice:

Place the letter corresponding to the correct answer in the space provided.

OBJ. 1 ____ 1. The layer of vascular tissue that consists of an endothelial lining and an underlying layer of connective tissue dominated by elastic fibers is the:

    a. tunica interna
    b. tunica media
    c. tunica externa
    d. tunica adventitia

OBJ. 1 ____ 2. Smooth muscle fibers in arteries and veins are found in the:

    a. endothelial lining
    b. tunica externa
    c. tunica interna
    d. tunica media

OBJ. 1 ____ 3. One of the major characteristics of the arteries supplying peripheral tissues is that they are:

    a. elastic
    b. muscular
    c. rigid
    d. a, b, and c are correct

OBJ. 2 ____ 4. The only blood vessels whose walls permit exchange between the blood and the surrounding interstitial fluids are:

    a. arterioles
    b. venules
    c. capillaries
    d. a, b, and c are correct

OBJ. 2 ____ 5. The unidirectional flow of blood in venules and medium-sized veins is maintained by:

    a. the muscular walls of the veins
    b. pressure from the left ventricle
    c. arterial pressure
    d. the presence of valves

OBJ. 2 ____ 6. The "specialized" arteries that are able to tolerate the pressure shock produced each time ventricular systole occurs and blood leaves the heart are:

    a. muscular arteries
    b. elastic arteries
    c. arterioles
    d. fenestrated arteries

OBJ. 2 ____ 7. Of the following blood vessels, the greatest resistance to blood flow occurs in the:

    a. veins
    b. capillaries
    c. venules
    d. arterioles

Level 1 Review of Chapter Objectives 215

[OBJ. 2] ____ 8. The distinctive sounds of Korotkoff heard when taking the blood pressure are produced by:

    a. turbulences as blood flows past the constricted portion of the artery
    b. the contraction and relaxation of the ventricles
    c. the opening and closing of the atrioventricular valves
    d. a, b, and c are correct

[OBJ. 3] ____ 9. The two major factors affecting blood flow rates are:

    a. diameter and length of blood vessels
    b. pressure and resistance
    c. neural and hormonal control mechanisms
    d. a, b, and c are correct

[OBJ. 4] ____ 10. The most important determinant of peripheral resistance is:

    a. a combination of neural and hormonal mechanisms
    b. differences in the length of the blood vessels
    c. friction between the blood and the vessel walls
    d. the diameter of the arterioles

[OBJ. 4] ____ 11. From the following selections, choose the answer that correctly identifies all the factors which would increase blood pressure. (Note: CO = cardiac output; SV = stroke volume; VR = venous return; PR = peripheral resistance; BV = blood volume.)

    a. increasing CO, increasing SV, decreasing VR, decreasing PR, increasing BV
    b. increasing CO, increasing SV, increasing VR, increasing PR, increasing BV
    c. increasing CO, increasing SV, decreasing VR, increasing PR, decreasing BV
    d. increasing CO, decreasing SV, increasing VR, decreasing PR, increasing BV

[OBJ. 5] ____ 12. Atrial natriuretic peptide (ANP) reduces blood volume and pressure by:

    a. blocking release of ADH
    b. stimulating peripheral vasodilation
    c. increased water loss by kidneys
    d. a, b, and c are correct

[OBJ. 5] ____ 13. The central regulation of cardiac output primarily involves the activities of the:

    a. somatic nervous system
    b. autonomic nervous system
    c. central nervous system
    d. a, b, and c are correct

[OBJ. 6] ____ 14. An increase in cardiac output normally occurs during:

    a. widespread sympathetic stimulation
    b. widespread parasympathetic stimulation
    c. the process of vasomotion
    d. stimulation of the vasomotor center

216 **Chapter 14 Blood Vessels and Circulation**

OBJ. 6 ___ 15. Stimulation of the vasomotor center in the medulla causes _____ and inhibition of the vasomotor center causes _____.

    a. vasodilation; vasoconstriction

    b. increasing diameter of arteriole; decreasing diameter of arteriole

    c. hyperemia; ischemia

    d. vasoconstriction; vasodilation

OBJ. 7 ___ 16. The three primary interrelated changes that occur as exercise begins are:

    a. decreasing vasodilation, increasing venous return, increasing cardiac output

    b. increasing vasodilation, decreasing venous return, increasing cardiac output

    c. increasing vasodilation, increasing venous return, increasing cardiac output

    d. decreasing vasodilation, decreasing venous return, decreasing cardiac output

OBJ. 7 ___ 17. The only area of the body where the blood supply is unaffected while exercising at maximum levels is the:

    a. hepatic portal circulation

    b. pulmonary circulation

    c. brain

    d. peripheral circulation

OBJ. 8 ___ 18. The three elastic arteries that originate along the aortic arch and deliver blood to the head, neck, shoulders, and arms are the:

    a. axillary, R. common carotid, right subclavian

    b. R. dorsal, R. thoracic, R. vertebral

    c. R. axillary, R. brachial, L. internal carotid

    d. brachiocephalic, L. common carotid, left subclavian

OBJ. 8 ___ 19. The large blood vessel that collects most of the venous blood from organs below the diaphragm is the:

    a. superior vena cava

    b. inferior vena cava

    c. hepatic portal vein

    d. superior mesenteric vein

OBJ. 8 ___ 20. The three blood vessels that provide blood to all of the digestive organs in the abdominopelvic cavity are the:

    a. thoracic aorta, abdominal aorta, superior phrenic artery

    b. intercostal, esophageal, and bronchial arteries

    c. celiac artery and the superior and inferior mesenteric arteries

    d. suprarenal, renal, and lumbar arteries

Level -1-

Level 1 Review of Chapter Objectives 217

OBJ. 8   ___ 21. The four large blood vessels, two from each lung, that empty into the left atrium, completing the pulmonary circuit, are the:

       a. venae cava
       b. pulmonary arteries
       c. pulmonary veins
       d. subclavian veins

OBJ. 8   ___ 22. The blood vessels that provide blood to capillary networks that surround the alveoli in the lungs are:

       a. pulmonary arterioles
       b. pulmonary venules
       c. left and right pulmonary arteries
       d. left and right pulmonary veins

OBJ. 9   ___ 23. The primary effect of a decrease in the hematocrit of elderly individuals is:

       a. thrombus formation in the blood vessels
       b. a lowering of the oxygen-carrying capacity of the blood
       c. a reduction in the maximum cardiac output
       d. damage to ventricular cardiac muscle fibers

OBJ. 9   ___ 24. The primary cause of varicose veins is:

       a. improper diet
       b. age
       c. swelling due to edema in veins
       d. inefficient venous valves

[L1] Completion:

Using the terms below, complete the following statements.

hydrostatic pressure	aortic arch	sphygmomanometer
autoregulation	vasomotion	total peripheral resistance
venules	shock	
vasoconstriction	hepatic portal system	pulse pressure
precapillary sphincter	arteriosclerosis	arterioles
osmotic pressure		

OBJ. 1   25. The smallest vessels of the arterial system are the _____.

OBJ. 1   26. Blood flowing out of the capillary complex first enters small _____.

OBJ. 2   27. The entrance to each capillary is guarded by a band of smooth muscle, the _____.

OBJ. 3   28. The blood flow within any one capillary occurs in a series of pulses called _____.

OBJ. 3   29. The force that pushes water "out" of solution is _____.

OBJ. 3   30. A force that pulls water "into" a solution is _____.

OBJ. 4   31. The difference between the systolic and diastolic pressures is the _____.

OBJ. 4   32. The instrument used to determine blood pressure is called a _____.

OBJ. 4   33. For circulation to occur, the circulatory pressure must be greater than the _____.

218   Chapter 14   Blood Vessels and Circulation

[OBJ. 5] 34. The regulation of blood flow at the tissue level is called _____.

[OBJ. 6] 35. Stimulation of the vasomotor center in the medulla causes _____.

[OBJ. 7] 36. An acute circulatory crisis marked by low blood pressure and inadequate peripheral resistance is referred to as _____.

[OBJ. 8] 37. Blood leaving the capillaries supplied by the celiac, superior and inferior mesenteric arteries flows into the _____.

[OBJ. 8] 38. The part of the vascular system that connects the ascending aorta with the caudally-directed descending aorta is the _____.

[OBJ. 9] 39. Most of the age-related changes in the circulatory system are related to _____.

[L1]   Matching:

Match the terms in column "B" with the terms in column "A." Use the letters for answers in the spaces provided.

		COLUMN "A"	COLUMN "B"
OBJ. 1	___ 40.	Tunica externa	A. Changes in blood pressure
OBJ. 2	___ 41.	Respiratory pump	B. Increasing blood flow to skin
OBJ. 3	___ 42.	Peripheral Resistance	C. Vasomotor center
OBJ. 4	___ 43.	Systole	D. Weakened vascular wall
OBJ. 4	___ 44.	Diastole	E. Vasodilation
OBJ. 5	___ 45.	Baroreceptors	F. Receives blood from arm
OBJ. 5	___ 46.	Atrial natriuretic peptide	G. Connective tissue sheath
OBJ. 6	___ 47.	Medulla	H. Brain circulation
OBJ. 7	___ 48.	Rise in body temperature	I. Venous return
OBJ. 8	___ 49.	Circle of Willis	J. Peak blood pressure
OBJ. 8	___ 50.	Axillary vein	K. Blood clot in lungs
OBJ. 9	___ 51.	Pulmonary embolism	L. Diameter of arterioles
OBJ. 9	___ 52.	Aneurysm	M. Minimum blood pressue

Level 1 Review of Chapter Objectives 219

[L1] **Drawing/Illustration Labeling:**

OBJ. 8 **FIGURE 14.1** The Arterial System

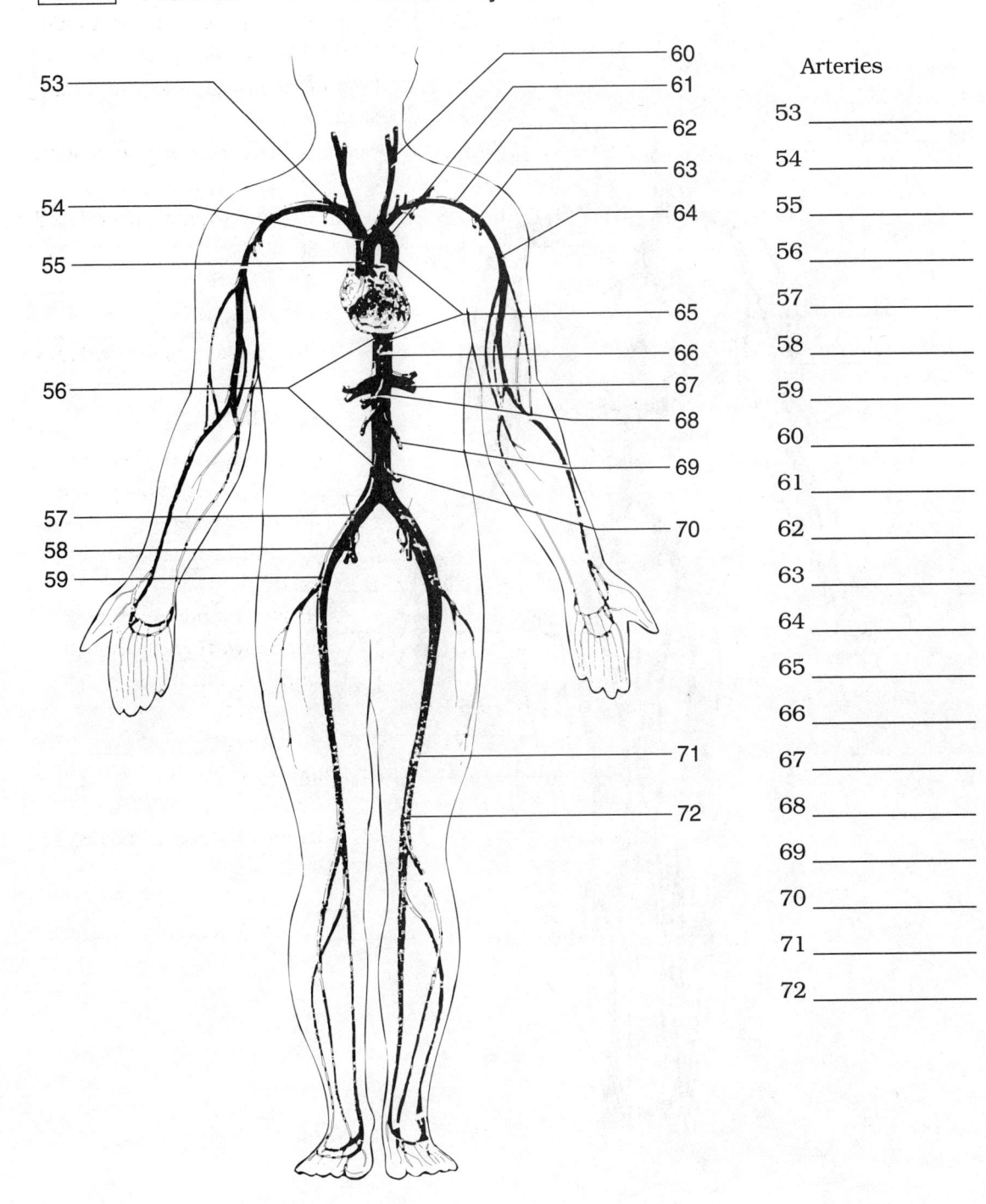

Arteries

53 _____
54 _____
55 _____
56 _____
57 _____
58 _____
59 _____
60 _____
61 _____
62 _____
63 _____
64 _____
65 _____
66 _____
67 _____
68 _____
69 _____
70 _____
71 _____
72 _____

Level
-1-

220 Chapter 14 Blood Vessels and Circulation

OBJ. 8 **FIGURE 14.2** The Venous System

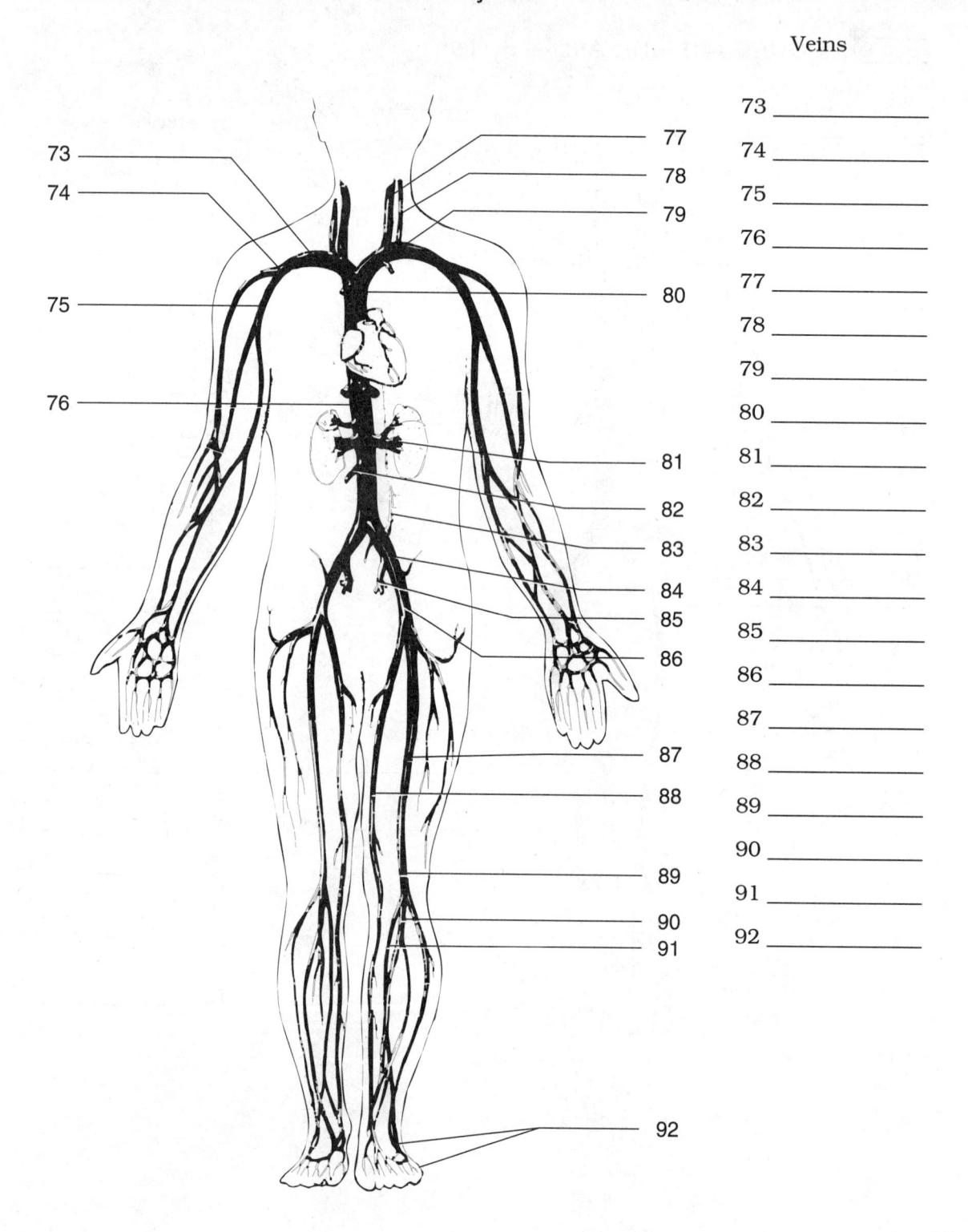

Veins

73 _____
74 _____
75 _____
76 _____
77 _____
78 _____
79 _____
80 _____
81 _____
82 _____
83 _____
84 _____
85 _____
86 _____
87 _____
88 _____
89 _____
90 _____
91 _____
92 _____

Level -1-

Level 1 Review of Chapter Objectives 221

OBJ. 8   FIGURE 14.3   Major Arteries of the Head and Neck

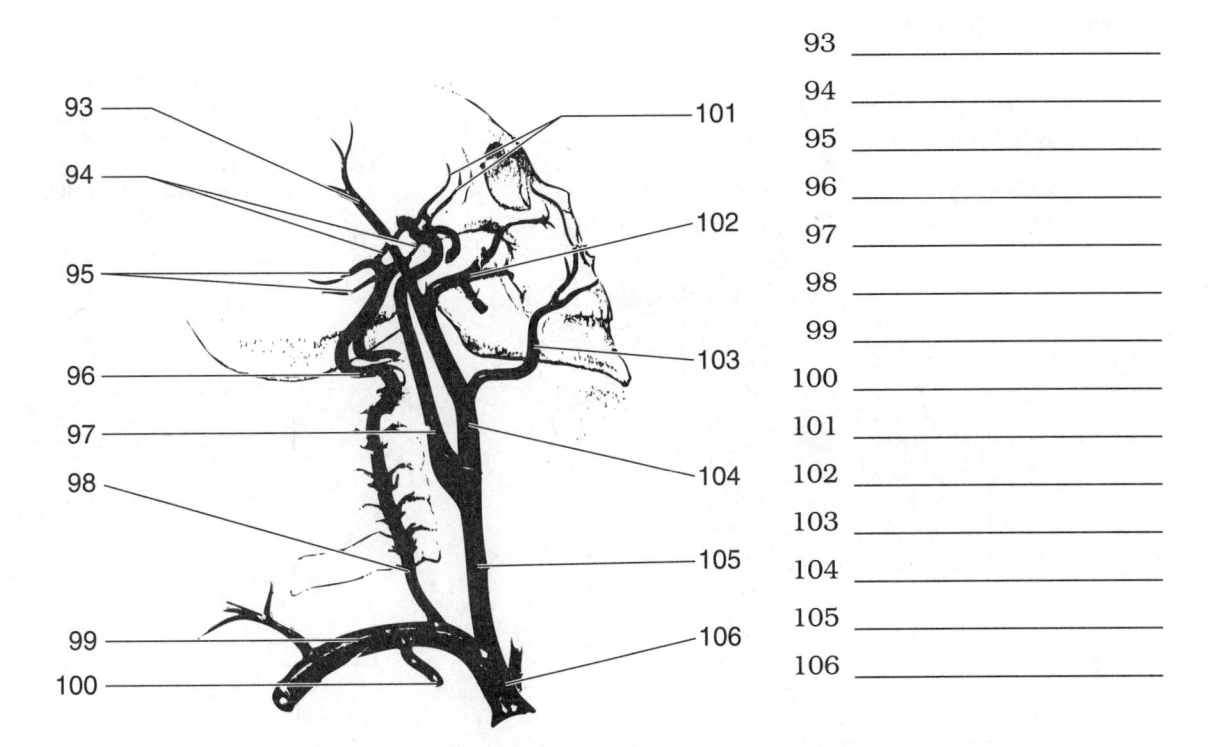

93 _____
94 _____
95 _____
96 _____
97 _____
98 _____
99 _____
100 _____
101 _____
102 _____
103 _____
104 _____
105 _____
106 _____

OBJ. 8   FIGURE 14.4   Major Veins Draining the Head and Neck

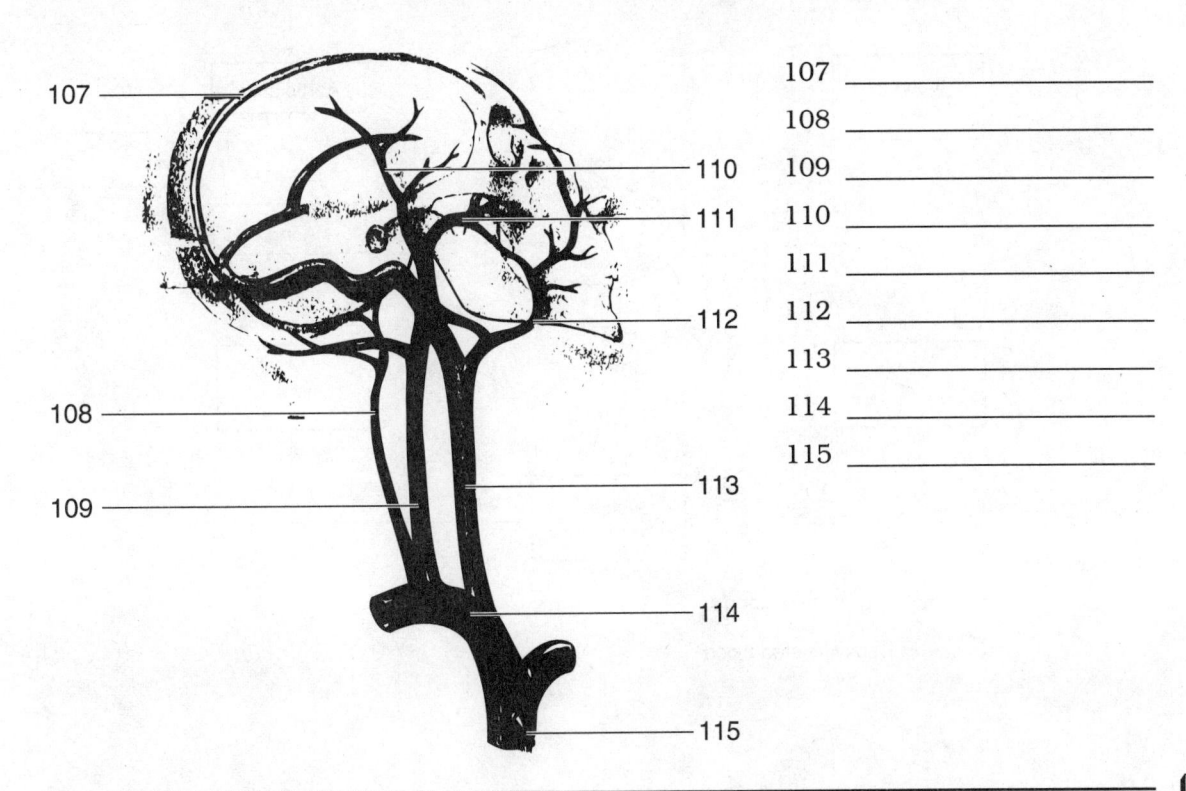

107 _____
108 _____
109 _____
110 _____
111 _____
112 _____
113 _____
114 _____
115 _____

When you have successfully completed the exercises in L1 proceed to L2.

Chapter 14 Blood Vessels and Circulation

☐ LEVEL 2   CONCEPT SYNTHESIS

Concept Map I:

Using the following terms, fill in the numbered, blank spaces to complete the concept map. Follow the numbers that comply with the organization of the map, moving in a "clock-wise" direction from top to bottom and back to top.

- Systemic circuit
- Veins and venules
- Pulmonary arteries
- Pulmonary veins
- Arteries and arterioles

The cardiovascular system

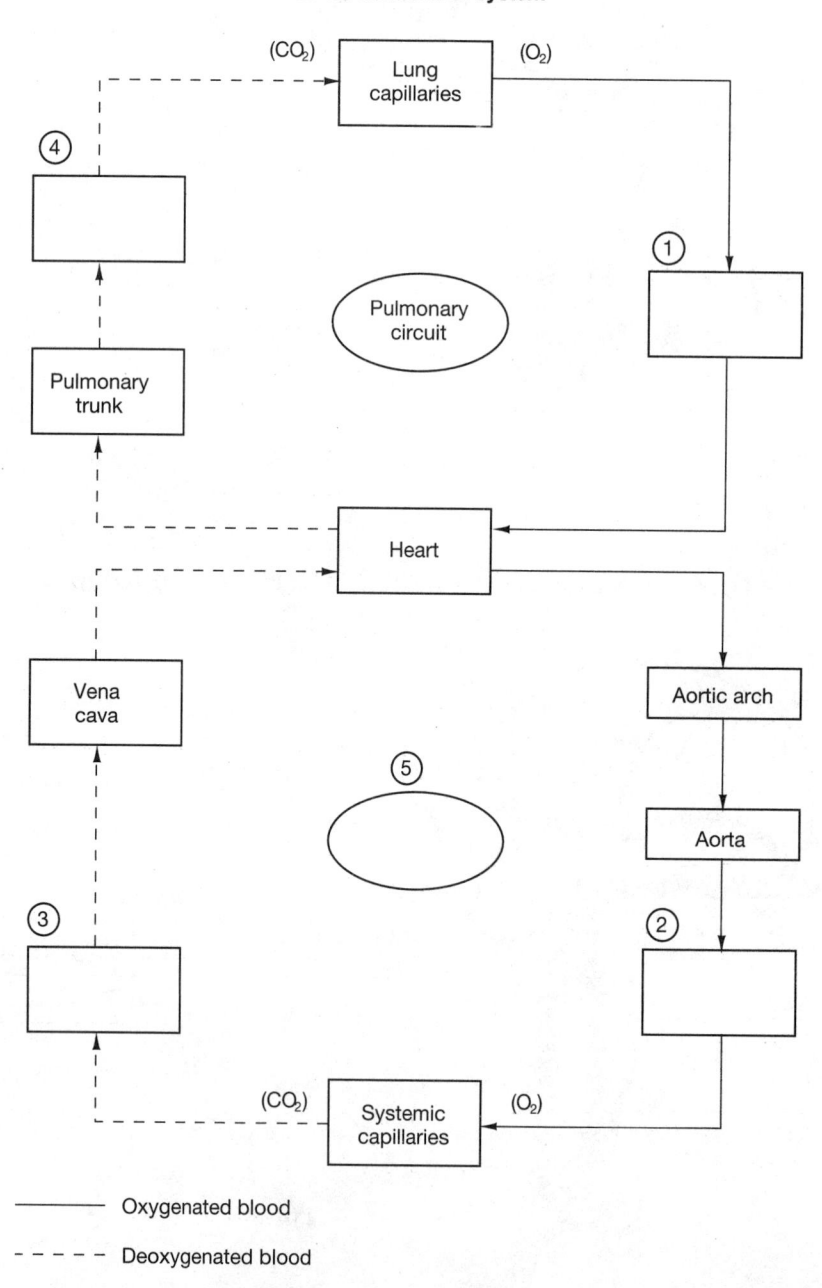

Level 2 Concept Synthesis

Concept Map II:

Using the following terms, fill in the numbered, blank spaces to complete the concept map. Follow the numbers that comply with the organization of the map.

- Superior mesenteric artery
- Brachiocephalic artery
- Ascending aorta
- Thoracic aorta
- L. Subclavian artery
- Celiac trunk
- R. gonadal artery
- L. common iliac artery

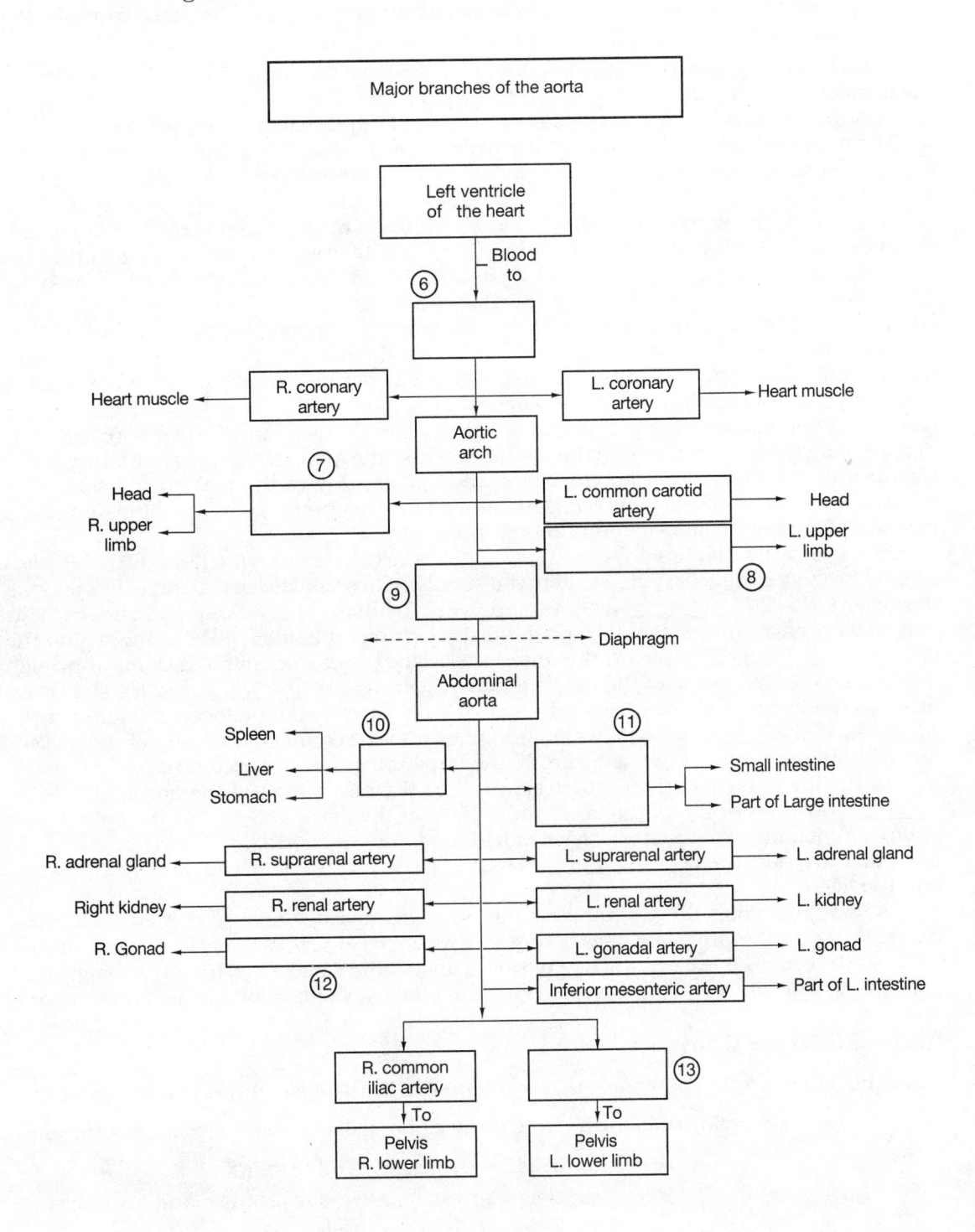

[Concept map: Major branches of the aorta]

- Left ventricle of the heart → Blood to → (6) → Aortic arch
  - R. coronary artery → Heart muscle
  - L. coronary artery → Heart muscle
- Aortic arch branches:
  - (7) → Head, R. upper limb
  - L. common carotid artery → Head
  - (8) → L. upper limb
- (9) → Diaphragm → Abdominal aorta
- Abdominal aorta branches:
  - (10) → Spleen, Liver, Stomach
  - (11) → Small intestine, Part of Large intestine
  - R. suprarenal artery → R. adrenal gland; L. suprarenal artery → L. adrenal gland
  - R. renal artery → Right kidney; L. renal artery → L. kidney
  - (12) → R. Gonad; L. gonadal artery → L. gonad
  - Inferior mesenteric artery → Part of L. intestine
- Terminal branches:
  - R. common iliac artery → To Pelvis, R. lower limb
  - (13) → To Pelvis, L. lower limb

Chapter 14 Blood Vessels and Circulation

Body Trek:

Using the terms below, fill in the blanks to complete a trek through the "major arteries" of the body.

lumbar	phrenic	L. subclavian
common iliacs	brachiocephalic	aortic valve
inferior mesenteric	L. common carotid	celiac
renal	superior mesenteric	descending aorta
gonadal	aortic arch	

Robo has been "charged" and "programmed" to take an "aortic trek." The objective of the mission is to identify the regions and major arteries that branch off the aorta from its superior position in the thorax to its inferior location in the abdominopelvic region.

The micro-robot is catheterized directly into the left ventricle of the heart, via a technique devised exclusively for introducing high-tech devices directly into the heart. A ventricular contraction "swooshes" the robot through the (14) _____ into the (15) _____, which curves across the superior surface of the heart, connecting the ascending aorta with the caudally-directed (16) _____. The first artery branching off the aortic arch, the (17) _____, serves as a passageway for blood to arteries that serve the arms, neck, and head. As the robot continues its ascent, the (18) _____ and the (19) _____ artery arise separately from the aortic arch, both supplying arterial blood to vessels that provide blood to regions that include the neck, head, shoulders, and arms. All of a sudden the robot is directed downward to begin its descent into the descending aorta. Proceeding caudally, near the diaphragm, a pair of (20) _____ arteries deliver blood to the muscular diaphragm that separates the thoracic and abdominoplevic cavities. Leaving the thoracic aorta Robo continues trekking along the same circulatory pathway into the abdominal aorta, which descends posteriorly to the peritoneal cavity. The robot's "thermosensors" detect record high temperatures in the area, probably due to the cushion of adipose tissue surrounding the aorta in this region.

Just below the diaphragm, the (21) _____ artery arises, which supplies blood to arterial branches that circulate blood to the stomach, liver, spleen and pancreas. Trekking downward, the (22) _____ arteries supplying the kidneys arise along the posteriolateral surface of the abdominal aorta behind the peritoneal lining. In the same region the (23) _____ arteries arise on the anterior surface of the abdominal aorta and branch into the connective tissue of the mesenteries. A pair of (24) _____ arteries supplying blood to the testicles in the male and the ovaries in the female are located slightly superior to the (25) _____ artery, which branches into the connective tissues of the mesenteries supplying blood to the last third of the large intestine, colon, and rectum.

On the final phase of the aortic trek, prior to the bifurcation of the aorta, small (26) _____ arteries begin on the posterior surface of the aorta and supply the spinal cord and the abdominal wall. Near the level of L4 the abdominal aorta divides to form a pair of muscular arteries, the (27) _____, which are the major blood suppliers to the pelvis and the legs.

As Robo completes the programmed mission, the message relayed to Mission Control reads, "Mission accomplished, please remove." Mission Control instructs the robot to continue its descent into the femoral artery where an arterial removal technique for high-tech gadgetry will facilitate Robo's exit and return to Mission Control for the next assignment.

[L2] Multiple Choice:

Place the letter corresponding to the correct answer in the space provided.

_____ 28. In traveling from the heart to the peripheral capillaries, blood passes through:

    a. arteries, arterioles, and venules
    b. elastic arteries, muscular arteries, and arterioles
    c. veins, venules, arterioles
    d. a, b, and c are correct

_____ 29. The goal of cardiovascular regulation is:
- a. to equalize the stroke volume with the cardiac output
- b. to increase pressure and reduce resistance
- c. to equalize the blood flow with the pressure differences
- d. maintenance of adequate blood flow through peripheral tissues and organs

_____ 30. The average pressure in arteries is approximately:
- a. 120 mm Hg
- b. 100 mm Hg
- c. 140 mm Hg
- d. 80 mm Hg

_____ 31. The average pressure in veins is approximately:
- a. 2 mm Hg
- b. 10 mm Hg
- c. 15 mm Hg
- d. 80 mm Hg

_____ 32. When fluid moves across capillary membranes, the pressures forcing fluid "out" of the capillaries are:
- a. hydrostatic pressure; interstitial osmotic pressure
- b. interstitial fluid pressure; osmotic pressure of plasma
- c. hydrostatic pressure; interstitial fluid pressure
- d. interstitial osmotic pressure; osmotic pressure of plasma

_____ 33. Two arteries formed by the bifurcation of the brachiocephalic artery are the:
- a. aorta, subclavian
- b. common iliac, common carotid
- c. jugular, carotid
- d. common carotid, subclavian

_____ 34. The _____ return blood to the heart and the _____ transport blood away from the heart.
- a. arteries; veins
- b. venules; arterioles
- c. veins; arteries
- d. arterioles; venules

_____ 35. The large vein that drains the thorax is the:
- a. superior vena cava
- b. internal jugular
- c. vertebral vein
- d. azygous vein

_____ 36. The veins that drain the head, neck, and upper extremities are the:
- a. jugulars
- b. brachiocephalics
- c. subclavian
- d. azygous

Chapter 14 Blood Vessels and Circulation

_____ 37. The veins that drain venous blood from the legs and the pelvis are:
- a. posterior tibials
- b. femorals
- c. great saphenous
- d. common iliacs

_____ 38. The vein that drains the knee region of the body is the:
- a. femoral
- b. popliteal
- c. external iliacs
- d. great saphenous

_____ 39. The large artery that serves the brain is the:
- a. internal carotid
- b. external carotid
- c. subclavian
- d. cephalic

_____ 40. The "link" between the subclavian and brachial artery is the:
- a. brachiocephalic
- b. vertebral
- c. cephalic
- d. axillary

_____ 41. The three arterial branches of the celiac trunk are the:
- a. splenic, pancreatic, mesenteric
- b. phrenic, intercostal, adrenolumbar
- c. gastric, splenic, hepatic
- d. brachial, ulnar, radial

_____ 42. The artery that supplies most of the small intestine and the first half of the large intestine is the:
- a. suprarenal artery
- b. superior mesenteric
- c. hepatic
- d. inferior mesenteric

_____ 43. The artery that supplies the pelvic organs is the:
- a. internal iliac artery
- b. external iliac artery
- c. common iliacs
- d. femoral artery

_____ 44. The subdivision(s) of the popliteal artery is (are):
- a. great saphenous artery
- b. anterior and posterior tibial arteries
- c. peroneal artery
- d. femoral and deep femoral arteries

Level 2

[L2] Completion:

Using the terms below, complete the following statements.

- radial
- edema
- precapillary sphincters
- great saphenous
- brachial
- circle of Willis
- venous return
- endothelium
- veins

45. The anastomosis that encircles the infundibulum of the pituitary gland, supplying blood to the brain, is the _____.
46. The abnormal accumulation of interstitial fluid is called _____.
47. Rhythmic alterations in blood flow in capillary beds are controlled by _____.
48. The lining of the lumen of blood vessels is comprised of a tissue layer called the _____.
49. The blood vessels that contain valves are the _____.
50. Changes in thoracic pressure during breathing and the action of skeletal muscles serve to aid in _____.
51. The artery generally auscultated to determine the blood pressure in the arm is the _____ artery.
52. The artery generally used to take the pulse at the wrist is the _____ artery.
53. The longest vein in the body is the _____.

[L2] Short Essay:

Briefly answer the following questions in the spaces provided below.

54. List the types of blood vessels in the cardiovascular tree and briefly describe their anatomical associations (use arrows to show this relationship).

55. Relative to gaseous exchange, what is the primary difference between the pulmonary circuit and the systemic circuit?

56. What are the three (3) primary sources of peripheral resistance?

57. What are the important functions of continual movement of fluid from the plasma into tissues and lymphatic vessels?

58. What are the three (3) primary factors that influence blood pressure and blood flow?

59. What three (3) major baroreceptor populations enable the cardiovascular system to respond to alterations in blood pressure?

60. What hormones are responsible for long-term and short-term regulation of cardiovascular performance?

61. How does arteriosclerosis affect blood vessels?

When you have successfully completed the exercises in L2 proceed to L3.

☐ LEVEL 3   CRITICAL THINKING/APPLICATION

Using principles and concepts learned about blood vessels and circulation, answer the following questions. Write your answers on a separate sheet of paper.

1. Trace the circulatory pathway a drop of blood would take if it begins in the L. ventricle, travels down the left arm, and returns to the R. atrium. (Use arrows to indicate direction of flow.)
2. Suppose you are lying down and quickly rise to a standing position. What would cause dizziness or a loss of consciousness to occur as a result of standing up quickly?
3. While pedalling an exercycle, Mary periodically takes her pulse by applying pressure to the carotid artery in the upper neck. Why might this method give her an erroneous perception of her pulse rate while exercising?

CHAPTER 15

The Lymphatic System and Immunity

■ Overview

The lymphatic system includes lymphoid organs and tissues, a network of lymphatic vessels that contain a fluid called lymph, and a dominant population of individual cells, the lymphocytes. The cells, tissues, organs, and vessels containing lymph perform three major functions:

1. The lymphoid organs and tissues serve as operating sites for the phagocytes and cells of the immune system that provide the body with protection from pathogens;
2. the lymphatic vessels containing lymph help to maintain blood volume in the cardiovascular system and absorb fats and other substances from the digestive tract; and
3. the lymphocytes are the "defensive specialists" that protect the body from pathogenic microorganisms, foreign tissue cells, and diseased or infected cells in the body that pose a threat to the normal cell population.

Chapter 15 provides exercises focusing on topics that include the organization of the lymphatic system, the body's defense mechanisms, patterns of immune response, and interactions between the lymphatic system and other physiological systems.

☐ LEVEL 1   REVIEW OF CHAPTER OBJECTIVES

1. Identify the major components of the lymphatic system and explain their functions.
2. Discuss the importance of lymphocytes and describe where they are found in the body.
3. List the body's nonspecific defenses and explain how each functions.
4. Define specific resistance and identify the forms and properties of immunity.
5. Distinguish between cell-mediated immunity and antibody-mediated (humoral) immunity.
6. Discuss the different types of T cells and the role played by each in the immune response.
7. Describe the structure of antibody molecules and explain how they function.
8. Describe the primary and secondary responses to antigen exposure.
9. Relate allergic reactions and autoimmune disorders to immune mechanisms.
10. Describe the changes in the immune system that occur with aging.

[L1] Multiple Choice:

Place the letter corresponding to the correct answer in the space provided.

OBJ. 1 ____ 1. The major components of the lymphatic system include:
   a. lymph nodes, lymph, lymphocytes
   b. spleen, thymus, tonsils
   c. thoracic duct, R. lymphatic duct, lymph nodes
   d. lymphatic vessels, lymph, lymphatic organs

OBJ. 1 ____ 2. Lymphatic organs found in the lymphatic system include:
   a. thoracic duct, R. lymphatic duct, lymph nodes
   b. lymphatic vessels, tonsils, lymph nodes
   c. spleen, thymus, lymph nodes
   d. a, b, and c are correct

OBJ. 1 ____ 3. The primary function of the lymphatic system is:
   a. transporting of nutrients and oxygen to tissues
   b. removal of carbon dioxide and waste products from tissues
   c. regulation of temperature, fluid, electrolytes, and pH balance
   d. production, maintenance, and distribution of lymphocytes

OBJ. 2 ____ 4. Lymphocytes that assist in the regulation and coordination of the immune response are:
   a. plasma cells
   b. helper T and suppressor T cells
   c. B cells
   d. NK and B cells

OBJ. 2 ____ 5. Normal lymphocyte populations are maintained through lymphopoiesis in the:
   a. bone marrow and lymphatic tissues
   b. lymph in the lymphatic tissues
   c. blood and the lymph
   d. spleen and liver

OBJ. 2 ____ 6. The largest collection of lymphoid tissue in the body is contained within the:
   a. adult spleen
   b. thymus gland
   c. the tonsils
   d. the lymphatic nodules

OBJ. 3 ____ 7. Of the following selections, the one that includes only nonspecific defenses is:
   a. T- and B-cell activation, complement, inflammation, phagocytosis
   b. hair, skin, mucous membranes, antibodies
   c. hair, skin, complement, inflammation, phagocytosis
   d. antigens, antibodies, complement, macrophages

Level 1 Review of Chapter Objectives 231

OBJ. 3 ____ 8. The protective categories that prevent the approach of, deny entrance to, or limit the spread of microorganisms or other 10 environmental hazards are called:
   a. specific defenses
   b. nonspecific defenses
   c. specific immunity
   d. immunological surveillance

OBJ. 3 ____ 9. NK (natural killer) cells sensitive to the presence of abnormal cell membranes are primarily involved with:
   a. defenses against specific threats
   b. delayed defense mechanisms
   c. phagocytic activity for defense
   d. immunological surveillance

OBJ. 4 ____ 10. The four general characteristics of specific defenses include:
   a. specificity, versatility, memory, and tolerance
   b. innate, active, acquired, passive
   c. accessibility, recognition, compatibility, immunity
   d. a, b, and c are correct

OBJ. 4 ____ 11. The two major ways that the body "carries out" the immune response are:
   a. phagocytosis and the inflammatory response
   b. immunological surveillance and fever
   c. direct attack by T cells and attack by circulating antibodies
   d. physical barriers and the complement system

OBJ. 4 ____ 12. A "specific" defense mechanism is always activated by:
   a. an antigen
   b. an antibody
   c. inflammation
   d. fever

OBJ. 5 ____ 13. The type of immunity that develops as a result of natural exposure to an antigen in the environment is:
   a. naturally acquired immunity
   b. natural innate immunity
   c. naturally acquired active immunity
   d. naturally acquired passive immunity

OBJ. 5 ____ 14. When an antigen appears, the immune response begins with:
   a. the presence of immunoglobulins in body fluids
   b. the release of endogenous fever producing substances
   c. the activation of the complement system
   d. activation of specific T and B cells

232 Chapter 15 The Lymphatic System and Immunity

OBJ. 6 ____ 15. T-cell activation leads to the formation of cytotoxic T cells and memory T cells that provide:

    a. humoral immunity
    b. cellular immunity
    c. phagocytosis
    d. immunological surveillance

OBJ. 6 ____ 16. Before an antigen can stimulate a lymphocyte, it must first be processed by a:

    a. macrophage
    b. NK cell
    c. cytotoxic T cell
    d. neutrophil

OBJ. 7 ____ 17. An active antibody is shaped like a(n):

    a. T
    b. A
    c. Y
    d. B

OBJ. 7 ____ 18. Antibodies may promote inflammation through the stimulation of:

    a. basophils and mast cells
    b. plasma cells and memory B cells
    c. suppressor T cells
    d. cytotoxic T cells

OBJ. 8 ____ 19. The antigenic determinant site is the certain portion of the antigen's exposed surface where:

    a. the foreign "body" attacks
    b. phagocytosis occurs
    c. the antibody attacks
    d. immune surveillance is activated

OBJ. 8 ____ 20. In order for an antigenic molecule to be a complete antigen, it must:

    a. be a large molecule
    b. be immunogenic and reactive
    c. contain a hapten and a small organic molecule
    d. be subject to antibody activity

OBJ. 8 ____ 21. The major functions of interleukins in the immune system are to:

    a. increase T-cell sensitivity to antigens exposed on macrophage membranes
    b. stimulate B-cell activity, plasma-cell formation, and antibody production
    c. enhance nonspecific defenses
    d. a, b, and c are correct

Level -1-

Level 1 Review of Chapter Objectives 233

OBJ. 8 ___ 22. Fetal antibody production is uncommon because the developing fetus has:

    a. cell-mediated immunity
    b. natural passive immunity
    c. antibody mediated immunity
    d. endogenous fever producing substances

OBJ. 9 ___ 23. When an immune response mistakenly targets normal body cells and tissues, the result is:

    a. immune system failure
    b. the development of an allergy
    c. depression of the inflammatory response
    d. an autoimmune disorder

OBJ. 10 ___ 24. With advancing age the immune system becomes:

    a. increasingly susceptible to viral infection
    b. increasingly susceptible to bacterial infection
    c. less effective at combatting disease
    d. a, b, and c are correct

[L1] Completion:

Using the terms below, complete the following statements.

lymphokines	immunological competence	helper T
plasma cells	diapedesis	lymph capillaries
active	lacteals	passive
immunodeficiency disease	vaccinated	cell-mediated
cytotoxic T cells	suppressor T	phagocytes
IgG		

OBJ. 1   25. The special lymphatic vessels in the lining of the small intestines are the _____.

OBJ. 1   26. The lymphatic system begins in the tissues as _____.

OBJ. 2   27. Lymphocytes that attack foreign cells or body cells infected by viruses are called _____ cells.

OBJ. 3   28. Cells that represent the "first line" of cellular defense against pathogens are the _____.

OBJ. 3   29. The process during which macrophages move through adjacent endothelial cells of capillary walls is called _____.

OBJ. 4   30. An immunization where antibodies are administered to fight infection or prevent disease is _____.

OBJ. 5   31. Cytotoxic T cells are responsible for the type of immunity referred to as _____.

OBJ. 5   32. Immunity that appears following exposure to an antigen as a consequence of the immune response is referred to as _____.

OBJ. 6   33. The types of cells that inhibit the responses of other T cells and B cells are called _____ cells.

OBJ. 6   34. Before B cells can respond to an antigen, they must receive a signal from _____ cells.

234 Chapter 15 The Lymphatic System and Immunity

OBJ. 7 — 35. Antibodies are produced and secreted by _____.

OBJ. 8 — 36. The ability to demonstrate an immune response upon exposure to an antigen is called _____.

OBJ. 8 — 37. Chemical messengers secreted by lymphocytes are called _____.

OBJ. 8 — 38. The only antibodies that cross the placenta from the maternal blood stream are _____ antibodies.

OBJ. 9 — 39. When the immune system fails to develop normally or the immune response is blocked in some way, the condition is termed _____.

OBJ. 10 — 40. Because of increased susceptibility of acute viral infection in the elderly, it is recommended that they be _____.

[L1] Matching:

Match the terms in column "A" with the terms in column "B." Use letters for answers in the spaces provided.

	COLUMN "A"	COLUMN "B"
OBJ. 1 — 41.	Peyer's patches	A. Decline in immune surveillance
OBJ. 2 — 42.	Macrophages	B. Cellular immunity
OBJ. 2 — 43.	Microphages	C. Innate or acquired
OBJ. 3 — 44.	Mast cells	D. Nonspecific immune response
OBJ. 4 — 45.	Acquired immunity	E. Activation of B cells
OBJ. 4 — 46.	Specific immunity	F. Monocytes
OBJ. 5 — 47.	B cells	G. Lymph nodues in small intestine
OBJ. 6 — 48.	Cytotoxic T cells	H. Resistance to viral infections
OBJ. 6 — 49.	T lymphocytes	I. Active and passive
OBJ. 7 — 50.	Antibody	J. Activation of T cells
OBJ. 8 — 51.	Interferons	K. Humoral immunity
OBJ. 8 — 52.	Lymphokines	L. Neutrophils and eosinophils
OBJ. 9 — 53.	Cytotoxic reactions	M. Cell-mediated immunity
OBJ. 10 — 54.	Cancer	N. Two parallel pairs of polypeptide chains

Level -1-

Level 1 Review of Chapter Objectives 235

[L1] Drawing/Illustration Labeling:

OBJ. 3   **FIGURE 15.1**   Nonspecific Defenses

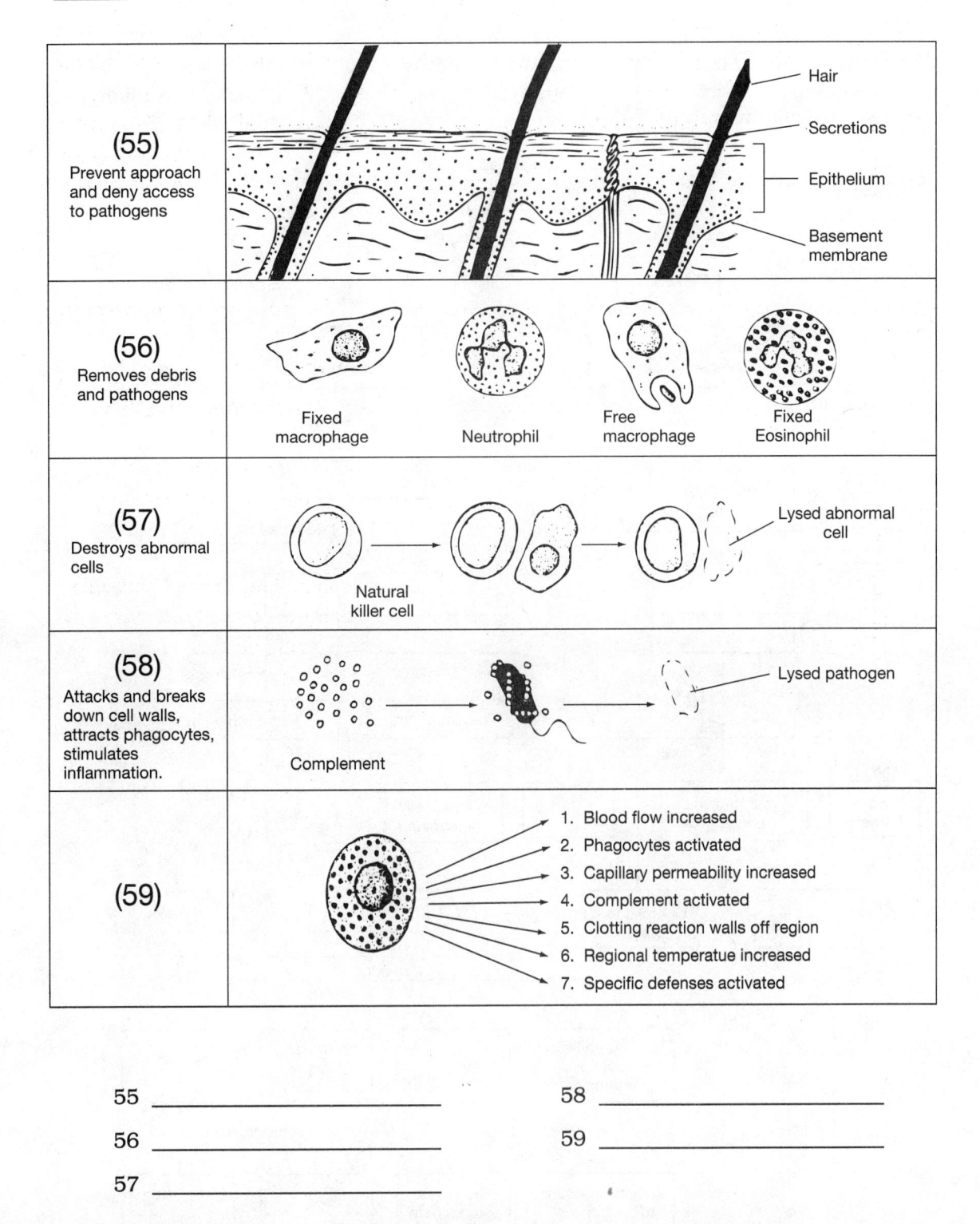

Label	Description	Illustration details
(55)	Prevent approach and deny access to pathogens	Hair, Secretions, Epithelium, Basement membrane
(56)	Removes debris and pathogens	Fixed macrophage, Neutrophil, Free macrophage, Fixed Eosinophil
(57)	Destroys abnormal cells	Natural killer cell → Lysed abnormal cell
(58)	Attacks and breaks down cell walls, attracts phagocytes, stimulates inflammation.	Complement → Lysed pathogen
(59)		1. Blood flow increased 2. Phagocytes activated 3. Capillary permeability increased 4. Complement activated 5. Clotting reaction walls off region 6. Regional temperatue increased 7. Specific defenses activated

55 _____   58 _____

56 _____   59 _____

57 _____

When you have successfully completed the exercises in L1 proceed to L2.

Level -1-

236 Chapter 15 The Lymphatic System and Immunity

☐ LEVEL 2   CONCEPT SYNTHESIS

Using the following terms, fill in the numbered, blank spaces to complete the concept map. Follow the numbers that comply with the organization of the map.

- Active immunization
- Passive immunization
- Acquired
- Nonspecific-immunity
- Inflammation
- Specific immunity
- Active
- Phagocytic cells
- Innate
- Transfer of antibodies via placenta

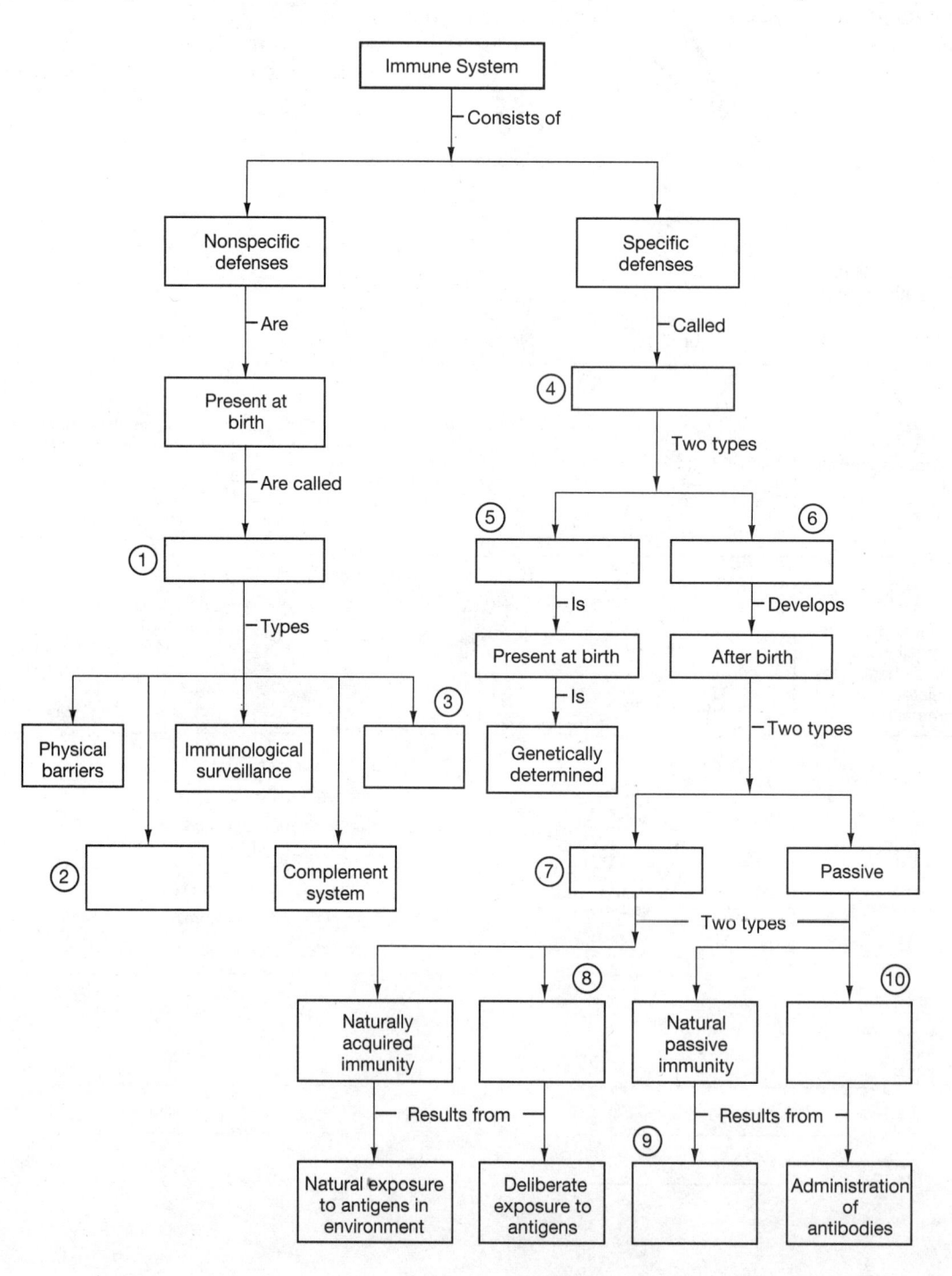

Level 2 Concept Synthesis 237

Body Trek:

Using the terms below, fill in the blanks to complete a trek through the body's department of defense.

killer T cells	viruses	B cells
antibodies	helper T cells	macrophages
natural killer cells	suppressor T cells	memory T and B cells

Robo has been programmed to guide you on a trek through the body's department of defense-the immune system. You will proceed with the micro-robot from statement 1 (question 11) to statement 9 (question 19). At each site you will complete the event that is taking place by identifying the type of cells or proteins participating in the specific immune response.

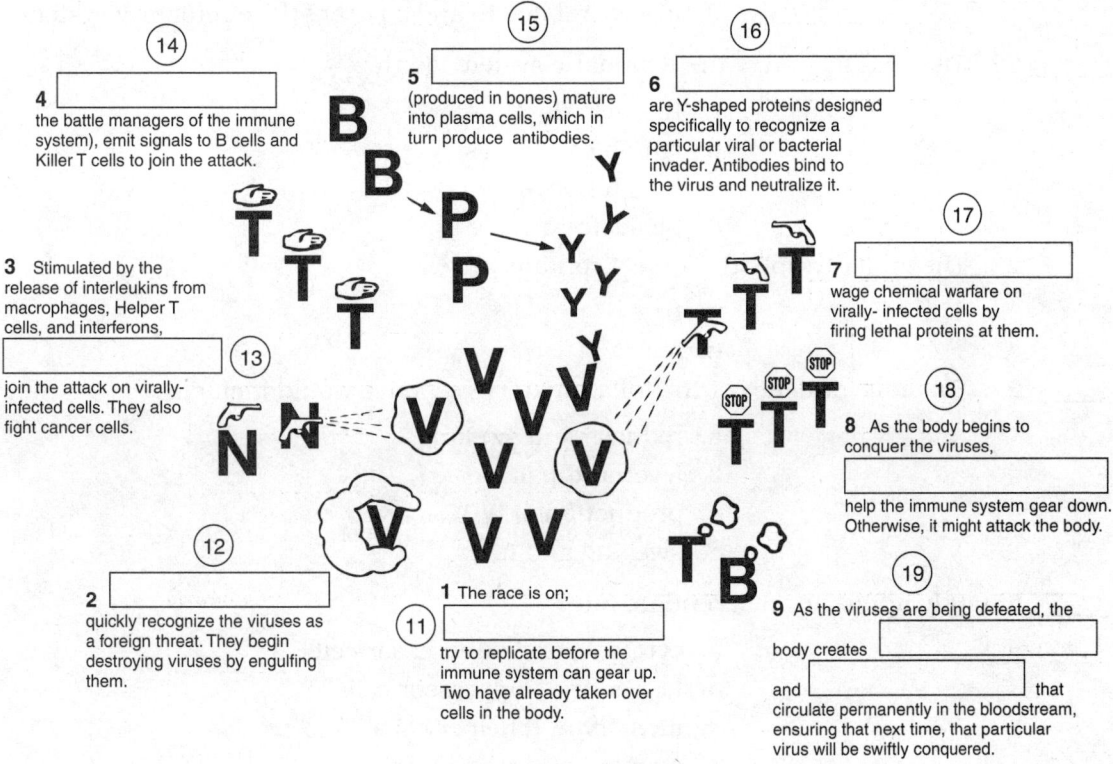

The body's department of defense

4. (14) _____ the battle managers of the immune system), emit signals to B cells and Killer T cells to join the attack.

5. (15) _____ (produced in bones) mature into plasma cells, which in turn produce antibodies.

6. (16) _____ are Y-shaped proteins designed specifically to recognize a particular viral or bacterial invader. Antibodies bind to the virus and neutralize it.

3. Stimulated by the release of interleukins from macrophages, Helper T cells, and interferons, (13) _____ join the attack on virally-infected cells. They also fight cancer cells.

7. (17) _____ wage chemical warfare on virally-infected cells by firing lethal proteins at them.

8. As the body begins to conquer the viruses, (18) _____ help the immune system gear down. Otherwise, it might attack the body.

2. (12) _____ quickly recognize the viruses as a foreign threat. They begin destroying viruses by engulfing them.

1. The race is on; (11) _____ try to replicate before the immune system can gear up. Two have already taken over cells in the body.

9. As the viruses are being defeated, the body creates (19) _____ and _____ that circulate permanently in the bloodstream, ensuring that next time, that particular virus will be swiftly conquered.

Level 2

[L2] Multiple Choice:

Place the letter corresponding to the correct answer in the space provided.

_____ 20. The three different classes of lymphocytes in the blood are:
- a. cytotoxic cells, helper cells, suppressor cells
- b. T cells, B cells, NK cells
- c. plasma cells, B cells, cytotoxic cells
- d. antigens, antibodies, immunoglobulins

_____ 21. Of the following selections, the one that best defines the lymphatic system is that it is:
- a. an integral part of the circulatory system
- b. a one-way route from the blood to the interstitial fluid
- c. a one-way route from the interstitial fluid to the blood
- d. closely related to and a part of the circulatory system

_____ 22. Tissue fluid enters the lymphatic system via the:
- a. thoracic duct
- b. lymph capillaries
- c. lymph nodes
- d. bloodstream

_____ 23. The larger lymphatic vessels contain valves.
- a. true
- b. false

_____ 24. Systemic evidence of the inflammatory response would include:
- a. redness and swelling
- b. fever and pain
- c. production of WBCs, fever
- d. swelling and fever

_____ 25. B lymphocytes differentiate into:
- a. cytotoxic and suppressor cells
- b. helper and suppressor cells
- c. memory and helper cells
- d. memory and plasma cells

_____ 26. _____ cells may activate B cells while _____ cells inhibit the activity of B cells.
- a. memory; plasma
- b. macrophages; microphages
- c. memory; cytotoxic
- d. helper T; suppressor T

_____ 27. The primary response of T-cell differentiation in cell-mediated immunity is the production of _____ cells.
- a. helper T
- b. suppressor T
- c. cytotoxic T
- d. memory

____ 28. The vaccination of antigenic materials into the body is called:
   a. naturally acquired active immunity
   b. artificially acquired active immunity
   c. naturally acquired passive immunity
   d. artificially acquired passive immunity

____ 29. The antibodies produced and secreted by B lymphocytes are soluble proteins called:
   a. lymphokines
   b. agglutinins
   c. immunoglobulins
   d. leukotrines

____ 30. Memory B cells do not differentiate into plasma cells unless they:
   a. are initially subjected to a specific antigen
   b. are stimulated by active immunization
   c. are exposed to the same antigen a second time
   d. are stimulated by passive immunization

____ 31. The three-dimensional "fit" between the variable segments of the antibody molecule and the corresponding antigenic determinant site is referred to as the:
   a. immunodeficiency complex
   b. antibody-antigen complex
   c. protein-complement complex
   d. a, b, and c are correct

____ 32. One of the primary nonspecific effects that glucocorticoids have on the immune response is:
   a. inhibition of interleukin secretion
   b. increased release of T and B cells
   c. decreased activity of cytotoxic T cells
   d. depression of the inflammatory response

[L2] Completion:

Using the terms below, complete the following statements.

cytokines	mast	interferon	NK cells
helper T cells	IgG	IgM	tumor necrosis factor
Langerhans cells			

33. Macrophages that reside within the epithelia of the skin and digestive tract are _____.
34. Hormones of the immune system released by tissue cells to coordinate local activities are classified as _____.
35. Cells that play a pivotal role in the inflammatory process are called _____ cells.
36. The substance that slows tumor growth is _____.
37. Immunological surveillance involves specific lymphocytes called _____.
38. The protein that is effective against viruses is called _____.
39. Antibodies that comprise approximately 80 percent of all antibodies in the body are _____.
40. Antibodies that occur naturally in blood plasma and are used to determine an individual's blood type are _____.
41. The human immunodeficiency virus (HIV) attacks _____ cells in humans.

[L2] Short Essay:

Briefly answer the following questions in the spaces provided below.

42. What three (3) major functions are performed by the lymphatic system?

43. What is the primary function of stimulated B cells and what are they ultimately responsible for?

44. What are the six (6) defenses that provide the body with a defensive capability known as nonspecific immunity?

45. What are the primary differences between the "recognition" mechanisms of NK (natural killer) cells and T and B cells?

46. What are the four (4) general characteristics of specific defenses?

47. What is the primary difference between active and passive immunity?

48. What five (5) different classes of antibodies (immunoglobulins) are found in body fluids? Describe each.

When you have successfully completed the exercises in L2 proceed to L3.

LEVEL 3 CRITICAL THINKING/APPLICATION

Using principles and concepts learned about the lymphatic system and immunity, answer the following questions. Write your answers on a separate sheet of paper.

1. Organ transplants are common surgical procedures in a number of hospitals throughout the United States. What happens if the donor and recipient are not compatible?
2. Via a diagram, draw a schematic model to illustrate your understanding of the immune system as a whole. (Hint: Begin with the antigen and show the interactions that result in cell-mediated and antibody-mediated immunity.)
3. Why are NK cells effective in fighting viral infections?
4. We usually associate a fever with illness or disease. In what ways may a fever be beneficial?

CHAPTER 16

The Respiratory System

■ Overview

The human body can survive without food for several weeks, without water for several days, but if the oxygen supply is cut off for more than several minutes, the possibility of death is imminent. All cells in the body require a continuous supply of oxygen and must continuously get rid of carbon dioxide, a major waste product.

The respiratory system delivers oxygen from air to the blood and removes carbon dioxide, the gaseous waste product of cellular metabolism. It also plays an important role in regulating the pH of the body fluids.

The respiratory system consists of the lungs (which contain air sacs with moist membranes), a number of accessory structures, and a system of passageways that conduct inspired air from the atmosphere to the membranous sacs of the lungs, and expired air from the sacs in the lungs back to the atmosphere.

Chapter 16 includes exercises that examine the functional anatomy and organization of the respiratory system, respiratory physiology, the control of respiration, and respiratory interactions with other systems.

☐ LEVEL 1   REVIEW OF CHAPTER OBJECTIVES

1. Describe the primary functions of the respiratory system.
2. Explain how the delicate respiratory exchange surfaces are protected from pathogens, debris and other hazards.
3. Relate respiratory functions to the structural specializations of the the tissues and organs of the system.
4. Describe the physical principles governing the movement of air into the lungs and the diffusion of gases into and out of the blood.
5. Describe the actions of muscles responsible for respiratory movements.
6. Describe how oxygen and carbon dioxide are transported in the blood.
7. Describe the major factors that influence the rate of respiration.
8. Identify the reflexes that regulate respiration.
9. Describe the changes that occur in the respiratory sytem at birth and with aging.

[L1] Multiple Choice:

Place the letter corresponding to the correct answer in the space provided.

OBJ. 1 ____ 1. The primary functions of the respiratory system is (are):
   a. to move air to and from the exchange surfaces
   b. to provide an area for gas exchange between air and circulating blood
   c. to protect respiratory surfaces from dehydration and environmental variations
   d. a, b, and c are correct

OBJ. 2 ____ 2. Pulmonary surfactant is a phospholipid secretion produced by alveolar cells to:
   a. increase the surface area of the alveoli
   b. reduce the cohesive force of H_2O molecules and lower surface tension
   c. increase the cohesive force of air molecules and raise surface tension
   d. reduce the attractive forces of O_2 molecules and increase surface tension

OBJ. 2 ____ 3. The "patrol force" of the alveolar epithelium involved with phagocytosis is comprised primarily of:
   a. alveolar NK cells
   b. alveolar cytotoxic cells
   c. alveolar macrophages
   d. alveolar plasma cells

OBJ. 3 ____ 4. The respiratory system consists of structures that:
   a. provide defense from pathogenic invasion
   b. permit vocalization and production of other sounds
   c. regulate blood volume and pressure
   d. a, b, and c are correct

OBJ. 3 ____ 5. The difference between the true and false vocal cords is that the false vocal cords:
   a. are highly elastic
   b. are involved with the production of sound
   c. play no part in sound production
   d. articulate with the laryngeal cartilages

OBJ. 3 ____ 6. Structures in the trachea that prevent its collapse or overexpansion as pressures change in the respiratory system are the:
   a. O-ringed tracheal cartilages
   b. C-shaped tracheal cartilages
   c. irregular circular bones
   d. b and c are correct

OBJ. 3   ____ 7. If food particles or liquids manage to touch the surfaces of the ventricular or vocal folds the:

    a. individual will choke to death
    b. coughing reflex will be triggered
    c. glottis will remain open
    d. epiglottis will not function

OBJ. 3   ____ 8. The trachea allows for the passage of large masses of food through the esophagus due to:

    a. the C-shaped tracheal cartilages
    b. the elasticity of the ringed tracheal cartilages
    c. distortion of the esophageal wall
    d. a, b, and c are correct

OBJ. 3   ____ 9. The purpose of the hilus along the medial surface of the lung at the level of the branching primary bronchi is to:

    a. mark the line of separation between the two bronchi
    b. provide access for entry to pulmonary vessels and nerves
    c. prevent foreign objects from entering the trachea
    d. a, b, and c are correct

OBJ. 3   ____ 10. Dilation and relaxation of the bronchioles are possible because of the presence of:

    a. bands of smooth muscle encircling the lumen
    b. the presence of C-shaped cartilaginous rings
    c. cuboidal epithelial cells containing cilia
    d. bands of skeletal muscles in the submucosa

OBJ. 3   ____ 11. After passing through the trachea, the correct pathway a molecule of inspired air would take to reach an alveolus is:

    a. primary bronchus → secondary bronchus → bronchioles → respiratory bronchioles → terminal bronchioles → alveolus
    b. primary bronchus → bronchioles → terminal bronchioles → respiratory bronchioles → alveolus
    c. primary bronchus → secondary bronchus → bronchioles → terminal bronchioles → respiratory bronchioles → alveolus
    d. bronchi → secondary bronchus → bronchioles → terminal bronchioles → alveolus

OBJ. 3   ____ 12. The serous membrane in contact with the lung is the:

    a. visceral pleura
    b. parietal pleura
    c. pulmonary mediastinum
    d. pulmonary mesentery

Level 1   Review of Chapter Objectives   245

OBJ. 4 ___ 13. A necessary feature for normal gas exchange in the alveoli is:
  a. for the alveoli to remain dry
  b. an increase in pressure in pulmonary circulation
  c. for fluid to move into the pulmonary capillaries
  d. an increase in lung volume

OBJ. 4 ___ 14. The movement of air into and out of the lungs is primarily dependent on:
  a. pressure differences between the air in the atmosphere and air in the lungs
  b. pressure differences between the air in the atmosphere and the anatomic dead space
  c. pressure differences between the air in the atmosphere and individual cells
  d. a, b, and c are correct

OBJ. 4 ___ 15. During inspiration there will be an increase in the volume of the thoracic cavity and a(n):
  a. decreasing lung volume, increasing intrapulmonary pressure
  b. decreasing lung volume, decreasing intrapulmonary pressure
  c. increasing lung volume, decreasing intrapulmonary pressure
  d. increasing lung volume, increasing intrapulmonary pressure

OBJ. 4 ___ 16. During expiration there is a(n):
  a. decrease in intrapulmonary pressure
  b. increase in intrapulmonary pressure
  c. increase in atmospheric pressure
  d. increase in the volume of the lungs

OBJ. 4 ___ 17. Each molecule of hemoglobin has the capacity to carry ___ molecules of O_2.
  a. 6
  b. 8
  c. 4
  d. 2

OBJ. 4 ___ 18. What percentage of total oxygen (O_2) is carried within red blood cells chemically bound to hemoglobin?
  a. 5 %
  b. 68 %
  c. 98 %
  d. 100 %

OBJ. 5 ___ 19. During expiration the diaphragm:
  a. contracts and progresses inferiorly toward the stomach
  b. contracts and the dome rises into the thoracic cage
  c. relaxes and the dome rises into the thoracic cage
  d. relaxes and progresses inferiorly toward the stomach

Chapter 16 The Respiratory System

OBJ. 5 ____ 20. Alveolar ventilation can be calculated by:
- a. adding the tidal volume to the inspiratory reserve volume
- b. adding the expiratory reserve volume and the residual volume
- c. subtracting the tidal volume from the inspiratory reserve
- d. subtracting the dead space from the tidal volume

OBJ. 5 ____ 21. Pulmonary ventilation refers to the:
- a. gas exchange between the blood and the alveoli
- b. amount of air in the anatomic dead space
- c. movement of air in and out of the lungs
- d. movement of air in the upper respiratory tract

OBJ. 6 ____ 22. A developing fetus obtains its oxygen from the:
- a. ductus arteriosus
- b. atmosphere
- c. ductus venosus
- d. maternal bloodstream

OBJ. 7 ____ 23. The output from baroreceptors affects the respiratory centers causing:
- a. the respiratory rate to decrease with an increase in blood pressure
- b. the respiratory rate to increase with an increase in blood pressure
- c. the respiratory rate to decrease with a decrease in blood pressure
- d. the respiratory rate to increase with a decrease in blood pressure

OBJ. 7 ____ 24. Under normal conditions the greatest effect on the respiratory centers is initiated by:
- a. decreases in P_{O2}
- b. increases and decreases in P_{O2} and P_{CO2}
- c. increases and decreases in P_{CO2}
- d. increases in P_{O2}

OBJ. 7 ____ 25. An elevated body temperature will:
- a. decrease respiration
- b. increase depth of respiration
- c. accelerate respiration
- d. not affect the respiratory rate

OBJ. 8 ____ 26. The initiation of inspiration originates with discharge of inspiratory neurons in the:
- a. diaphragm
- b. medulla
- c. pons
- d. lungs

Level -1-

Level 1 Review of Chapter Objectives 247

OBJ. 8 ___ 27. As the volume of the lungs increases, the:

    a. inspiratory center is stimulated, the expiration center inhibited
    b. the inspiratory center is inhibited, the expiratory center stimulated
    c. the inspiratory and expiratory centers are stimulated
    d. the inspiratory and expiratory centers are inhibited

OBJ. 9 ___ 28. The respiratory system is generally less efficient in the elderly because:

    a. some degree of emphysema is normal in the elderly
    b. elastic tissue deteriorates, lowering the vital capacity of lungs
    c. movements of the rib cage are restricted
    d. a, b, and c are correct

[L1] Completion:

Using the terms below, complete the following statements.

chemoreceptor	glottis	carbaminohemoglobin
apnea	external respiration	inspiration
vital capacity	expiration	mechanoreceptor
internal respiration	surfactant	larynx
alveolar ventilation	bronchioles	exercise performance

OBJ. 1   29. The movement of air out of the lungs is referred to as _____.

OBJ. 1   30. The movement of air into the lungs is called _____.

OBJ. 2   31. The oily phospholipid secretion that coats the alveolar epithelium and keeps the alveoli from collapsing is called _____.

OBJ. 3   32. Inspired air leaves the pharynx by passing through a narrow opening called the _____.

OBJ. 3   33. The glottis is surrounded and protected by the _____.

OBJ. 3   34. The part of the bronchial tree dominated by smooth muscle tissue is the _____.

OBJ. 4   35. The diffusion of gases between the alveoli and the circulating blood is termed _____.

OBJ. 4   36. The exchange of dissolved gases between the blood and the interstitial fluids in peripheral tissues is called _____.

OBJ. 5   37. With increasing age, deterioration of elastic tissue reduces lung elasticity, lowering the _____.

OBJ. 5   38. The primary function of pulmonary ventilation is to maintain adequate _____.

OBJ. 6   39. CO_2 molecules bound to hemoglobin molecules form _____.

OBJ. 7   40. When respiration is suspended due to exposure to toxic vapors or chemical irritants, reflex activity may result in _____.

OBJ. 8   41. Reflexes that are a response to changes in the volume of the lungs or in changes in arterial blood pressure are _____ reflexes.

248 Chapter 16 The Respiratory System

OBJ. 8   42. Reflexes that are a response to changes in the P_{O2} and P_{CO2} of the blood and cerebrospinal fluid are _____ reflexes.

OBJ. 9   43. The decrease in the ability of the rib cage to expand in the elderly leads directly to reduction in _____.

[L1] Matching:

Match the terms in column "B" with the terms in column "A." Use letters for answers in the spaces provided.

COLUMN "A"   **COLUMN "B"**

OBJ. 1	____ 44. Upper respiratory tract	A.	Carbon dioxide
OBJ. 2	____ 45. Alveolar macrophages	B.	Emphysema
OBJ. 3	____ 46. Larynx	C.	Loss of alveolar spaces
OBJ. 3	____ 47. Trachea	D.	Delivers air to lungs
OBJ. 3	____ 48. Lower respiratory tract	E.	Dust cells
OBJ. 4	____ 49. Hyperventilation	F.	Windpipe
OBJ. 4	____ 50. Hypoventilation	G.	Abnormal decreasing arterial P_{CO2}
OBJ. 5	____ 51. External intercostals	H.	Rise in arterial P_{CO2}
OBJ. 6	____ 52. Bicarbonate ion	I.	Prevents overexpansion of lungs
OBJ. 7	____ 53. Smoking	J.	Sound production
OBJ. 8	____ 54. Inflation reflex	K.	Stimulates inspiratory center
OBJ. 8	____ 55. Deflation reflex	L.	Lungs
OBJ. 9	____ 56. Emphysema	M.	Elevation of ribs

Level -1-

Level 1 Review of Chapter Objectives **249**

[L1] Drawing/Illustration Labeling:

Identify each numbered structure by labeling the following figures:

OBJ. 3 **FIGURE 16.1** Upper Respiratory Tract

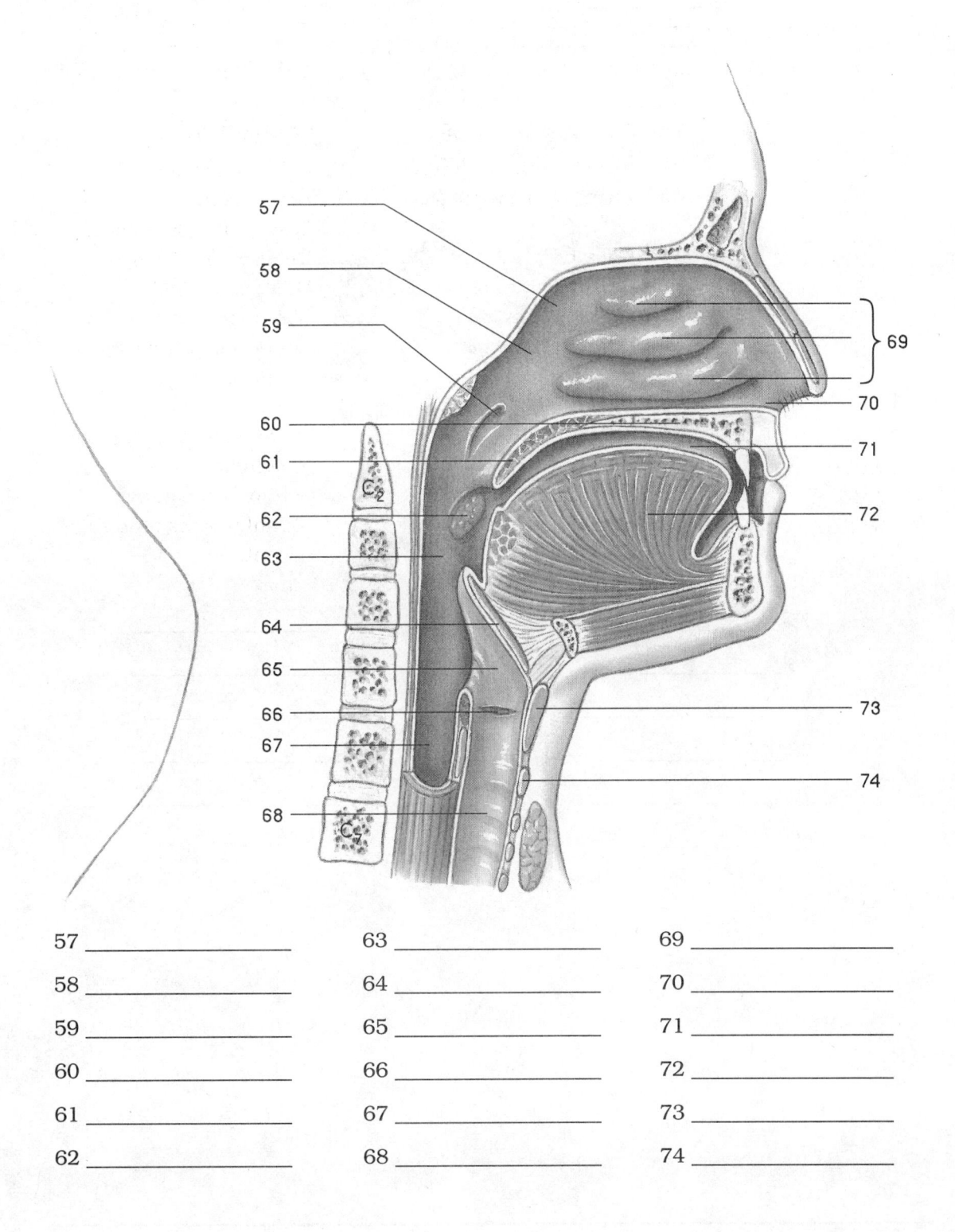

57 _____	63 _____	69 _____
58 _____	64 _____	70 _____
59 _____	65 _____	71 _____
60 _____	66 _____	72 _____
61 _____	67 _____	73 _____
62 _____	68 _____	74 _____

Chapter 16 The Respiratory System

OBJ. 3 **FIGURE 16.2** Lower Respiratory Tract

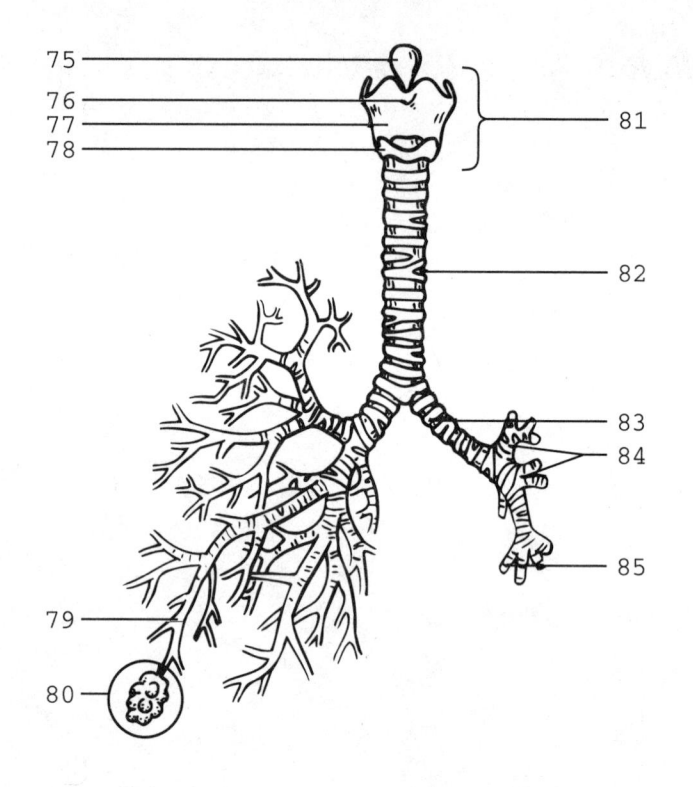

75 _____	81 _____
76 _____	82 _____
77 _____	83 _____
78 _____	84 _____
79 _____	85 _____
80 _____	

When you have successfully completed the exercises in L1 proceed to L2.

☐ LEVEL 2   CONCEPT SYNTHESIS

Concept Map I:

Using the following terms, fill in the numbered, blank spaces to complete the concept map. Follow the numbers that comply with the organization of the map.

    Lungs   Upper respiratory tract   Paranasal sinuses
    Blood   Ciliated mucous membrane   Pharynx & Larynx
    Alveoli CO_2 from alveoli into blood   Speech production

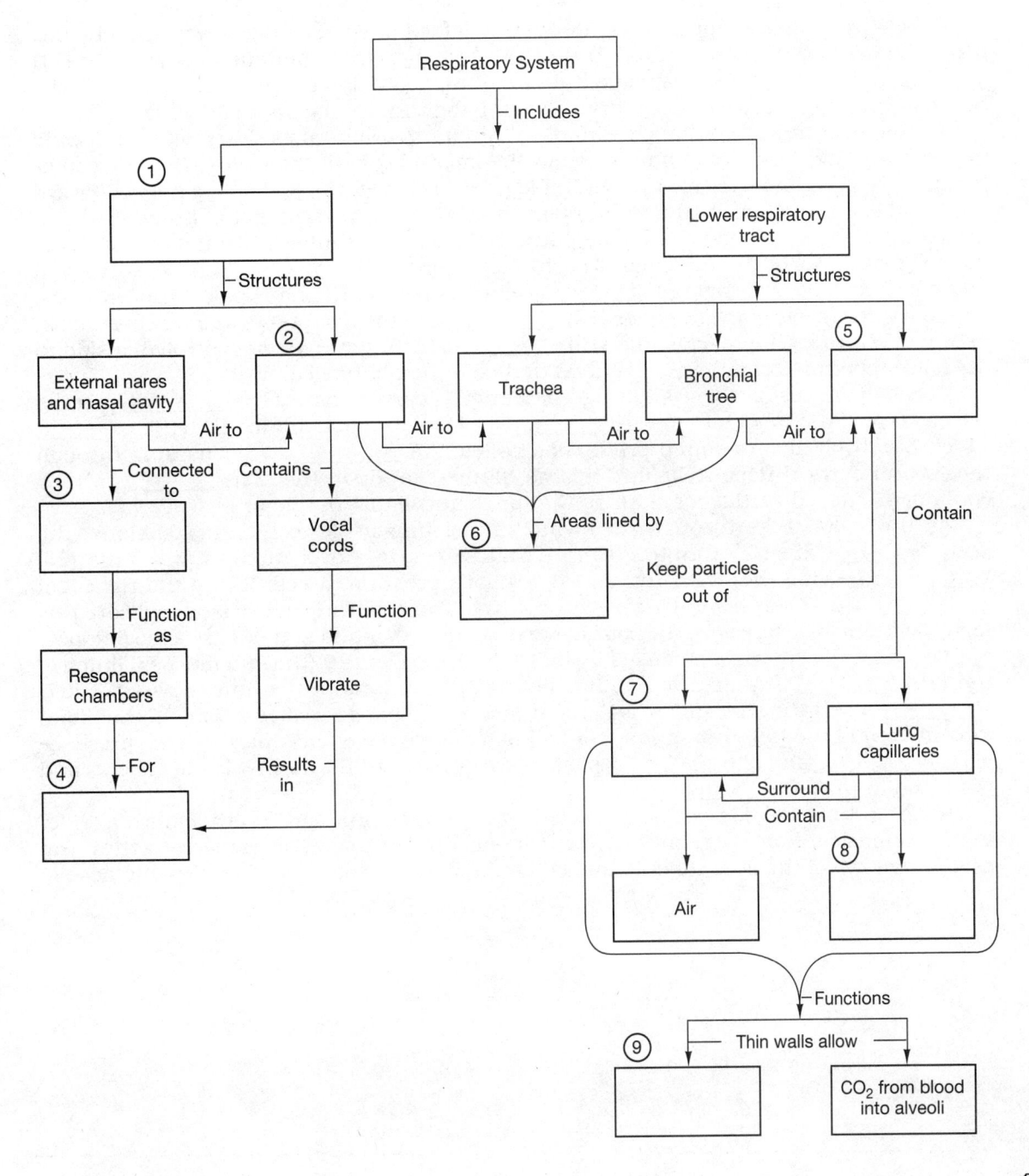

252 Chapter 16 The Respiratory System

Body Trek:

Using the terms below, fill in the blanks to complete a trek through the respiratory system.

primary bronchus	nasal cavity	nasopharynx
epiglottis	smooth muscle	oral cavity
hard palate	cilia	oxygen
alveolus	pharynx	carbon dioxide
larynx	nasal conchae	trachea
soft palate	bronchioles	external nares
vocal folds	pulmonary capillaries	phonation

Robo's trek into the upper respiratory tract is facilitated via a deep inhalation by the host. The micro-robot enters through the (10) _____ that communicate with the (11) _____. The reception area, called the vestibule, contains coarse hairs that trap airborne particles and prevent them from entering the respiratory tract.

As the robot treks into the "cavernous arena" its "thermosensors" are activated owing to the warm and humid conditions. From the lateral walls of the cavity, the "air-conditioning" system, consisting of superior, middle, and inferior (12) _____, project toward the nasal septum. As air bounces off these projections it is warmed and humidified and induces turbulence, causing airborne particles to come in contact with the mucous covering the surfaces of these lobular structures. A bony (13) _____ separates the oral and nasal cavities. A fleshy (14) _____ extends behind the hard palate, marking the boundary line between the superior (15) _____ and the rest of the pharyngeal regions. As the micro-robot approaches the (16) _____, it goes into an uncontrollable skid to the bottom because of mucus secretions that coat the pharyngeal walls.

Because the host is not swallowing, the elongate, cartilaginous (17) _____ permits the passage of the robot into the (18) _____, a region that contains the (19) _____, which are involved with sound production called (20) _____. After passing through the "sound barrier" Robo treks into a large "flume-like" duct, the (21) _____, which contains C-shaped cartilaginous rings that prevent collapse of the air passageway.

As the robot treks through the "wind tunnel" finger-like cellular extensions, the (22) _____ cause a "countercurrent" that serves to move mucus toward the (23) _____. Leaving the "wind tunnel," the robot's program directs it into the right (24) _____, a decision made by mission control. The robot's descent is complicated by increased "trek resistance" as the passageways get narrower and at times are almost impossible because of constriction caused by (25) _____ tissue in the sub mucosal lining of the (26) _____. After a few minor delays the trek continues into a sac-like (27) _____, where the atmosphere is dry and gaseous exchange creates a "breeze" that flows into and out of the "see-through" spheres. Robo's chemoreceptors "pick up" the presence of (28) _____ and (29) _____ passing freely between the air inside the spheres and the blood in the (30) _____.

Robo's return trek for exit is facilitated by a "reverse program" that includes a "ride" up the mucus, making the robot's ascent fast, smooth, and easy. Upon reaching the nasal cavity, removal of the little robot is immediate, due to the host's need to blow his nose.

Level 2

Level 2 Concept Synthesis

[L2] Multiple Choice:

Place the letter corresponding to the correct answer in the space provided.

_____ 31. The paranasal sinuses include:

    a. occipital, parietal, temporal, and mandibular
    b. ethmoid, parietal, sphenoid, and temporal
    c. frontal, sphenoid, ethmoid, and maxillary
    d. mandibular, maxillary, frontal, temporal

_____ 32. A rise in arterial P_{CO_2} elevates cerebrospinal fluid (CSF) carbon dioxide levels and stimulates the chemoreceptive neurons of the medulla to produce:

    a. hypoventilation
    b. hyperventilation

_____ 33. The primary function of pulmonary ventilation is to maintain adequate:

    a. air in the anatomic dead space
    b. pulmonary surfactant
    c. vital capacity
    d. alveolar ventilation

_____ 34. The purpose of the fluid in the pleural cavity is to:

    a. provide a medium for the exchange of O_2 and CO_2
    b. reduce friction between the parietal and visceral pleura
    c. allow for the exchange of electrolytes during respiratory movements
    d. provide lubrication for diaphragmatic constriction

_____ 35. The most important factor determining air-way resistance is:

    a. interactions between flowing gas molecules
    b. length of the airway
    c. thickness of the wall of the airway radius
    d. airway radius

_____ 36. The sympathetic division of the ANS causes _____ of airway smooth muscle, therefore, resistance is _____.

    a. relaxation; decreased
    b. relaxation; increased
    c. constriction; increased
    d. constriction; decreased

_____ 37. If a person is breathing 15 times a minute and has a tidal volume of 500 ml, the total minute respiratory volume is:

    a. 7500 min/ml
    b. 515 ml
    c. 7500 ml/min
    d. 5150 ml

_____ 38. The most effective means of increasing alveolar ventilation is:

    a. increase rapid shallow breathing
    b. breathe normally
    c. breathe slowly and deeper
    d. increase total pulmonary circulation

254 Chapter 16 The Respiratory System

_____ 39. As the number of the molecules of gas dissolved in a liquid increases:
- a. the pressure of the gas decreases
- b. the pressure of the gas increases
- c. the pressure of the gas is not affected
- d. none of these

_____ 40. The correct sequential transport of O_2 from the tissue capillaries to O_2 consumption in cells is:
- a. lung, alveoli, plasma, erythrocytes, cells
- b. erythrocytes, plasma, interstitial fluid, cells
- c. plasma, erythrocytes, alveoli, cells
- d. erythrocytes, interstitial fluid, plasma, cells

_____ 41. It is important that free H^+ resulting from dissociation of H_2CO_3 combine with hemoglobin to reduce the possibility of:
- a. CO_2 escaping from the RBC
- b. recombining with H_2O
- c. an acidic condition within the blood
- d. maintaining a constant pH in the blood

_____ 42. One of the early symptoms of emphysema is:
- a. a reduced expiratory volume
- b. the lung becomes solid and airless
- c. the lungs become inflamed
- d. the vital capacity is reduced

[L2] Completion:

Using the terms below, complete the following statements.

thyroid cartilage	intrapleural	pneumothorax
epiglottis	alveolar ventilation	anatomic dead space
laryngopharynx	cribiform plate	hypoxia

43. The portion of the pharynx lying between the hyoid and entrance to the esophagus is the _____.

44. The elastic cartilage that prevents the entry of liquids or solid food into the respiratory passageway is the _____.

45. The "Adam's apple" is the prominent ridge on the anterior surface of the _____.

46. The roof of the nasal cavity is formed primarily by the _____.

47. A decline in oxygen content causes affected tissues to suffer from _____.

48. An injury to the chest wall that penetrates the parietal pleura or damages the alveoli and the visceral pleura is called a _____.

49. The pressure measured in the slender space between the parietal and visceral pleura is the _____ pressure.

50. The volume of air in the conducting passages is known as the _____.

51. The amount of air reaching the alveoli each minute is the _____.

[L2] Short Essay:

Briefly answer the following questions in the spaces provided below.

52. What are the primary functions of the respiratory system?

53. How is the inhaled air warmed and humidified in the nasal cavities, and why is this type of environmental condition necessary?

54. What protective mechanisms comprise the respiratory defense system?

55. What is the relationship between the volume and the pressure of a gas?

56. What is the relationship between rise in arterial P_{CO_2} and hyperventilation?

When you have successfully completed the exercises in L2 proceed to L3.

☐ LEVEL 3   CRITICAL THINKING/APPLICATION

Using principles and concepts learned about the respiratory system, answer the following questions. Write your answers on a separate sheet of paper.

1. I. M. Good decides to run outside all winter long in spite of the cold weather. How does running in cold weather affect the respiratory passageways and the lungs?
2. C. U. Later's son is the victim of a tracheal defect that resulted in the formation of complete cartilaginous rings instead of the normal C-shaped tracheal rings. After eating a meal he experiences difficulty when swallowing and feels pain in the thoracic region. Why?
3. M. I. Right has been a two-pack-a-day smoker for the last 20 years. Recently, he has experienced difficulty breathing. After a series of pulmonary tests his doctor informs Mr. Right that he has emphysema. What is the relationship between his condition and his breathing difficulties?

CHAPTER 17

The Digestive System

■ Overview

The digestive system is the "food processor" in the human body. The system works at two levels—one mechanical, the other chemical. The mechanical processes include ingestion, mastication (chewing), deglutition (swallowing), peristalsis, compaction, and defecation, while chemical digestion and absorption serve as chemical mechanisms.

By the time you are 65 years old, you will have consumed more than 70,000 meals and disposed of 50 tons of food, most of which has to be converted into chemical forms that cells can utilize for their metabolic functions.

After ingestion and mastication, the food is propelled through the muscular gastrointestinal (GI) tract where it is chemically split into smaller molecular substances. The products of the digestive process are then absorbed from the GI tract into the circulating blood and transported wherever they are needed in the body or, if undigested, are eliminated from the body. As the food is processed through the GI tract, accessory organs such as the salivary glands, liver, and pancreas assist in the "breakdown" process.

Chapter 17 includes exercises organized to guide your study of the structure and function of the digestive tract and accessory organs, hormonal and nervous system influences on the digestive process, and the chemical and mechanical events that occur during absorption.

☐ LEVEL 1   REVIEW OF CHAPTER OBJECTIVES

1. Identify the organs of the digestive tract and the accessory organs of digestion.
2. List the primary functions of the digestive system.
3. Describe the histological characteristics of each segment of the digestive tract in relation to the function.
4. Describe the characteristics of smooth muscle and explain how ingested materials are propelled through the digestive tract.
5. Describe how food is processed in the mouth and describe the key events of the swallowing process.
6. Describe the anatomy of the stomach, its histological features, and its roles in digestion and absorption.
7. Explain the functions of the intestinal secretions and discuss the relative significance of digestion in the small intestine.

Level 1 Review of Chapter Objectives 257

8. Describe the structure and functions of the pancreas, liver, and gall bladder and explain how their activities are regulated.
9. Describe the structure of the large intestine, its movements, and its absorptive processes.
10. Describe the digestion and absorption of carbohydrates, lipids, and proteins.
11. Describe the changes in the digestive system that occur with aging.

[L1] Multiple Choice:

Place the letter corresponding to the correct answer in the space provided.

OBJ. 1 ___ 1. Which one of the following organs is not a part of the digestive system?
- a. liver
- b. gall bladder
- c. spleen
- d. pancreas

OBJ. 1 ___ 2. Of the following selections, the one which contains only accessory structures is:
- a. pharynx, esophagus, small and large intestine
- b. oral cavity, stomach, pancreas and liver
- c. salivary glands, pancreas, liver, gall bladder
- d. tongue, teeth, stomach, small and large intestine

OBJ. 2 ___ 3. The lining of the digestive tract plays a defensive role by protecting surrounding tissues against:
- a. corrosive effects of digestive acids and enzymes
- b. mechanical stresses
- c. pathogenic organisms swallowed with food
- d. a, b, and c are correct

OBJ. 3 ___ 4. The mucous-producing, unicellular glands found in the mucosal epithelium of the stomach and small and large intestine are:
- a. enteroendocrine cells
- b. parietal cells
- c. chief cells
- d. goblet cells

OBJ. 4 ___ 5. Which of the layers of the digestive tube is (are) most responsible for peristalsis along the esophagus?
- a. tunica mucosa
- b. circular and longitudinal layers
- c. tunica submucosa
- d. a, b, and c are correct

OBJ. 4 ___ 6. Which of the following is true about peristalsis in the esophagus?
- a. The rate of peristaltic waves in the esophagus is constant.
- b. The peristalsis is controlled by the nervous system.
- c. The peristalsis is controlled by the endocrine system.
- d. Peristalsis is controlled by the nervous and the endocrine systems.

Chapter 17 The Digestive System

OBJ. 4 ___ 7. Swirling, mixing, and churning motions of the digestive tract provide:

    a. action of acids, enzymes, and buffers
    b. enhanced mechanical processing after ingestion
    c. chemical breakdown of food into small fragments
    d. a, b, and c are correct

OBJ. 5 ___ 8. The three pairs of salivary glands that secrete into the oral cavity include the:

    a. pharyngeal, palatoglossal, palatopharyngeal
    b. lingual, labial, frenulum
    c. uvular, ankyloglossal, hypoglossal
    d. parotid, sublingual, submandibular

OBJ. 5 ___ 9. Crushing, mashing, and grinding of food is best accomplished by the action of the:

    a. incisors
    b. bicuspids
    c. cuspids
    d. molars

OBJ. 6 ___ 10. Stomach emptying occurs more rapidly when:

    a. there is a greater volume of stomach contents
    b. there is a greater volume of duodenal contents
    c. there is more fat in the stomach
    d. the material in the stomach is hyperosmotic to the plasma

OBJ. 6 ___ 11. The hormone gastrin:

    a. is produced in response to sympathetic stimulation
    b. is secreted by the pancreatic islets
    c. increases the activity of parietal and chief cells
    d. inhibits the activity of the muscularis externa of the stomach

OBJ. 7 ___ 12. The three divisions of the small intestine are:

    a. cephalic, gastric, intestinal
    b. buccal, pharyngeal, esophageal
    c. duodenum, jejunum, ileum
    d. fundus, body, pylorus

OBJ. 7 ___ 13. The three phases of gastric function include:

    a. parotid, sublingual, submandicular
    b. duodenal, jejunal, iliocecal
    c. cephalic, gastric, intestinal
    d. buccal, pharyngeal, esophageal

OBJ. 8 ___ 14. The functions of the gall bladder involve:

    a. contraction and synthesis
    b. contraction and absorption
    c. synthesis and absorption
    d. absorption and digestion

Level 1 Review of Chapter Objectives 259

OBJ. 8 ___ 15. The primary function(s) of the liver is (are):

    a. metabolic regulation
    b. hematological regulation
    c. bile production
    d. a, b, and c are correct

OBJ. 8 ___ 16. The hormone that promotes the flow of bile and of pancreatic juice containing enzymes is:

    a. secretin
    b. gastrin
    c. enterogastrone
    d. cholecystokinin

OBJ. 8 ___ 17. The secretion of parietal cells that facilitate absorption of vitamin B12 across the intestinal lining is:

    a. intrinsic factor
    b. hydrochloric acid
    c. gastrin
    d. secretin

OBJ. 8 ___ 18. The central mechanisms regulating gastric function are:

    a. direct control by the endocrine system, indirect regulation by the ANS
    b. direct control by the CNS, and indirect regulation by local hormones
    c. direct control by the CNS and the ANS
    d. direct control by local homeostatic mechanisms

OBJ. 9 ___ 19. Undigested food residues are moved through the large intestine in the following sequence:

    a. cecum, colon, and rectum
    b. colon, cecum, rectum
    c. ileum, colon, rectum
    d. duodenum, jejunum, ileum

OBJ. 10 ___ 20. Hydrochloric acid in the stomach functions primarily to:

    a. facilitate protein digestion
    b. facilitate lipid digestion
    c. facilitate carbohydrate digestion
    d. hydrolyze peptide bonds

OBJ. 10 ___ 21. A molecule absorbed into the lacteals of the lymphatic system within the walls of the small intestine is:

    a. glucose
    b. fat
    c. vitamin B12
    d. amino acids

OBJ. 11 ___ 22. One age-related change in the digestive system is that smooth muscle tone of the digestive tract wall decreases with age.

    a. true
    b. false

Chapter 17 The Digestive System

[L1] Completion:

Using the terms below, complete the following statements.

gastrin	cuspids	carbohydrates	diarrhea and constipation
chyme	esophagus	peristalsis	pyloric sphincter
haustrae	lamina propria	lipase	pepsin
acini	digestion	duodenum	cholecystokinin

OBJ. 1   23. The digestive tube between the pharynx and the stomach is the _____.

OBJ. 2   24. The chemical breakdown of food into small organic fragments suitable for absorption by the digestive epithelium refers to _____.

OBJ. 3   25. The layer of loose connective tissue in the mucosa that contains blood vessels, glands, and lymph nodes is the _____.

OBJ. 4   26. The muscularis externa propels materials from one portion of the digestive tract to another by waves of muscular contractions referred to as _____.

OBJ. 4   27. Stimulation of stretch receptors in the stomach wall and chemoreceptors in the mucosa trigger the release of _____.

OBJ. 5   28. The conical teeth used for tearing or slashing are the _____.

OBJ. 5   29. Salivary enzymes in the oral cavity begin with the digestive process by acting on _____.

OBJ. 6   30. The agitation of ingested materials with the gastric juices secreted by the glands of the stomach produces a viscous, soupy mixture called _____.

OBJ. 7   31. The portion of the small intestine that receives chyme from the stomach and exocrine secretions from the pancreas and liver is the _____.

OBJ. 7   32. The two intestinal hormones that inhibit gastric secretion to some degree are secretin and _____.

OBJ. 7   33. The ring of muscle tissue that regulates the flow of chyme between the stomach and small intestine is the _____.

OBJ. 8   34. The blind pockets lined by simple cuboidal epithelium that produce pancreatic juice are called _____.

OBJ. 9   35. The series of pouches that form the wall of colon permitting considerable distension and elongation are called _____.

OBJ. 10   36. The pancreatic enzyme that hydrolyzes triglycerides into glycerol and fatty acids is pancreatic _____.

OBJ. 10   37. The gastric secretion that digests protein into smaller peptide chains is _____.

OBJ. 11   38. Gastric disturbances that increase with age are _____.

Level 1 Review of Chapter Objectives

[L1] Matching:

Match the terms in column "A" with the terms in column "B." Use letters for answers in the spaces provided.

		COLUMN "A"	COLUMN "B"
OBJ. 1	____	39. Stomach	A. Starch digestion
OBJ. 2	____	40. Mechanical processing	B. Mucosal chemoreceptors
OBJ. 3	____	41. Swallowing	C. Fat digestion
OBJ. 4	____	42. Secretin	D. Deglutition
OBJ. 5	____	43. Chewing	E. Hepatocytes
OBJ. 5	____	44. Parotid gland	F. Small intestine
OBJ. 6	____	45. Chief cells	G. Vagus nerve
OBJ. 6	____	46. Distention of stomach	H. Liver Disease
OBJ. 6	____	47. Cephalic phase	I. Haustra
OBJ. 6	____	48. Gastric phase	J. Emulsification of fats
OBJ. 7	____	49. Villi	K. Effect of aging
OBJ. 8	____	50. Liver cells	L. Mastication
OBJ. 8	____	51. Cirrhosis	M. Salivary amylase
OBJ. 9	____	52. Colon	N. Gastroenteric reflex
OBJ. 10	____	53. Salivary amylase	O. Pepsinogen
OBJ. 10	____	54. Trypsin	P. Protein digestion
OBJ. 10	____	55. Bile salts	Q. Rugae
OBJ. 10	____	56. Lipases	R. Tearing with teeth
OBJ. 10	____	57. Colonic bacteria	S. Peptide hormone
OBJ. 11	____	58. Thinning of GI tract lining	T. Produce vitamin K

262 Chapter 17 The Digestive System

[L1] Drawing/Illustration Labeling:

Identify each numbered structure by labeling the following figure:

FIGURE 17.1 The Digestive Tract

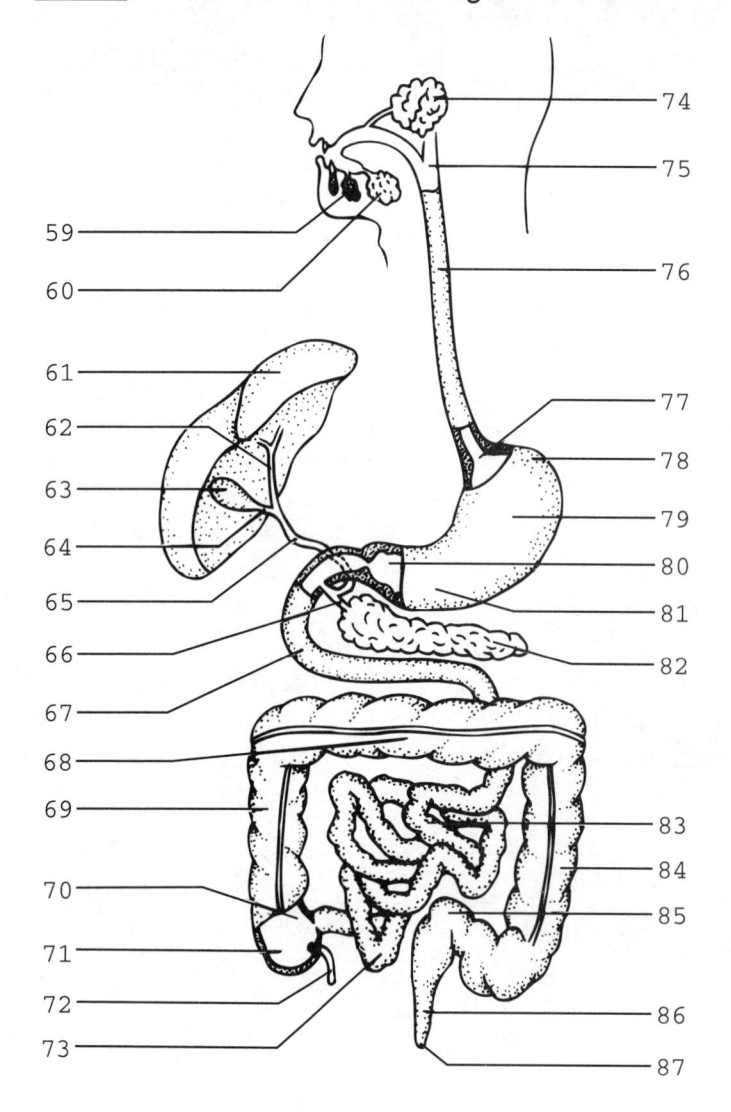

59 _____
60 _____
61 _____
62 _____
63 _____
64 _____
65 _____
66 _____
67 _____
68 _____
69 _____
70 _____
71 _____
72 _____
73 _____
74 _____
75 _____
76 _____
77 _____
78 _____
79 _____
80 _____
81 _____
82 _____
83 _____
84 _____
85 _____
86 _____
87 _____

Level 1

When you have successfully completed the exercises in L1 proceed to L2.

LEVEL 2 CONCEPT SYNTHESIS

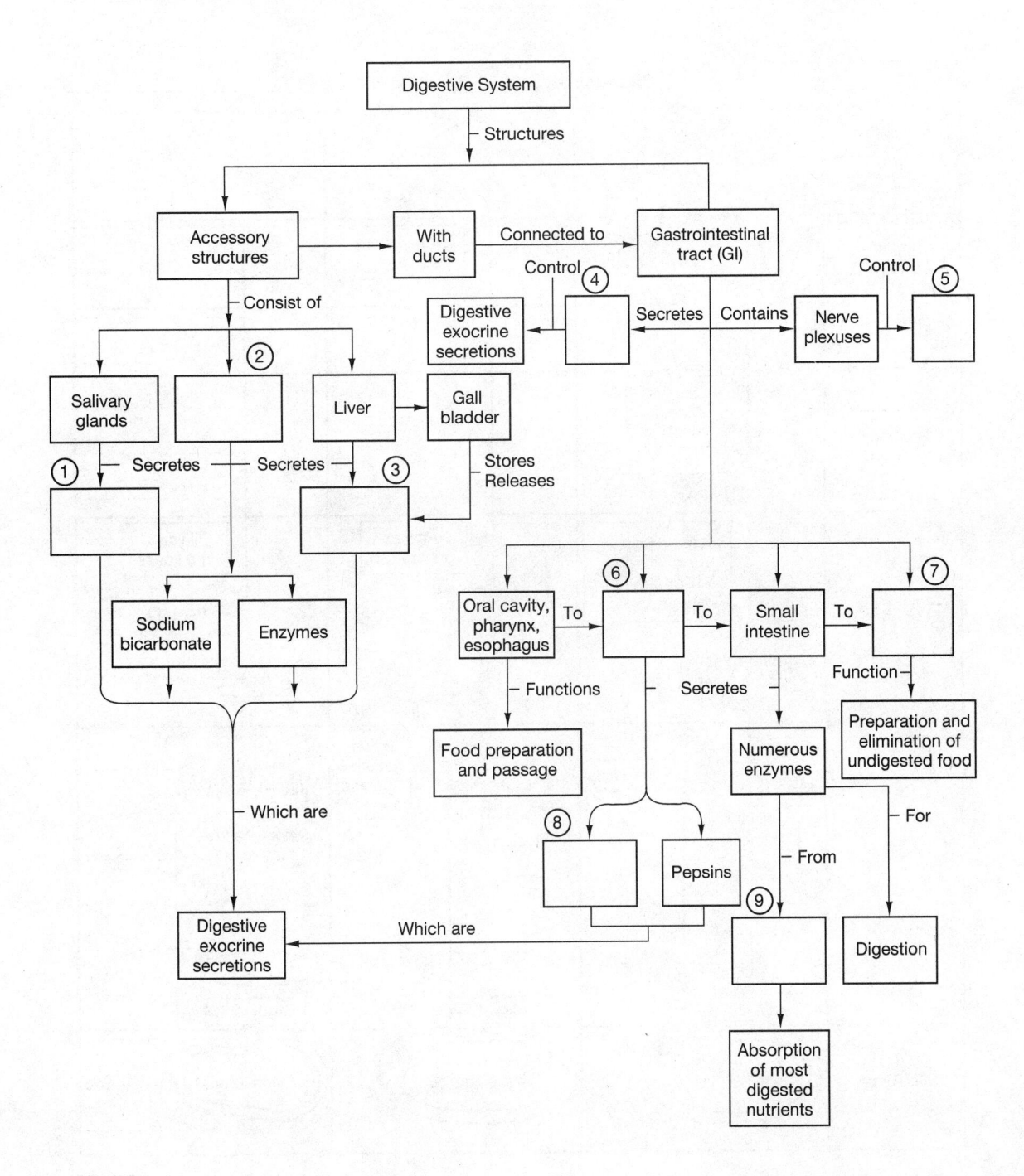

Concept Map I:

Using the following terms, fill in the numbered, blank spaces to complete the concept map. Follow the numbers that comply with the organization of the map.

- Digestive tract movements
- Hydrochloric acid
- Intestinal mucosa
- Stomach
- Large intestine
- Bile
- Hormones
- Pancreas
- Amylase

264 Chapter 17 The Digestive System

Concept Map II:

Using the following terms, fill in the circled, numbered, blank spaces to complete the concept map. Follow the numbers that comply with the organization of the map.

- Monoglycerides, fatty acids in micelles
- Polypeptides
- Lacteal
- Triglycerides
- Small intestine
- Simple sugars
- Amino acids
- Esophagus
- Complex sugars and starches
- Disaccharides, trisaccharides

Chemical events in digestion

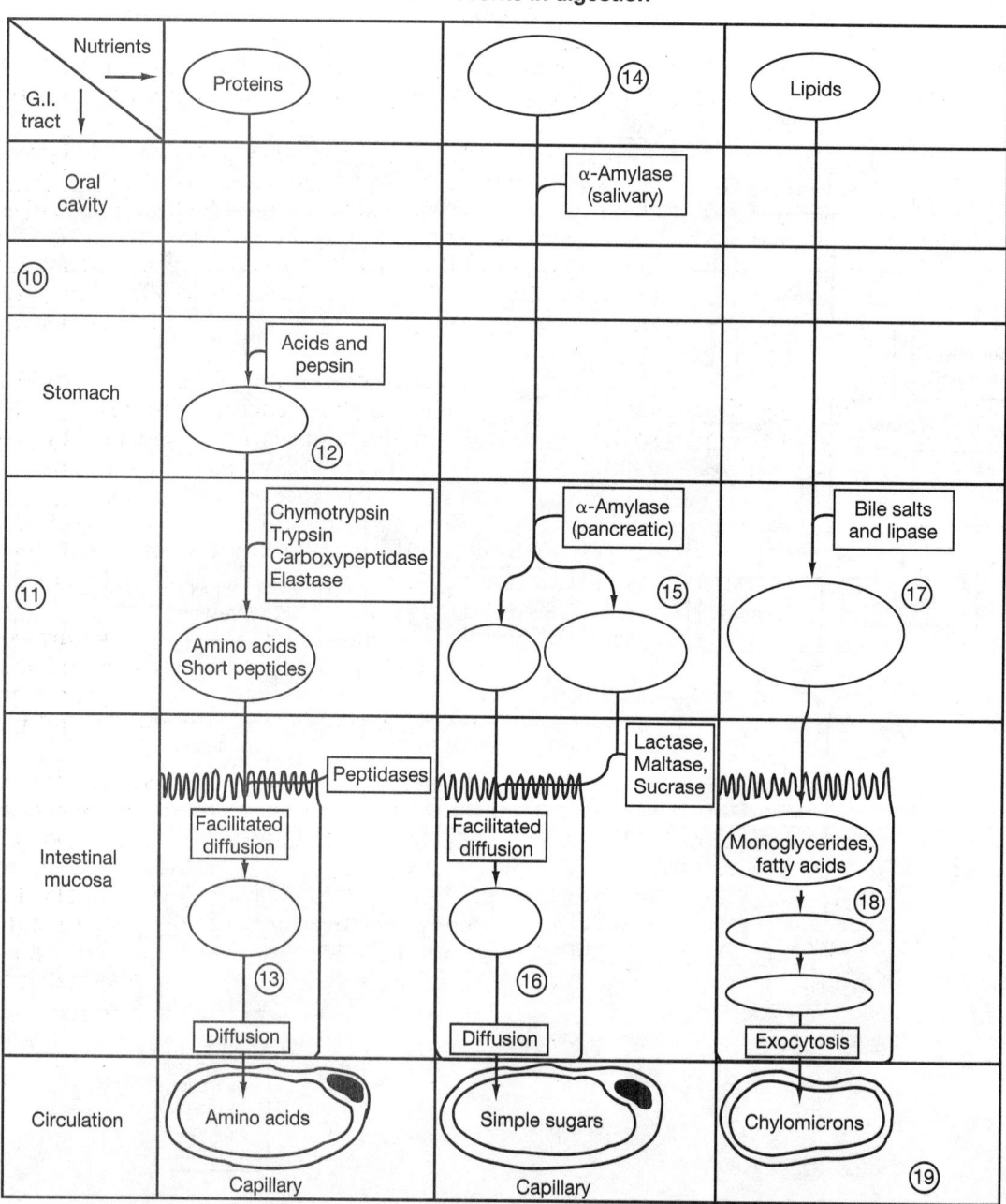

Nutrients → G.I. tract ↓	Proteins	(14)	Lipids
Oral cavity		α-Amylase (salivary)	
(10)			
Stomach	Acids and pepsin → (12)		
(11)	Chymotrypsin, Trypsin, Carboxypeptidase, Elastase → Amino acids, Short peptides	α-Amylase (pancreatic) → (15)	Bile salts and lipase → (17)
Intestinal mucosa	Peptidases → Facilitated diffusion → (13) → Diffusion	Lactase, Maltase, Sucrase → Facilitated diffusion → (16) → Diffusion	Monoglycerides, fatty acids → (18) → Exocytosis
Circulation	Amino acids (Capillary)	Simple sugars (Capillary)	Chylomicrons (19)

Level 2

Level 2 Concept Synthesis 265

Body Trek:

Using the terms below, fill in the blanks to complete the trek through the digestive system.

chyme	pancreas	mastication
saliva	hydrochloric	tongue
stomach	large intestine	protein
palates	swallowing	feces
pharynx	gastric juices	teeth
lubrication	gingivae (gums)	rugae
carbohydrates	peristalsis	uvula
mucus	duodenum	pylorus
pepsin	mechanical processing	lipase
salivary amylase	esophagus	oral cavity

On this trek, Robo will follow a bolus of food as it passes through the GI tract. The micro-robot's metallic construction provides protection from the acids and enzymes that are a part of the digestive process.

Robo's entry through the mouth into the (20) _____ is quick and easy. Food preparation via analysis, (21) _____, digestion by salivary amylase, and (22) _____ occurs in this region of the processing system. Noticeable features include pink ridges, the (23) _____ that surround the base of the glistening white (24) _____ used in handling and (25) _____ of food. The roof of the cavity is formed by hard and soft (26) _____ while the floor is comprised of the (27) _____. Three pairs of salivary glands secrete (28) _____ which contains the enzyme (29) _____, a part of the digestive process that acts on (30) _____.

After food preparation and the start of the digestive process, the food bolus with Robo trekking along passes into the (31) _____, past a dangling structure, the (32) _____ supported by the posterior part of the soft palate. Additional movement is provided by powerful constrictor muscles involved in (33) _____, causing propulsion into an elongated, flattened tube, the (34) _____. Alternating wave-like contractions called (35) _____ facilitate passage to a region that "looks" like a ring of muscle, the gastro-esophageal sphincter, which serves as the entry "gate" into the (36) _____. In this enlarged chamber the robot's sensors and the food bolus are "agitated" because of glandular secretions called (37) _____ that produce a viscous, soupy mixture referred to as (38) _____. The walls of the chamber look "wrinkled" due to folds called (39) _____ that are covered with a slippery, slimy (40) _____ coat that offers protection from erosion and other potential damage. Robo's chemosensors detect the presence of (41) _____ acid and an enzyme called (52) _____, both of which are involved in the preparation and partial digestion of (43) _____.

Following the digestive delay, the chyme-covered robot is squirted through the (44) _____ into the (45) _____ of the small intestine. The presence of fats and other partially digested food, including the chyme, creates a rather crowded condition. Some of the fat begins to "break up" owing to the action of (46) _____, which has been released from the (47) _____ where it is secreted. Robo's descent continues into the (48) _____ where the micro-robot becomes a part of the compacted, undigestible residue that comprises the (49) _____. The remainder of the trek involves important "movements" that eventually return Robo to mission control for cleanup and re-energizing for the next adventure.

[L2] Multiple Choice:

Place the letter corresponding to the correct answer in the space provided.

_____ 50. Many visceral smooth muscle networks show rhythmic cycles of activity in the absence of neural stimulation due to the presence of:

    a. direct contact with motor neurons carrying impulses to the CNS

    b. an action potential generated and conducted over the sarcolemma

    c. the single motor units that contract independently of each other

    d. pacesetter cells that spontaneously depolarize and trigger contraction of entire muscular sheets

_____ 51. The reason a completely dry food bolus cannot be swallowed is:

    a. the dry food inhibits parasympathetic activity in the esophagus

    b. friction with the walls of the esophagus makes peristalsis ineffective

    c. the dry food stimulates sympathetic activity, inhibiting peristalsis

    d. a, b, and c are correct

_____ 52. The two factors that play an important part in the movement of chyme from the stomach to the small intestine are:

    a. CNS and ANS regulation

    b. release of HCl and gastric juice

    c. stomach distension and gastrin release

    d. sympathetic and parasympathetic stimulation

_____ 53. The plicae of the intestinal mucosa, which bears the intestinal villi, are structural features that provide for:

    a. increased total surface area for absorption

    b. stabilizing the mesenteries attached to the dorsal body wall

    c. gastric contractions that chum and swirl the gastric contents

    d. initiating enterogastric reflexes

_____ 54. Most intestinal absorption occurs in the:

    a. distal end of the duodenum

    b. body of the stomach

    c. proximal half of the duodenum

    d. proximal half of the jejunum

_____ 55. The primary function(s) of the gastrointestinal juice is (are) to:

    a. moisten the chyme

    b. assist in buffering acids

    c. dissolve digestive enzymes and products of digestion

    d. a, b, and c are correct

_____ 56. The average composition of the fecal waste material is:
   a. 20% water, 5% bacteria, 75% indigestible remains and inorganic matter
   b. 45% water, 45% indigestible and inorganic matter, 10% bacteria
   c. 60% water, 10% bacteria, 30% indigestible and inorganic matter
   d. 75% water, 5% bacteria, 20% indigestible materials, inorganic matter, and epithelial remains

_____ 57. The external anal sphincter is under voluntary control.
   a. true
   b. false

_____ 58. The "doorway to the liver" (porta hepatis) is a complex that includes the:
   a. hilus, bile duct, cystic duct
   b. bile duct, hepatic portal vein, hepatic artery
   c. caudate lobe, quadrate lobe, and hepatic duct
   d. left lobe, right lobe, and round ligament

[L2] Completion:

Using the terms below, complete the following statements.

| lacteals | enamel | mesenteries | visceral peritoneum |
| cephalic | adventitia | intestinal | segmentation |

59. The serosa that lines the inner surfaces of the body wall is called the _____.
60. Double sheets of peritoneal membrane that connect the parietal peritoneum with the visceral peritoneum are called _____.
61. The muscularis externa is surrounded by a layer of loose connective tissue called the _____.
62. Movements that churn and fragment digested materials in the small intestine are termed _____.
63. Terminal lymphatics contained within each villus are called _____.
64. Cavities in one's teeth are due to erosions in the _____ layer of the tooth.
65. The _____ phase of gastric activity controls the rate of gastric emptying.
66. The _____ phase of gastric activity prepares the stomach to receive ingested materials.

268 Chapter 17   The Digestive System

[L2]   Short Essay:

Briefly answer the following questions in the spaces provided below.

67. What seven (7) integrated steps comprise the digestive functions?

68. What four (4) types of teeth are found in the oral cavity and what is the function of each type?

69. What three (3) phases are involved in the regulation of gastric function? What regulatory mechanism(s) dominate each phase?

70. What three (3) basic categories describe the functions of the liver?

71. What two (2) distinct functions are performed by the pancreas?

When you have successfully completed the exercises in L2 proceed to L3.

☐ LEVEL 3   CRITICAL THINKING/APPLICATION

Using principles and concepts learned about the digestive system, answer the following questions. Write your answers on a separate sheet of paper.

1. A 19-year-old male walks into a hospital emergency room and reports the following symptoms: fever (103 degrees F), pain in the neck, headache, and swelling in front of and below the ear. What is your diagnosis and what should be done to relieve the condition and to avoid the problem in the future?

2. O. B. Good likes his four to six cups of caffeinated coffee daily, and he relieves his thirst by drinking a few alcoholic beverages during the day. He constantly complains of heartburn. What is happening in his GI tract to cause the "burning" sensation?

3. After studying anatomy and physiology for a year, I. M. Nervous complains of recurring abdominal pains, usually 2 to 3 hours after eating. Additional eating seems to relieve the pain. She finally agrees to see her doctor, who diagnoses her condition as a duodenal ulcer. Use your knowledge of anatomy and physiology to explain the diagnosis to this patient.

CHAPTER 18

Nutrition and Metabolism

■ Overview

The processes of metabolism and energetics are intriguing to most students of anatomy and physiology because of the mystique associated with the "fate of absorbed nutrients." This mysterious phrase raises questions such as:

- What happens to the food we eat?
- What determines the "fate" of the food and the way it will be used?
- How are the nutrients from the food utilized by the body?

All cells require energy for anabolic processes and breakdown mechanisms involving catabolic processes. Provisions for these cellular activities are made by the food we eat; these activities provide energy, promote tissue growth and repair, and serve as regulatory mechanisms for the body's metabolic machinery.

The exercises in Chapter 18 provide for study and review of cellular metabolism; metabolic interactions; diet and nutrition; and bioenergetics. Much of the material you have learned in previous chapters will be of value as you "see" the integrated forces of the digestive and cardiovascular system exert a coordinated effort to initiate and advance the work of metabolism.

☐ LEVEL 1   REVIEW OF CHAPTER OBJECTIVES

1. Define metabolism and explain why cells need to synthesize new organic components.
2. Describe the basic steps in glycolysis, the TCA cycle, and the electron transport SYSTEM.
3. Describe the pathways involved in lipid metabolism.
4. Discuss protein metabolism and the use of proteins as an energy source.
5. Discuss nucleic acid metabolism.
6. Explain what constitutes a balanced diet, and why it is important.
7. Discuss the functions of vitamins, minerals and other important nutrients.
8. Describe the significance of the caloric value of foods.
9. Define metabolic rate and discuss the factors involved in determining an individual's metabolic rate.
10. Discuss the homeostatic mechanisms that maintain a constant body temperature.

Chapter 18 Nutrition and Metabolism

[L1] Multiple Choice:

Place the letter corresponding to the correct answer in the space provided.

OBJ. 1   ____ 1. Neurons must be provided with a reliable supply of glucose because they are:
- a. usually unable to metabolize other molecules
- b. involved primarily with transmitting nerve impulses
- c. primarily located in the brain
- d. covered with myelinated fibrous sheaths

OBJ. 1   ____ 2. In resting skeletal muscles, a significant portion of the metabolic demand is met through the:
- a. catabolism of glucose
- b. catabolism of fatty acids
- c. catabolism of glycogen
- d. anabolism of ADP to ATP

OBJ. 1   ____ 3. The process that breaks down organic substrates, releasing energy that can be used to synthesize ATP or other high energy compounds is:
- a. metabolism
- b. anabolism
- c. catabolism
- d. oxidation

OBJ. 2   ____ 4. In glycolysis, six carbon glucose molecules are broken down into 2 three-carbon molecules of:
- a. pyruvic acid
- b. acetyl-CoA
- c. citric acid
- d. oxaloacetic acid

OBJ. 2   ____ 5. The first step in a sequence of enzymatic reactions in the tricarboxylic acid cycle is the formation of:
- a. acetyl-CoA
- b. citric acid
- c. oxaloacetate
- d. pyruvic acid

OBJ. 2   ____ 6. For each glucose molecule converted to 2 pyruvates, the anaerobic reaction sequence in glycolysis provides a net gain of ____ molecules of ATP for the cell.
- a. 2
- b. 4
- c. 1
- d. 6

OBJ. 2   ____ 7. For each glucose molecule processed during aerobic cellular respiration the cell gains ____ molecules of ATP.
- a. 4
- b. 32
- c. 36
- d. 24

Level 1 Review of Chapter Objectives 271

OBJ. 3 ___ 8. Although small quantities of lipids are normally stored in the liver, most of the synthesized triglycerides are bound to:
   a. glucose molecules
   b. transport proteins
   c. adipocytes
   d. hepatocytes in the liver

OBJ. 4 ___ 9. The factor(s) that make protein catabolism an impractical source of quick energy is (are):
   a. their energy yield is less than that of lipids
   b. one of the byproducts, ammonia, is a toxin that can damage cells
   c. proteins are important structural and functional cellular components
   d. a, b, and c are correct

OBJ. 4 ___ 10. The first step in amino acid catabolism is the removal of the:
   a. carboxyl group
   b. amino group
   c. keto acid
   d. hydrogen from the central carbon

OBJ. 5 ___ 11. All cells synthesize RNA, but DNA synthesis occurs only:
   a. in red blood cells
   b. in cells that are preparing for mitosis
   c. in lymph and cerebrospinal fluid
   d. in the bone marrow

OBJ. 6 ___ 12. Minerals, vitamins, and water are classified as essential nutrients because:
   a. they are used by the body in large quantities
   b. the body cannot synthesize the nutrients in sufficient quantities
   c. they are the major providers of calories for the body
   d. a, b, and c are correct

OBJ. 6 ___ 13. The "trace" minerals found in extremely small quantities in the body include:
   a. sodium, potassium, chloride, calcium
   b. phosphorus, magnesium, calcium, iron
   c. iron, zinc, copper, manganese
   d. phosphorus, zinc, copper, potassium

OBJ. 7 ___ 14. Hypervitaminosis involving water-soluble vitamins is relatively uncommon because:
   a. excessive amounts are stored in adipose tissue
   b. excessive amounts are readily excreted in the urine
   c. the excess amount is stored in the bones
   d. excesses are readily absorbed into skeletal muscle

272 Chapter 18   Nutrition and Metabolism

OBJ. 7 ___ 15. Before the large vitamin B12 molecule can be absorbed, it must be bound to:
- a. the gastric epithelium
- b. a water-insoluble vitamin
- c. vitamin C
- d. intrinsic factor

OBJ. 8 ___ 16. Which of the following provides the most calories per gram when metabolized?
- a. carbohydrates
- b. proteins
- c. neutral fats
- d. nucleic acids

OBJ. 9 ___ 17. An individual's basal metabolic rate ideally represents:
- a. the minimum, resting energy expenditure of an alert person
- b. genetic differences among ethnic groups
- c. the amounts of circulating hormone levels in the body
- d. a measurement of the daily energy expenditures for a given individual

OBJ. 10 ___ 18. The greatest amount of the daily water intake is obtained by:
- a. consumption of food
- b. drinking fluids
- c. metabolic processes
- d. decreased urination

[L1]   Completion:

Using the terms below, complete the following statements.

glucagon	triglycerides	essential	basal metabolic rate
minerals	hypervitaminosis	avitaminosis	liver
nutrition	thermoregulation	insulin	beta oxidation
anabolism	TCA cycle	calorie	oxidative
niacin	iron	sodium ion	phosphorylation
vitamin D	cobalamin	vitamin C	vitamin K
vitamin B1			

OBJ. 1   19. The synthesis of new organic compounds which involves the formation of new chemical bonds is _____.

OBJ. 2   20. The process that produces over 90% of the ATP used by our cells is _____.

OBJ. 2   21. The focal point for metabolic regulation and control in the body is the _____.

OBJ. 2   22. Following a large meal, increased glucose uptake and utilization is affected by the hormone _____.

OBJ. 2   23. Between meals, decreased levels of stored glycogen are affected by the hormone _____.

OBJ. 3   24. The most abundant lipids in the body are the _____.

Level 1   Review of Chapter Objectives   273

OBJ. 3   25. Fatty acid molecules are broken down into two-carbon fragments by means of a sequence of reactions known as _____.

OBJ. 4   26. Amino acids which must be acquired from the diet are called _____.

OBJ. 5   27. During RNA catabolism the nitrogen bases, cytosine and uracil, are converted to acetyl-CoA and metabolized via the _____.

OBJ. 6   28. The absorption of nutrients from food is called _____.

OBJ. 6   29. Inorganic ions released through the dissociation of electrolytes are called _____.

OBJ. 6   30. The deficiency disease resulting from a vitamin deficiency is referred to as _____.

OBJ. 6   31. The dietary intake of vitamins that exceeds the ability to store, utilize or excrete a particular vitamin is called _____.

OBJ. 7   32. The major positive ion in body fluids is _____.

OBJ. 7   33. The mineral component of hemoglobin and myoglobin is _____.

OBJ. 7   34. The vitamin that forms a component of nicatinamide-adenine-dinucleotide is _____.

OBJ. 7   35. The vitamin, when present in excess, that results in polycythemia is _____.

OBJ. 7   36. The vitamin, when not included in the diet, that results in scurvy is _____.

OBJ. 7   37. The vitamin, when not included in the diet, that results in rickets is _____.

OBJ. 7   38. The vitamin necessary for the production of clotting factors by the liver is _____.

OBJ. 7   39. The vitamin, when not included in the diet, that results in beri beri is _____.

OBJ. 8   40. The amount of energy required to raise the temperature of one (1) gram of water one degree centigrade is the _____.

OBJ. 9   41. The minimum resting energy expenditure of an awake, alert person is the individual's _____.

OBJ. 10   42. The homeostatic process that keeps body temperatures within acceptable limits regardless of environmental conditions is called _____.

274 Chapter 18 Nutrition and Metabolism

[L1] Matching:

Match the terms in column "B" with the terms in column "A." Use letters for answers in the spaces provided.

		COLUMN "A"	COLUMN "B"
OBJ. 1	___ 43.	Catabolism	A. Protein catabolism
OBJ. 1	___ 44.	Anabolism	B. ADEK
OBJ. 2	___ 45.	Glycolysis	C. Release of hormones; increasing metabolism
OBJ. 2	___ 46.	Gluconeogenesis	D. Glycogen reserves
OBJ. 2	___ 47.	Glycogenesis	E. Glucose synthesis
OBJ. 2	___ 48.	Skeletal muscle	F. B complex and C
OBJ. 3	___ 49.	Lipolysis	G. Lipid synthesis
OBJ. 3	___ 50.	Lipogenesis	H. Increasing muscle tone
OBJ. 3	___ 51.	Adipose tissue	I. Glycogen formation
OBJ. 4	___ 52.	Ketone bodies	J. Protein sparing
OBJ. 4	___ 53.	Amino acid metabolism	K. Lipid metabolism
OBJ. 4	___ 54.	Carbohydrates	L. Urea formation
OBJ. 5	___ 55.	Purines and pyrimidines	M. Lipid storage
OBJ. 6	___ 56.	Fat-soluble vitamins	N. Nitrogen compounds
OBJ. 7	___ 57.	Water-soluble vitamins	O. Energy release
OBJ. 8	___ 58.	Energy content of food	P. Synthesis
OBJ. 9	___ 59.	Basal metabolic rate	Q. Anaerobic reaction sequence
OBJ. 10	___ 60.	Shivering thermogenesis	R. Calories/gram
OBJ. 10	___ 61.	Nonshivering thermogenesis	S. Resting energy expenditure

When you have successfully completed the exercises in L1 proceed to L2.

☐ LEVEL 2   CONCEPT SYNTHESIS

Concept Map I:

Using the following terms, fill in the circled, numbered, blank spaces to complete the concept map. Follow the numbers that comply with the organization of the map.

| Gluconeogenesis | Lipogenesis | Lipolysis |
| Amino acids | Beta oxidation | Glycolysis |

Anabolism & Catabolism of Carbohydrates Lipids and Proteins

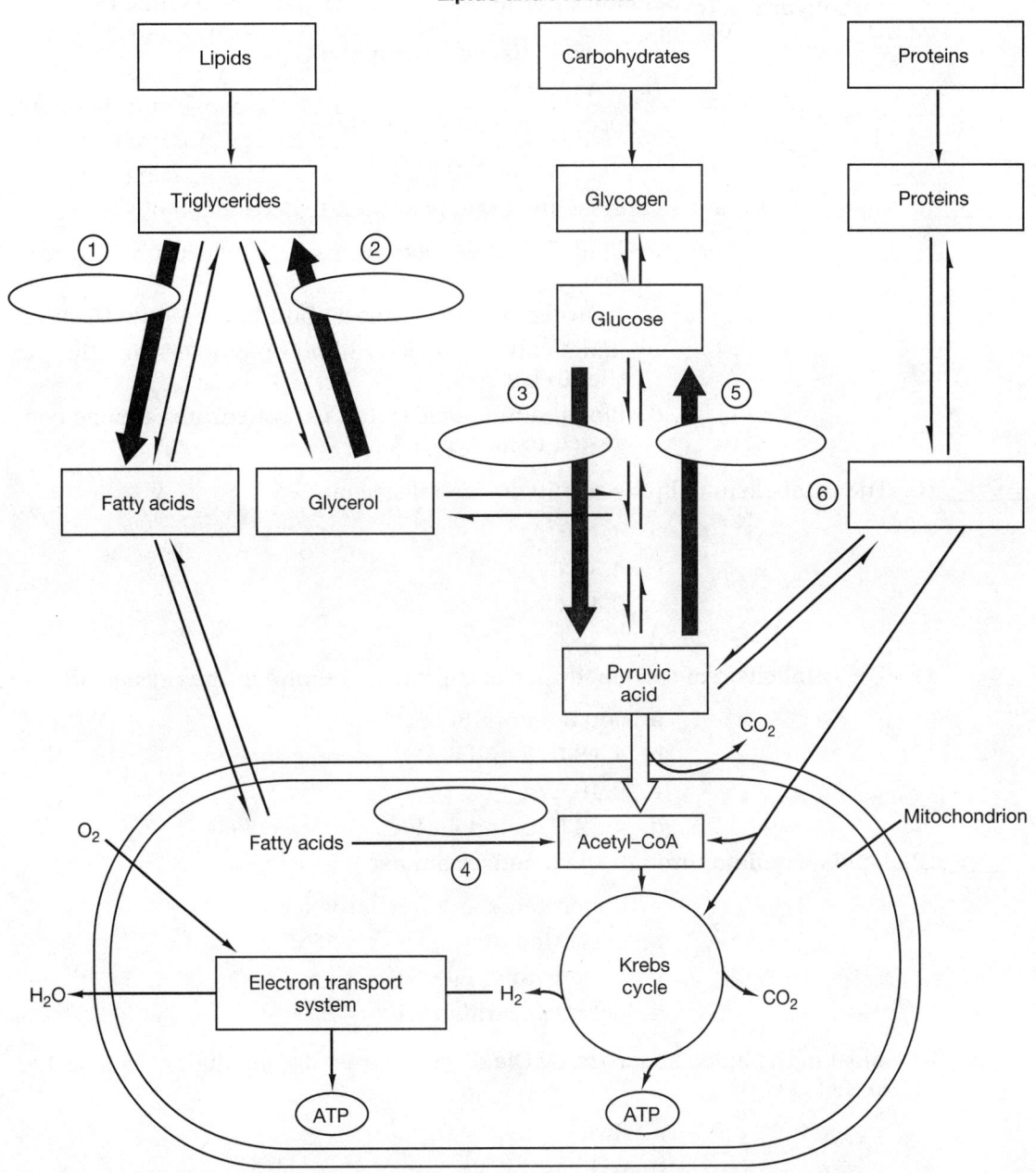

[L2] Multiple Choice:

Place the letter corresponding to the correct answer in the space provided.

_____ 7. The major metabolic pathways that provide most of the ATP used by typical cells are:

      a. anabolism and catabolism
      b. gluconeogenesis and glycogenesis
      c. glycolysis and aerobic respiration
      d. lipolysis and lipogenesis

_____ 8. A cell with excess carbohydrates, lipids, and amino acids will break down carbohydrates to:

      a. provide tissue growth and repair
      b. obtain energy
      c. provide metabolic regulation
      d. a, b, and c are correct

_____ 9. Lipogenesis can use almost any organic substrate because:

      a. lipid molecules contain carbon, hydrogen, and oxygen
      b. triglycerides are the most abundant lipids in the body
      c. lipids can be converted and channeled directly into the Kreb's cycle
      d. lipids, amino acids, and carbohydrates can be converted to acetyl-CoA

_____ 10. The catabolism of lipids results in the release of:

      a. 4.18 C/g
      b. 4.32 C/g
      c. 9.46 C/g
      d. 7.38 C/g

_____ 11. The catabolism of carbohydrates and proteins results in the release of:

      a. equal amounts of C/g
      b. 4.18 C/g and 4.32 C/g, respectively
      c. 9.46 C/g
      d. 4.32 C/g and 4.18 C/g, respectively

_____ 12. Lipids circulate through the bloodstream as:

      a. lipoproteins and free fatty acids
      b. saturated fats
      c. unsaturated fats
      d. polyunsaturated fat

_____ 13. Most of the lipids absorbed by the digestive tract are imediately transferred to the:

      a. liver
      b. red blood cells
      c. venous circulation via the left lymphatic duct
      d. hepatocytes for storage

_____ 14. An important energy source during periods of starvation, when glucose supplies are limited, is:
   a. glycerol
   b. lipoproteins
   c. cholesterol
   d. free fatty acids

_____ 15. Milk and eggs are complete proteins because they contain:
   a. more protein than fat
   b. the recommended intake for vitamin B12
   c. all the essential amino acids in sufficient quantities
   d. all the essential fatty acids and amino acids

[L2] Completion:

Using the terms below, complete the following statements.

| nutrient pool | lipoproteins | HDLs | chylomicrons | metabolic rate |
| uric acid | deamination | LDLs | acclimatization | |

16. All of the anabolic and catabolic pathways in the cell utilize a collection of organic substances known as the _____.
17. Complexes that contain large insoluble glycerides and cholesterol and a coating dominated by phospholipids and protein are called _____.
18. The largest lipoproteins in the body that are produced by the intestinal epithelial cells are the _____.
19. Lipoproteins that deliver cholesterol to peripheral tissues are the _____.
20. Lipoproteins that transport excess cholesterol from peripheral tissues back to the liver are _____.
21. The removal of an amino group in a reaction that generates an ammonia molecule is called _____.
22. The nitrogen bases adenine and guanine cannot be catabolized for energy but are deaminated and excreted as _____.
23. The value of the sum total of the anabolic and catabolic proceses occurring in the body is the _____.
24. Making physiological adjustment to a particular environment over time is referred to as _____.

[L2] Short Essay:

Briefly answer the following questions in the spaces provided below.

25. What factors make protein catabolism an impractical source of quick energy?

26. Why are nucleic acids insignificant contributors to the total energy reserves of the cell?

27. From a metabolic standpoint, what five (5) distinctive components are found in the human body?

28. What four (4) food groups in sufficient quantity and quality provide the basis for a balanced diet?

29. Even though minerals do not contain calories, why are they important in good nutrition?

30. (a) List the fat-soluble vitamins. (b) List the water-soluble vitamins.

When you have successfully completed the exercises in L2 proceed to L3.

☐ LEVEL 3   CRITICAL THINKING/APPLICATION

Using principles and concepts learned about metabolism and energetics, answer the following questions. Write your answers on a separate sheet of paper.

1. Greg S. received a blood test assessment that reported the following values: *total cholesterol*-200 mg/dl (normal); *HDL cholesterol*-21 mg/dl (below normal), *triglycerides*-125 mg/dl (normal). If the minimal normal value for HDLs is 35 mg/dl, what are the physiological implications of his test results?

2. Charlene S. expresses a desire to lose weight. She decides to go on a diet, selecting food from the four food groups; however, she limits her total caloric intake to approximately 300-400 calories daily. Within a few weeks Charlene begins to experience symptoms marked by a fruity, sweetish breath odor, excessive thirst, weakness, and at times nausea accompanied by vomiting. What are the physiological implications of this low-calorie diet?

3. On a recent visit to her doctor, Renee C. complained that she felt sick. She had a temperature of 101 degrees F and was feeling nauseous. The doctor prescribed an antibiotic, advised her to go home, drink plenty of fluids, and rest in bed for a few days. What is the physiological basis for drinking plenty of fluids when one is sick?

CHAPTER 19

The Urinary System

■ Overview

As you have learned in previous chapters, the body's cells break down the food we eat, release energy from it, and produce chemical byproducts that collect in the bloodstream. The kidneys, playing a crucial homeostatic role, cleanse the blood of these waste products and excess water by forming urine, which is then transferred to the urinary bladder and eventually removed from the body via urination. The kidneys receive more blood from the heart than any other organ of the body. They handle 1½ quarts of blood every minute through a complex blood circulation housed in an organ 4 inches high, 2 inches wide, 1 inch thick, and weighing 5 to 6 ounces.

In addition to the kidneys, which produce the urine, the urinary system consists of the ureters, urinary bladder, and urethra, components that are responsible for transport, storage, and conduction of the urine to the exterior.

In many of the previous chapters we examined the various organ systems, focusing on the structural components and the functional activities necessary to *support* life. This chapter also deals with *maintaining* life in the billions of individual cells in the body. Early in the study of anatomy and physiology we established that the cell is the basic unit of structure and function of all living things, no matter how complex the organism is as a whole. The last few chapters concentrated on the necessity of meeting the nutrient needs of cells. To meet the nutrient needs of cells, substances must move in; and to get rid of wastes, materials must move out. The result is a constant movement of materials into and out of the cells.

Both the external environment (interstitial fluid) and the internal environment of the cell (intracellular fluid) comprise an "exchange system" operating within controlled and changing surroundings, producing a dynamic equilibrium by which homeostasis is maintained.

The activities for Chapter 19 focus on the structural and functional organization of the urinary system; the major regulatory mechanisms that control urine formation and modification; urine transport, storage, and elimination; the mechanics and dynamics of fluid balance, electrolyte balance, and acid-base balance; and the interrelationships of functional patterns that operate in the body to support and maintain a constant state of equilibrium.

Chapter 19 The Urinary System

☐ LEVEL 1   REVIEW OF CHAPTER OBJECTIVES

1. Identify the components of the urinary system and describe their functions.
2. Describe the structural features of the kidney.
3. Describe the structure of the nephron and the processes involved in urine formation.
4. Trace the path of blood flow through the kidney.
5. List and describe the factors that influence filtration pressure and the rate of filtrate formation.
6. Describe the changes that occur in the filtrate as it moves through the nephrons and exits as urine.
7. Describe the structures and functions of the ureters, urinary bladder and urethra.
8. Discuss the process of urination and how it is controlled.
9. Explain how the urinary system interacts with other body systems to maintain homeostasis in body fluids.
10. Describe how water and electrolytes are distributed within the body.
11. Explain the basic concepts involved in the control of fluid and electrolyte regulation.
12. Explain the buffering systems that balance the pH of the intracellular and extracellular fluid.
13. Describe the effects of aging on the urinary system.

[L1]   Multiple Choice:

Place the letter corresponding to the correct answer in the space provided.

OBJ. 1   ____   1. Urine leaving the kidneys travels along the following sequential pathway to the exterior:

      a. ureters, urinary bladder, urethra
      b. urethra, urinary bladder, ureters
      c. urinary bladder, ureters, urethra
      d. urinary bladder, urethra, ureters

OBJ. 1   ____   2. The openings of the urethra and the two ureters mark an area on the internal surface of the urinary bladder called the:

      a. internal urethral sphincter
      b. external urethral sphincter
      c. trigone
      d. renal sinus

OBJ. 1   ____   3. Along with the urinary system, the other systems of the body that affect the composition of body fluids are:

      a. nervous, endocrine, and cardiovascular
      b. lymphatic, cardiovascular, and respiratory
      c. integumentary, respiratory, and digestive
      d. muscular, digestive, and lymphatic

OBJ. 2   ____   4. Seen in section, the kidney is divided into:

      a. renal columns and renal pelves
      b. an outer cortex and an inner medulla
      c. major and minor calyces
      d. a renal tubule and renal corpuscle

Level 1   Review of Chapter Objectives

OBJ. 2 ___ 5. The basic functional unit in the kidney is the:
    a. glomerulus
    b. loop of Henle
    c. Bowman's capsule
    d. nephron

OBJ. 3 ___ 6. In a nephron, the long tubular passageway through which the filtrate passes includes:
    a. collecting tubule, collecting duct, papillary duct
    b. renal corpuscle, renal tubule, renal pelvis
    c. proximal and distal convoluted tubules and loop of Henle
    d. loop of Henle, collecting and papillary duct

OBJ. 3 ___ 7. The three processes involved in urine formation are:
    a. diffusion, osmosis, and filtration
    b. co-transport, countertransport, facilitated diffusion
    c. regulation, elimination, micturition
    d. filtration, reabsorption, secretion

OBJ. 3 ___ 8. The primary site for secretion of substances into the filtrate is the:
    a. renal corpuscle
    b. loop of Henle
    c. distal convoluted tubule
    d. proximal convoluted tubule

OBJ. 4 ___ 9. Dilation of the afferent arteriole and glomerular capillaries and constriction of the efferent arteriole causes:
    a. elevation of glomerular blood pressure to normal levels
    b. a decrease in glomerular blood pressure
    c. a decrease in the glomerular filtration rate
    d. an increase in the secretion of renin and erythropoietin

OBJ. 4 ___ 10. Blood supply to the proximal and distal convoluted tubules of the nephron is provided by the:
    a. peritubular capillaries
    b. afferent arterioles
    c. segmental veins
    d. interlobular veins

OBJ. 5 ___ 11. The glomerular filtration rate is regulated by:
    a. autoregulation
    b. hormonal regulation
    c. autonomic regulation
    d. a, b, and c are correct

282 Chapter 19 The Urinary System

[OBJ. 5] ____ 12. Dropping filtration pressure stimulates the juxtaglomerular apparatus to release angiotensin.
   a. true
   b. false

[OBJ. 6] ____ 13. The primary site of nutrient reabsorption in the nephron is the:
   a. proximal convoluted tubule
   b. distal convoluted tubule
   c. loop of Henle
   d. renal corpuscle

[OBJ. 6] ____ 14. In countercurrent multiplication, the countercurrent refers to the fact that an exchange occurs between:
   a. sodium ions and chloride ions
   b. fluids moving in opposite directions
   c. potassium and chloride ions
   d. solute concentrations in the loop of Henle

[OBJ. 6] ____ 15. When antidiuretic hormone levels rise the distal convoluted tubule becomes:
   a. less permeable to water; reabsorption of water decreases
   b. more permeable to water; water reabsorption increases
   c. less permeable to water; reabsorption of water increases
   d. more permeable to water; water reabsorption decreases

[OBJ. 6] ____ 16. The results of the effect of aldosterone along the DCT, the collecting tubule, and the collecting duct are:
   a. increased conservation of sodium ions and water
   b. increased sodium ion excretion
   c. decreased sodium ion reabsorption in the DCT
   d. increased sodium ion and water excretion

[OBJ. 6] ____ 17. The average pH for normal urine is about:
   a. 5.0
   b. 6.0
   c. 7.0
   d. 8.0

[OBJ. 7] ____ 18. When urine leaves the kidney it travels to the urinary bladder via the:
   a. urethra
   b. ureters
   c. renal hilus
   d. renal calyces

Level
-1-

Level 1 Review of Chapter Objectives 283

OBJ. 7 ___ 19. Contraction of the muscular bladder forces the urine out of the body through the:
    a. ureter
    b. urethra
    c. penis
    d. a, b, and c are correct

OBJ. 8 ___ 20. Urine reaches the urinary bladder by the:
    a. action of stretch receptors in the bladder wall
    b. fluid pressures in the renal pelvis
    c. peristaltic contractions of the ureters
    d. sustained contractions and relaxation of the urinary

OBJ. 9 ___ 21. The body system which provides bicarbonate buffers that assist in the regulation of pH is the _____ system.
    a. integumentary
    b. muscular
    c. digestive
    d. respiratory

OBJ. 10 ___ 22. Nearly two-thirds of the total body water content is:
    a. extracellular fluid (ECF)
    b. intracellular fluid (ICF)
    c. tissue fluid
    d. interstitial fluid (IF)

OBJ. 10 ___ 23. Extracellular fluids in the body consist of:
    a. interstitial fluid, blood plasma, lymph
    b. cerebrospinal fluid, synovial fluid, serous fluids
    c. aqueous humor, perilymph, endolymph
    d. a, b, and c are correct

OBJ. 10 ___ 24. The principal ions in the extracellular fluid (ECF) are:
    a. sodium, chloride, and bicarbonate
    b. potassium, magnesium, and phosphate
    c. phosphate, sulfate, magnesium
    d. potassium, ammonium, and chloride

OBJ. 11 ___ 25. If the ECF is hypertonic with respect to the ICF, water will move:
    a. from the ECF into the cell until osmotic equilibrium is restored
    b. from the cells into the ECF until osmotic equilibrium is restored
    c. in both directions until osmotic equilibrium is restored
    d. in response to the pressure of carrier molecules

284 Chapter 19 The Urinary System

OBJ. 11 ___ 26. When pure water is consumed, the extracellular fluid becomes:

    a. hypotonic with respect to the ICF
    b. hypertonic with respect to the ICF
    c. isotonic with respect to the ICF
    d. the ICF and the ECF are in equilibrium

OBJ. 11 ___ 27. Physiological adjustments affecting fluid and electrolyte balance are mediated primarily by:

    a. antidiuretic hormone (ADH)
    b. aldosterone
    c. atrial natriuretic peptide (ANP)
    d. a, b, and c are correct

OBJ. 11 ___ 28. The two important effects of increased release of ADH are:

    a. increased rate of sodium absorption and decreased thirst
    b. reduction of urinary water losses and stimulation of the thirst center
    c. decrease in the plasma volume and elimination of the source of stimulation
    d. decrease in plasma osmolarity and alteration of composition of tissue fluid

OBJ. 11 ___ 29. The concentration of potassium in the ECF is controlled by adjustments in the rate of active secretion:

    a. in the proximal convoluted tubule of the nephron
    b. in the loop of Henle
    c. along the distal convoluted tubule of the nephron
    d. along the collecting tubules

OBJ. 12 ___ 30. Pulmonary and renal mechanisms support the buffer systems by:

    a. secreting or generating hydrogen ions
    b. controlling the excretion of acids and bases
    c. generating additional buffers when necessary
    d. a, b, and c are correct

OBJ. 12 ___ 31. The lungs contribute to pH regulation by their effects on the:

    a. hemoglobin buffer system
    b. phosphate buffer system
    c. carbonic acid-bicarbonate buffer system
    d. protein buffer system

OBJ. 12 ___ 32. Increasing or decreasing the rate of respiration can have a profound effect on the buffering capacity of body fluids by:

    a. lowering or raising the P_{O_2}
    b. lowering or raising the P_{CO_2}
    c. increasing production of lactic acid
    d. a, b, and c are correct

Level -1-

Level 1 Review of Chapter Objectives 285

OBJ. 12 ___ 33. When carbon dioxide concentrations rise, additional hydrogen ions and bicarbonate ions are excreted and the:

    a. pH goes up
    b. pH goes down
    c. pH remains the same
    d. pH is not affected

OBJ. 12 ___ 34. The most frequent cause of metabolic acidosis is:

    a. production of a large number of fixed or organic acids
    b. a severe bicarbonate loss
    c. an impaired ability to excrete hydrogen ions at the kidneys
    d. generation of large quantities of ketone bodies

OBJ. 13 ___ 35. A reduction in the glomerular filtration rate (GFR) due to aging results from:

    a. decreased numbers of glomeruli
    b. cumulative damage to the filtration apparatus
    c. reductions in renal blood flow
    d. a, b, and c are correct

OBJ. 13 ___ 36. Reduced sensitivity to antidiuretic hormone (ADH) due to aging causes:

    a. decreasing reabsorption of water and sodium ions
    b. decreasing potassium ion loss in the urine
    c. decreasing numbers of glomeruli
    d. a, b, and c are correct

[L1] Completion:

Using the terms below, complete the following statements.

cerebral cortex	urethra	micturition reflex	composition
concentration	incontinence	filtrate	glomerulus
internal sphincter	kidneys	interlobar veins	antidiuretic hormone
fluid	osmoreceptors	alkalosis	glomerular hydrostatic
acidosis	aldosterone	electrolyte	integumentary

OBJ. 1   37. The excretory functions of the urinary system are performed by the _____.

OBJ. 2   38. The renal corpuscle contains a capillary knot referred to as the _____.

OBJ. 3   39. The outflow across the walls of the glomerulus produces a protein-free solution known as the _____.

OBJ. 4   40. In a mirror image of arterial distribution, the interlobular veins deliver blood to arcuate veins that empty into _____.

OBJ. 5   41. The pressure that tends to drive water and solute molecules across the glomerular wall is the _____ pressure.

OBJ. 6   42. Passive reabsorption of water from urine in the collecting system is regulated by circulating levels of _____.

OBJ. 6   43. The filtration, absorption, and secretion activities of the nephrons reflect the urine's _____.

OBJ. 6   44. The osmotic movement of water across the walls of the tubules and collecting ducts determines the urine's _____.

286 Chapter 19   The Urinary System

OBJ. 7 45. The structure that carries urine from the urinary bladder to the exterior of the body is the _____.

OBJ. 7 46. The muscular ring that provides involuntary control over the discharge of urine from the urinary bladder is the _____.

OBJ. 8 47. The process of urination is coordinated by the _____.

OBJ. 8 48. We become consciously aware of the fluid pressure in the urinary bladder because of sensations relayed to the _____.

OBJ. 9 49. The _____ is responsible for preventing excess fluid loss while eliminating excess salts, in particular sodium and chloride.

OBJ. 10 50. When the amount of water gained each day is equal to the amount lost to the environment a person is in _____ balance.

OBJ. 10 51. When there is neither a net gain nor a net loss of any ion in the body fluid, an _____ balance exists.

OBJ. 11 52. Osmotic concentrations of the plasma are monitored by special cells in the hypothalamus called _____.

OBJ. 11 53. The rate of sodium absorption along the distal convoluted tubule and collecting system of the kidneys is regulated by the secretion of _____.

OBJ. 12 54. When the pH in the body falls below 7.35, the condition is called _____.

OBJ. 12 55. When the pH in the body increases above 7.45, the condtion is called _____.

OBJ. 13 56. A slow leakage of urine due to the loss of sphincter muscle tone is refered to as _____.

[L1] Matching:

Match the terms in column "B" with the terms in column "A". Use letters for answers in the spaces provided.

	COLUMN "A"	COLUMN "B"
OBJ. 1 ____ 57.	Juxtaglomerular apparatus	A. Internal sphincter forced open
OBJ. 2 ____ 58.	Renal capsule	B. Vasomotor center
OBJ. 3 ____ 59.	Glomerular epithelium	C. ICF and ECF
OBJ. 4 ____ 60.	Renal artery	D. Interstitial fluid
OBJ. 5 ____ 61.	Lowers filtration rate	E. Podocytes
OBJ. 7 ____ 62.	Urinary bladder	F. Detrusor muscle
OBJ. 8 ____ 63.	200 ml of urine in bladder	G. No urine production
OBJ. 8 ____ 64.	500 ml of urine in bladder	H. Release of ANP
OBJ. 9 ____ 65.	Changes regional pattern of blood circulation	I. Renin and erythropoietin
OBJ. 10 ____ 66.	Tissue fluid	J. Buffers pH of ECF
OBJ. 10 ____ 67.	Fluid compartments	K. Urge to urinate
OBJ. 11 ____ 68.	Increased venous return	L. Kidney failure
OBJ. 12 ____ 69.	Phosphate buffer system	M. Buffers pH of ICF
OBJ. 12 ____ 70.	Carbonic acid-bicarbonate buffer	N. Sympathetic anctivation
		O. Fibrous tunic
OBJ. 13 ____ 71.	Uremia	P. Blood to kidney
OBJ. 13 ____ 72.	Anuria	

Level -1-

Level 1   Review of Chapter Objectives   287

[L1]   Drawing/Illustration Labeling:

Identify each numbered structure by labeling the following figures:

OBJ. 1   **FIGURE 19.1**   Components of the Urinary System

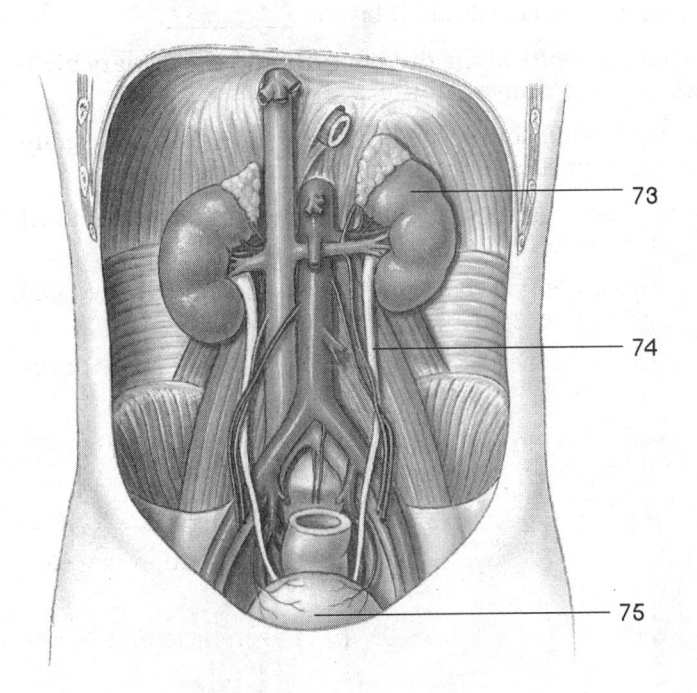

73 _____
74 _____
75 _____

OBJ. 2   **FIGURE 19.2**   Sectional Anatomy of the Kidney

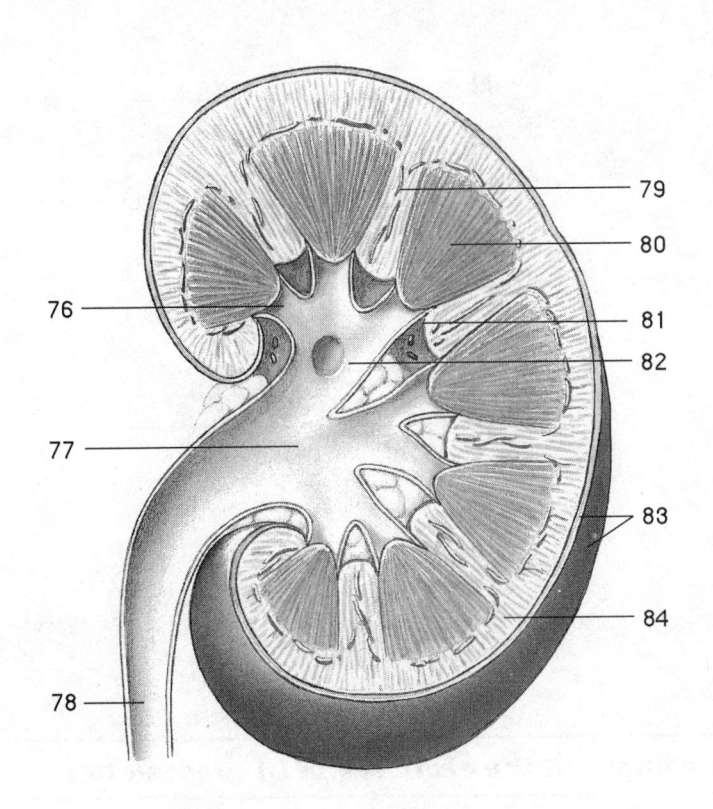

76 _____
77 _____
78 _____
79 _____
80 _____
81 _____
82 _____
83 _____
84 _____

Level 1

288 Chapter 19   The Urinary System

OBJ. 3   **FIGURE 19.3**   Structure of a Typical Nephron (Including Circulation)

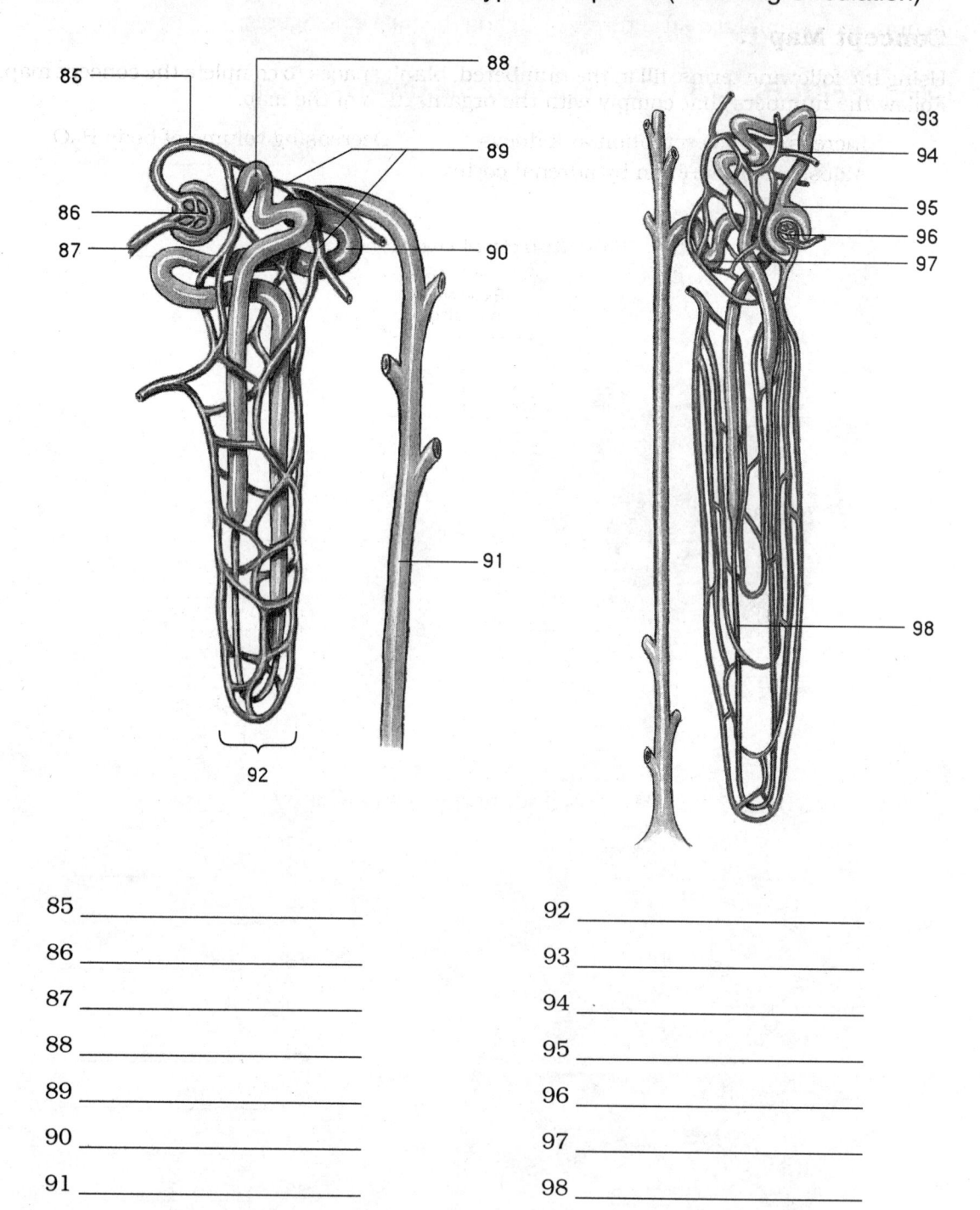

85 _____   92 _____
86 _____   93 _____
87 _____   94 _____
88 _____   95 _____
89 _____   96 _____
90 _____   97 _____
91 _____   98 _____

Level -1-   **When you have successfully completed the exercises in L1 proceed to L.**

☐ LEVEL 2 CONCEPT SYNTHESIS

Concept Map I:

Using the following terms, fill in the numbered, blank spaces to complete the concept map. Follow the numbers that comply with the organization of the map.

- Increasing H₂O retention at kidneys
- Decreasing volume of body H₂O
- Aldosterone secretion by adrenal cortex

Homeostasis of total volume of body water

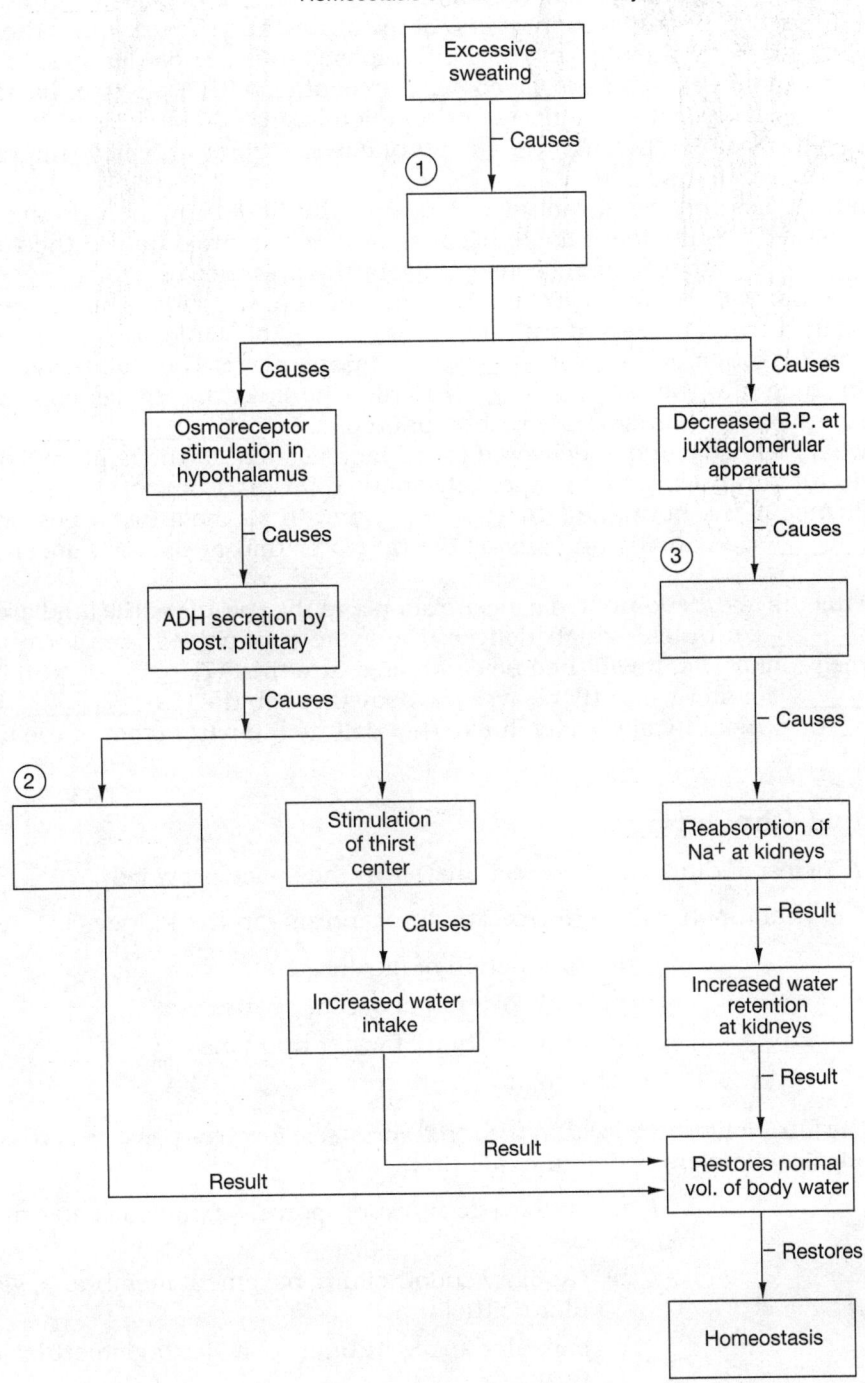

Excessive sweating
— Causes →
① [ ]

— Causes → Osmoreceptor stimulation in hypothalamus
— Causes → ADH secretion by post. pituitary
— Causes → ② [ ] and Stimulation of thirst center
— Causes → Increased water intake
— Result → Restores normal vol. of body water

— Causes → Decreased B.P. at juxtaglomerular apparatus
— Causes → ③ [ ]
— Causes → Reabsorption of Na⁺ at kidneys
— Result → Increased water retention at kidneys
— Result → Restores normal vol. of body water

— Restores → Homeostasis

Body Trek:

Using the terms below, fill in the blanks to complete the trek through the urinary system.

aldosterone	protein-free	ions	ascending limb
active transport	ADH	glomerulus	urine
urinary bladder	collecting	proximal	descending limb
urethra	filtrate	ureters	distal

Robo's trek through the urinary system begins as the tiny robot is inserted into the urethra and with the aid of two mini-rockets is propelled through the urinary tract into the region of the renal corpuscle in the cortex of the kidney. The use of the mini-rockets eliminates the threat of the countercurrent flow of the filtrate and the urine and the inability of the robot to penetrate the physical barriers imposed in the capsular space.

Rocket shutdown occurs just as Robo comes into contact with a physical barrier, the filtration membrane. The robot's energizers are completely turned off because the current produced by the fluid coming through the membrane is sufficient to "carry" the robot as it treks through the tubular system.

As the fluid crosses the membrane it enters into the first tubular conduit, the (4) _____ convoluted tubule, identifiable because of its close proximity to the vascular pole of the (5)_____. Robo's chemosensors detect the presence of a (6) _____ filtrate in this area. Using the current in the tubule to move on, the robot's speed increases because of a sharp turn and descent into the (7) _____ of Henle, where water reabsorption and concentration of the (8) _____ are taking place. The trek turns upward after a "hairpin" turn into the (9) _____ of Henle where, in the thickened area, (10) _____ mechanisms are causing the reabsorption of (11) _____.

The somewhat "refined" fluid is delivered to the last segment of the nephron, the (12) _____ convoluted tubule, which is specially adapted for reabsorption of sodium ions due to the influence of the hormone (13) _____, and in its most distal position, the effects of (14) _____, causing an osmotic flow of water that assists in concentrating the filtrate.

Final adjustments to the sodium ion concentration and the volume of the fluid are made in the (15) _____ tubules, which deliver the waste products in the form of (16) _____ to the renal pelvis. It will then be conducted into the (17) _____ on its way to the (18) _____ for storage until it leaves the body through the (19) _____ Robo's way of escaping the possibility of toxicity due to the "polluted" environment of the urinary tract.

[L2] Multiple Choice:

Place the letter corresponding to the correct answer in the space provided.

_____ 20. The vital function(s) performed by the nephrons in the kidneys is (are):

    a. production of filtrate
    b. reabsorption of organic substrates
    c. reabsorption of water and ions
    d. a, b, and c are correct

_____ 21. The filtration process within the renal corpuscle involves passage across three physical barriers, which include the:

    a. podocytes, filtration pores, juxtaglomerular apparatus
    b. capillary endothelium, basement membrane, glomerular epithelium
    c. capsular space, tubular pole, juxtaglomerular apparatus
    d. collecting tubules, collecting ducts, papillary ducts

_____ 22. The collecting system in the kidney is responsible for:
- a. active secretion and reabsorption of sodium ions
- b. absorption of nutrients, plasma proteins, and ions from the filtrate
- c. creation of the medullary concentration gradient
- d. making final adjustments to the sodium ion concentration and volume of urine

_____ 23. Sympathetic innervation into the kidney is responsible for:
- a. regulation of glomerular blood flow and pressure
- b. stimulation of renin release
- c. direct stimulation of water and sodium ion reabsorption
- d. a, b, and c are correct

_____ 24. Inadequate ADH secretion results in the inability to reclaim the water entering the filtrate, causing:
- a. blood in the urine
- b. dehydration
- c. lack of urine production
- d. excess glucose in the urine

_____ 25. Under normal circumstances virtually all the glucose, amino acids, and other nutrients are reabsorbed before the filtrate leaves the:
- a. distal convoluted tubule
- b. glomerulus
- c. collecting ducts
- d. proximal convoluted tubule

_____ 26. Aldosterone stimulates ion pumps along the distal convoluted tubule, the collecting tubule, and the collecting duct, causing a(n):
- a. increase in the number of sodium ions lost in the urine
- b. decrease in the concentration of the filtrate
- c. reduction in the number of sodium ions lost in the urine
- d. increase in the concentration of the filtrate

_____ 27. The hormones that affect the glomerular filtration rate (GFR) by regulating blood pressure and volume are:
- a. aldosterone, epinephrine, oxytocin
- b. insulin, glucagon, glucocorticoids
- c. renin, erythropoietin, ADH
- d. a, b, and c are correct

_____ 28. During periods of strenuous exercise sympathetic activation causes the blood flow to:
- a. decrease to skin and skeletal muscles; increase to kidneys
- b. cause an increase in GFR
- c. increase to skin and skeletal muscles; decrease to kidneys
- d. be shunted toward the kidneys

292 Chapter 19 The Urinary System

_____ 29. All of the homeostatic mechanisms that monitor and adjust the composition of body fluids respond to changes in the:

    a. intracellular fluid
    b. extracellular fluid
    c. regulatory hormones
    d. fluid balance

_____ 30. All water transport across cell membranes and epithelia occur passively, in response to:

    a. active transport and difusion
    b. active transport and facilitated diffusion
    c. osmotic gradients and hydrostatic pressure
    d. active transport and endocytosis

_____ 31. The most important factor affecting the pH in body tissues is:

    a. the protein buffer system
    b. carbon dioxide concentration
    c. the bicarbonate reserve
    d. the presence of ammonium ions

_____ 32. When an individual loses body water:

    a. plasma volume decreases and electrolyte concentrations rise
    b. plasma volume increases and electrolyte concentrations decrease
    c. plasma volume increases and electrolyte concentrations increase
    d. plasma volume decreases and electrolyte concentrations decrease

_____ 33. When the P_{CO2} increases and additional hydrogen ions and bicarbonate ions are released into the plasma, the:

    a. pH goes up; increasing alkalinity
    b. pH goes down; increasing acidity
    c. pH goes up; decreasing acidity
    d. pH is not affected

_____ 34. Under normal circumstances, during respiratory acidosis the chemoreceptors monitoring the P_{CO2} of the plasma and CSF will eliminate the problem by calling for:

    a. a decrease in the breathing rate
    b. a decrease in pulmonary ventilation rates
    c. an increase in pulmonary ventilation rates
    d. breathing into a small paper bag

_____ 35. When a normal pulmonary response does not reverse respiratory acidosis, the kidneys respond by:

    a. increasing the reabsorption of hydrogen ions
    b. increasing the rate of hydrogen ion secretion into the filtrate
    c. decreasing the rate of hydrogen ion secretion into the filtrate
    d. increased loss of bicarbonate ions

Level =2=

_____ 36. Chronic diarrhea causes a severe loss of bicarbonate ions resulting in:
   a. respiratory acidosis
   b. respiratory alkalosis
   c. metabolic acidosis
   d. metabolic alkalosis

[L2]   Short Essay:

Briefly answer the following questions in the spaces provided below.

37. What are the essential functions of the urinary system?

38. What known functions result from sympathetic innervation into the kidneys?

39. What control mechanisms are involved with regulation of the glomerular filtration rate (GFR)?

40. What four (4) hormones affect urine production? Describe the role of each.

41. What two (2) major effects does ADH have on maintaining homeostatic volumes of water in the body?

42. How do pulmonary and renal mechanisms support the chemical buffer system?

When you have successfully completed the exercises in L2 proceed to L 3.

☐ LEVEL 3   CRITICAL THINKING/APPLICATION

Using principles and concepts learned about the urinary system, answer the following questions. Write your answers on a separate sheet of paper.

1. I. O. Yew spends an evening with the boys at the local tavern. During the course of the night he makes numerous trips to the rest room to urinate. In addition to drinking an excessive amount of fluid, what effect does the consumption of alcohol have on the urinary system to cause urination?

2. On an anatomy and physiology examination your instructor asks the following question:

   What is the "principal function" associated with each of the following components of the nephron?

   a. renal corpuscle
   b. proximal convoluted tubule
   c. distal convoluted tubule
   d. loop of Henle and collecting system

Question number 3 will make use of the following information:

Normal arterial blood gas values:

pH: 7.35-7.45
P_{CO2}:   35 to 45 mm Hg
P_{O2}:   80 to 100 mm Hg
HCO_3^-:   22 to 26 mEq/liter

3. After analyzing the ABG values below, identify the condition in each one of the following four cases.

   a. pH 7.30; P_{CO2} 37 mm Hg; HCO_3^- 16 mEq/liter
   b. pH 7.52; P_{CO2} 32 mm Hg; HCO_3^- 25 mEq/liter
   c. pH 7.36; P_{CO2} 67 mm Hg; HCO_3^- 23 mEq/liter
   d. pH 7.58; P_{CO2} 43 mm Hg; HCO_3^- 42 mEq/liter

CHAPTER 20

The Reproductive System

■ Overview

The structures and functions of the reproductive system are notably different from any other organ system in the human body. The other systems of the body are functional at birth or shortly thereafter; however, the reproductive system does not become functional until it is acted on by hormones during puberty.

Most of the other body systems function to support and maintain the individual, but the reproductive system is specialized to ensure survival, not of the individual but of the species.

Even though major differences exist between the reproductive organs of the male and female, both are primarily concerned with propagation of the species and passing genetic material from one generation to another. In addition, the reproductive system produces hormones that allow for the development of secondary sex characteristics.

This chapter provides a series of exercises that will assist you in reviewing and reinforcing your understanding of the anatomy and physiology of the male and female reproductive systems, the effects of male and female hormones, and changes that occur during the aging process.

☐ LEVEL 1   REVIEW OF CHAPTER OBJECTIVES

1. Summarize the functions of the human reproductive system and its principal components.
2. Describe the components of the male reproductive system.
3. Describe the process of spermatogenesis.
4. Describe the roles the male reproductive tract and the accessory glands play in the maturation and transport of spermatozoa.
5. Describe the hormonal mechanisms that regulate male reproductive functions.
6. Describe the components of the female reproductive system.
7. Describe the process of oogenesis in the ovary.
8. Detail the physiological processes involved in the ovarian and menstrual cycles.
9. Discuss the physiology of sexual intercourse as it affects the reproductive systems of males and females.
10. Describe the changes in the reproductive system that occur with aging.
11. Explain how the reproductive system interacts with other body systems.

296 Chapter 20 The Reproductive System

[L1] Multiple Choice:

Place the letter corresponding to the correct answer in the space provided.

OBJ. 1 ____ 1. The systems involved in an adequate sperm count, correct pH and nutrients, and erection and ejaculation are:
- a. reproductive and digestive
- b. endocrine and nervous
- c. cardiovascular and urinary
- d. a, b, and c are correct

OBJ. 1 ____ 2. The reproductive organs that produce gametes and hormones are the:
- a. accessory glands
- b. gonads
- c. vagina and penis
- d. a, b, and c are correct

OBJ. 2 ____ 3. In the male the important function(s) of the epididymis is (are):
- a. monitors and adjusts the composition of the tubular fluid
- b. acts as a recycling center for damaged spermatozoa
- c. the site of physical maturation of spermatozoa
- d. a, b, and c are correct

OBJ. 3 ____ 4. In the process of spermatogenesis, the developmental sequence includes:
- a. spermatids, spermatozoon, spermatogonia, spermatocytes
- b. spermatogonia, spermatocytes, spermatids, spermatozoon
- c. spermatocytes, spermatogonia, spermatids, spermatozoon
- d. spermatogonia, spermatids, spermatocytes, spermatozoon

OBJ. 4 ____ 5. In the male, sperm cells, before leaving the body, travel from the testes to the:
- a. ductus deferens → epididymis → urethra → ejaculatory duct
- b. ejaculatory duct → epididymis → ductus deferens → urethra
- c. epididymis → ductus deferens → ejaculatory duct → urethra
- d. epididymis → ejaculatory duct → ductus deferens → urethra

OBJ. 4 ____ 6. The accessory organs in the male that secrete into the ejaculatory ducts and the urethra are:
- a. epididymis, seminal vesicles, vas deferens
- b. prostate gland, inguinal canals, testes
- c. adrenal glands, bulbourethral glands, seminal glands
- d. seminal vesicles, prostate gland, bulbourethral glands

Level -1-

Level 1 Review of Chapter Objectives

OBJ. 4 ___ 7. Semen, the volume of fluid called the ejaculate, contains:
   a. spermatozoa, seminal plasmin, and enzymes
   b. alkaline and acid secretions and sperm
   c. mucus, sperm, and enzymes
   d. spermatozoa, seminal fluid, and enzymes

OBJ. 4 ___ 8. The external genitalia of the male includes the:
   a. scrotum and penis
   b. urethra and bulbourethral glands
   c. inguinal ligament and dartos
   d. prepuce and glans

OBJ. 4 ___ 9. The three masses of erectile tissue that comprise the body of the penis are:
   a. two cylindrical corpora cavernosa and a slender corpus spongiosum
   b. two slender corpora spongiosa and a cylindrical corpus cavernosum
   c. preputial glands, a corpus cavernosum, and a corpus spongiosum
   d. two corpora cavernosa and a preputial gland

OBJ. 5 ___ 10. The hormone synthesized in the hypothalamus that initiates release of pituitary hormones is:
   a. FSH (follicle-stimulating hormone)
   b. ICSH (interstitial cell-stimulating hormone)
   c. LH (lutenizing hormone)
   d. GnRH (gonadotropin-releasing hormone)

OBJ. 5 ___ 11. The hormone that promotes spermatogenesis along the seminiferous tubules is:
   a. ICSH
   b. FSH
   c. GnRH
   d. a and b are correct

OBJ. 6 ___ 12. The function of the uterus in the female is to:
   a. move the sperm into the uterine tube for possible fertilization
   b. provide ovum transport via peristaltic contractions of the uterine wall
   c. provide mechanical protection and nutritional support to the developing embryo
   d. a, b, and c are correct

OBJ. 6 ___ 13. Starting at the superior end, the uterus in the female is divided into:
   a. body, isthmus, cervix
   b. isthmus, body, cervix
   c. body, cervix, isthmus
   d. cervix, body, isthmus

OBJ. 6 ___ 14. Ovum transport in the uterine tubes presumably involves a combination of:

    a. flagellar locomotion and ciliary movement
    b. active transport and ciliary movement
    c. ciliary movement and peristaltic contractions
    d. a, b, and c are correct

OBJ. 6 ___ 15. The reproductive function(s) of the vagina is (are):

    a. passageway for the elimination of menstrual fluids
    b. receives the penis during coitus
    c. forms the lower portion of the birth canal during childbirth
    d. a, b, and c are correct

OBJ. 6 ___ 16. The outer limits of the vulva are established by the:

    a. vestibule and the labia minora
    b. mons pubis and labia majora
    c. lesser and greater vestibular glands
    d. prepuce and vestibule

OBJ. 6 ___ 17. Engorgement of the erectile tissues of the clitoris and increased secretion of the greater vestibular glands involve neural activity that includes:

    a. somatic motor neurons
    b. sympathetic activation
    c. parasympathetic activation
    d. a, b, and c are correct

OBJ. 6 ___ 18. Hormones produced by the placenta include:

    a. estrogen and progesterone
    b. relaxin and human placental lactogen
    c. human chorionic gonadotropin
    d. a, b, and c are correct

OBJ. 7 ___ 19. The ovarian cycle begins as activated follicles develop into:

    a. ova
    b. primary follicles
    c. Graafian follicles
    d. primordial follicles

OBJ. 7 ___ 20. The process of oogenesis produces three non-functional polar bodies that eventually disintegrate and form:

    a. a primordial follicle
    b. a granulosa cell
    c. one functional ovum
    d. b and c are correct

Level -1-

Level 1 Review of Chapter Objectives 299

OBJ. 8 ___ 21. The proper sequence that describes the ovarian cycle involves the formation of:

   a. primary follicles, secondary follicles, tertiary follicles, ovulation, and formation and destruction of the corpus luteum
   b. primary follicles, secondary follicles, tertiary follicles, corpus luteum, and ovulation
   c. corpus luteum; primary, secondary, and tertiary follicles; and ovulation
   d. primary and tertiary follicles, secondary follicles, ovulation, and formation and destruction of the corpus luteum

OBJ. 8 ___ 22. Under normal circumstances, in a 28-day cycle, ovulation occurs on ____, and the menses begins on ____.

   a. day 1; day 14
   b. day 28; day 14
   c. day 14; day 1
   d. day 0; day 14

OBJ. 9 ___ 23. Peristaltic contractions of the ampulla, pushing fluid and spermatozoa into the prostatic urethra, is called:

   a. emission
   b. ejaculation
   c. detumescence
   d. subsidence

OBJ. 10 ___ 24. In the male, between the ages of 50 and 60 circulating _____ levels begin to decline, coupled with increases in circulating levels of _____.

   a. FSH and LH; testosterone
   b. FSH; testosterone and LH
   c. testosterone; FSH and LH
   d. a, b, and c are correct

OBJ. 11 ___ 25. Which of the following hormones may help maintain healthy blood vessels and slow development of atherosclerosis?

   a. estrogen
   b. testosterone
   c. progesterone
   d. a, b, and c are correct

300 Chapter 20 The Reproductive System

[L1] Completion:

Using the terms below, complete the following statements.

menopause	infundibulum	climacteric	ICSH
ovaries	fertilization	testes	placenta
implantation	ovulation	cardiovascular	seminiferous tubules
progesterone	ductus deferens	Graafian	fructose
spermiogenesis	areola	testosterone	

OBJ. 1 26. The fusion of a sperm from the father and an ovum from the mother is called _____.

OBJ. 2 27. Sperm production occurs within the slender, tightly coiled _____.

OBJ. 2 28. The male gonads are the _____.

OBJ. 3 29. The physical transformation of a spermatid to a spermatozoon is called _____.

OBJ. 4 30. After passing along the tail of the epididymis the spermatozoa arrive at the _____.

OBJ. 4 31. The primary energy source for the mobilization of sperm is _____.

OBJ. 5 32. A peptide hormone that causes the secretion of androgens by the interstitial cells of the testes is _____.

OBJ. 6 33. The female gonads are the _____.

OBJ. 6 34. The reddish-brown coloration surrounding the nipples of the breasts is referred to as the _____.

OBJ. 6 35. The principal hormone that prepares the uterus for pregnancy is _____.

OBJ. 6 36. Support for embryonic and fetal development occurs in a special organ called the _____.

OBJ. 7 37. By the tenth day of the ovarian cycle, the mature tertiary follicle is called the _____ follicle.

OBJ. 8 38. The release of ova from the ovary is called _____.

OBJ. 8 39. After ovulation the ovum passes from the ovary into the expanded funnel called the _____.

OBJ. 8 40. When the blastocyst contacts the endometrial wall, erodes the epithelium, and buries itself in the endometlium, the process is known as _____.

OBJ. 9 41. The major systems involved in the process of erection are the nervous and _____.

OBJ. 10 42. In females, the time that ovulation and menstruation cease is referred to as _____.

OBJ. 10 43. Changes in the male reproductive system that occur gradually over a period of time are known as the male _____.

OBJ. 11 44. Reproductive hormones, in particular _____, accelerate skeletal muscle growth.

Level -1-

Level 1 Review of Chapter Objectives

[L1] Matching:

Match the terms in column "B" with the terms in column "A." Use letters for answers in the spaces provided.

		COLUMN "A"	COLUMN "B"
OBJ. 1	___	45. Gonadotropin-releasing hormone	A. Sperm production
OBJ. 1	___	46. FSH, LH, ICSH	B. Nervous and endocrine systems
OBJ. 2	___	47. Interstitial cells	C. Anterior pituitary
OBJ. 3	___	48. Seminiferous tubules	D. Oocytes
OBJ. 3	___	49. Puberty in male	E. Zygote
OBJ. 4	___	50. Prostate glands	F. Produces testosterone
OBJ. 4	___	51. External genitalia	G. Hypothalamus
OBJ. 5	___	52. Testosterone	H. Milk ejection
OBJ. 6	___	53. Oviducts	I. Hormone-postovulatory period
OBJ. 6	___	54. Clitoris	J. Spermatogenesis
OBJ. 6	___	55. Human chorionic hormone	K. An estrogen
OBJ. 6	___	56. Oxytocin	L. Hormone-male secondary sexual characteristics
OBJ. 6	___	57. Progesterone	M. Indicates pregnancy
OBJ. 7	___	58. Ovaries	N. Ovum production
OBJ. 7	___	59. Immature ova	O. Produces alkaline secretion
OBJ. 8	___	60. Estradiol	P. Fallopian tubes
OBJ. 9	___	61. Fertilized ovum	Q. Female equivalent of penis
OBJ. 10	___	62. Menopause	R. Vulva
OBJ. 11	___	63. Controls sexual behavior	S. Cessation of ovulation and menstruation

Chapter 20 The Reproductive System

[L1] Drawing/Illustration Labeling:

Identify each numbered structure by labeling the following figures:

FIGURE 20.1 Male Reproductive Organs

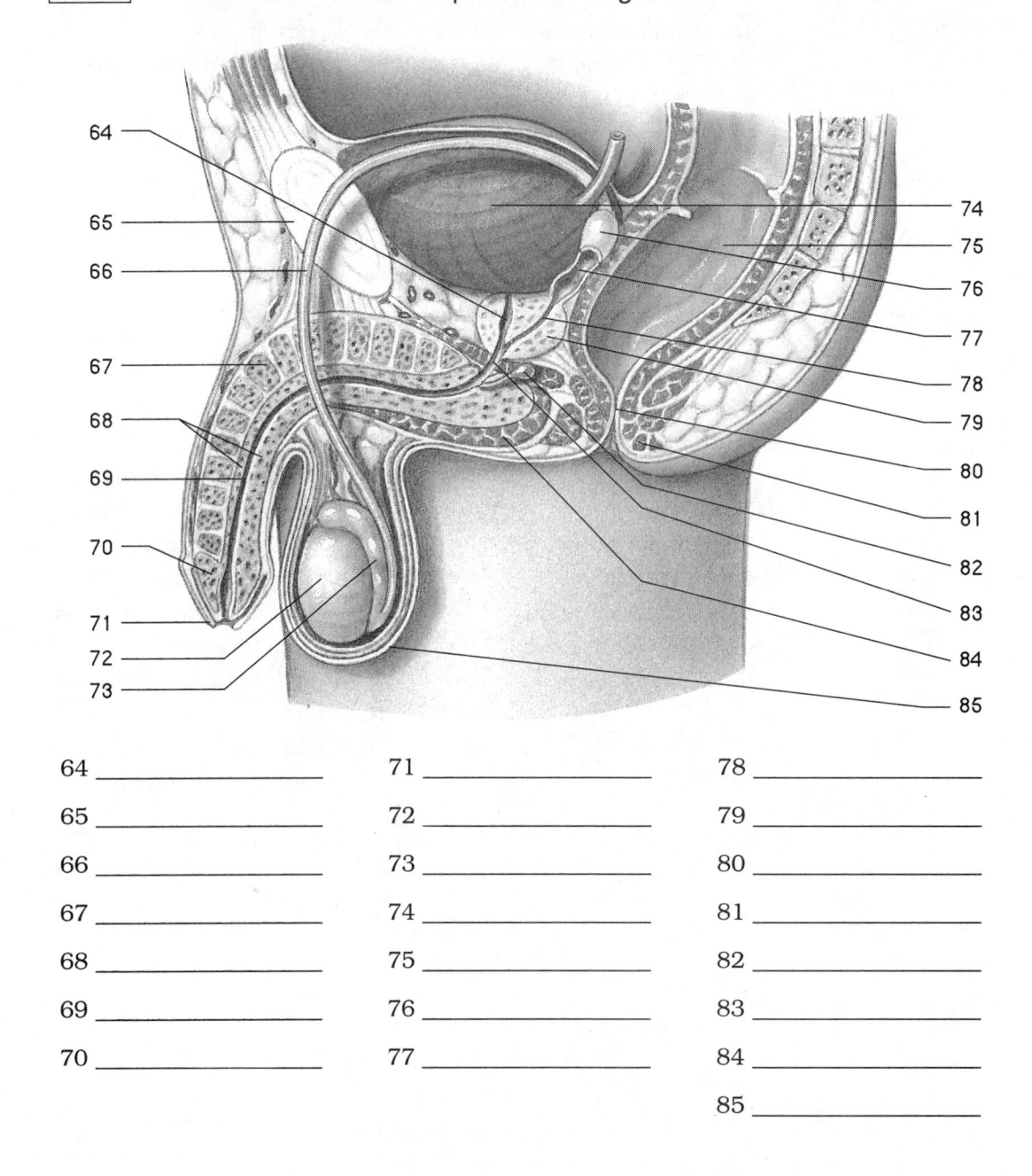

64 _____
65 _____
66 _____
67 _____
68 _____
69 _____
70 _____

71 _____
72 _____
73 _____
74 _____
75 _____
76 _____
77 _____

78 _____
79 _____
80 _____
81 _____
82 _____
83 _____
84 _____
85 _____

Level -1-

Level 1   Review of Chapter Objectives   303

OBJ. 2   **FIGURE 20.2**   The Testis

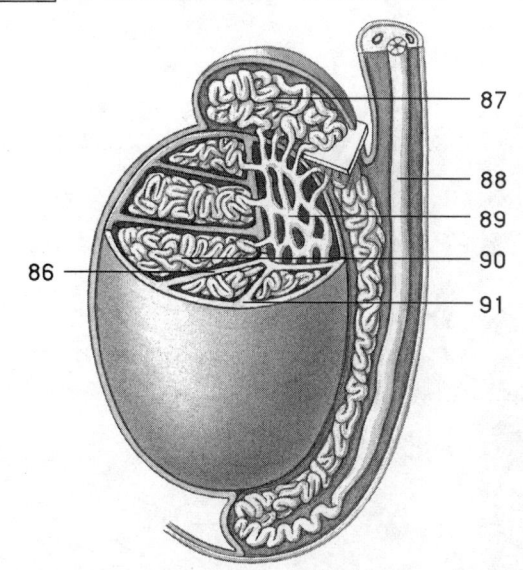

86 _____
87 _____
88 _____
89 _____
90 _____
91 _____

OBJ. 6   **FIGURE 20.3**   Female External Genitalia

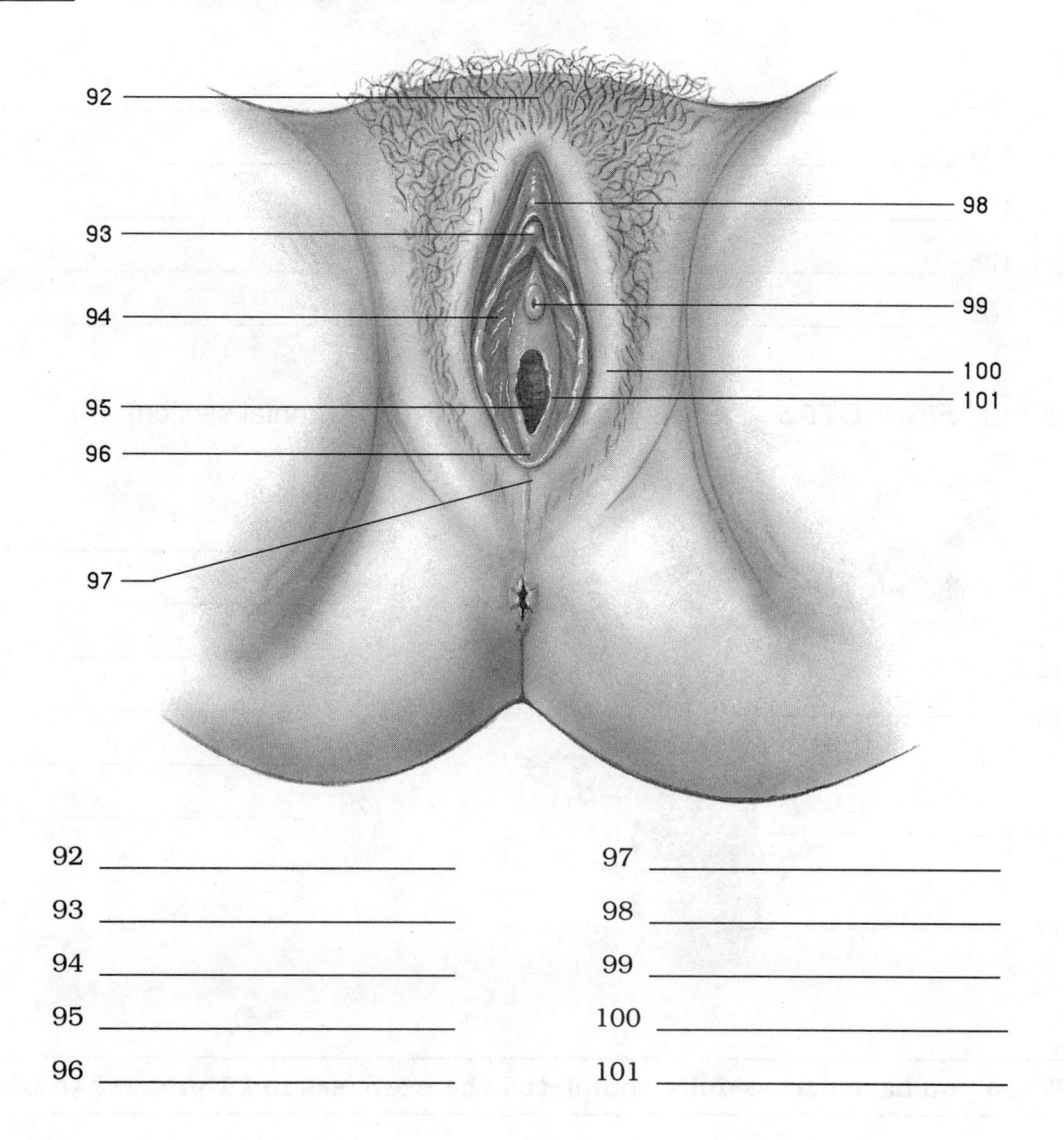

92 _____   97 _____
93 _____   98 _____
94 _____   99 _____
95 _____   100 _____
96 _____   101 _____

Level
-1-

304 **Chapter 20 The Reproductive System**

OBJ. 2   **FIGURE 20.4** Female Reproductive Organs (sagittal section)

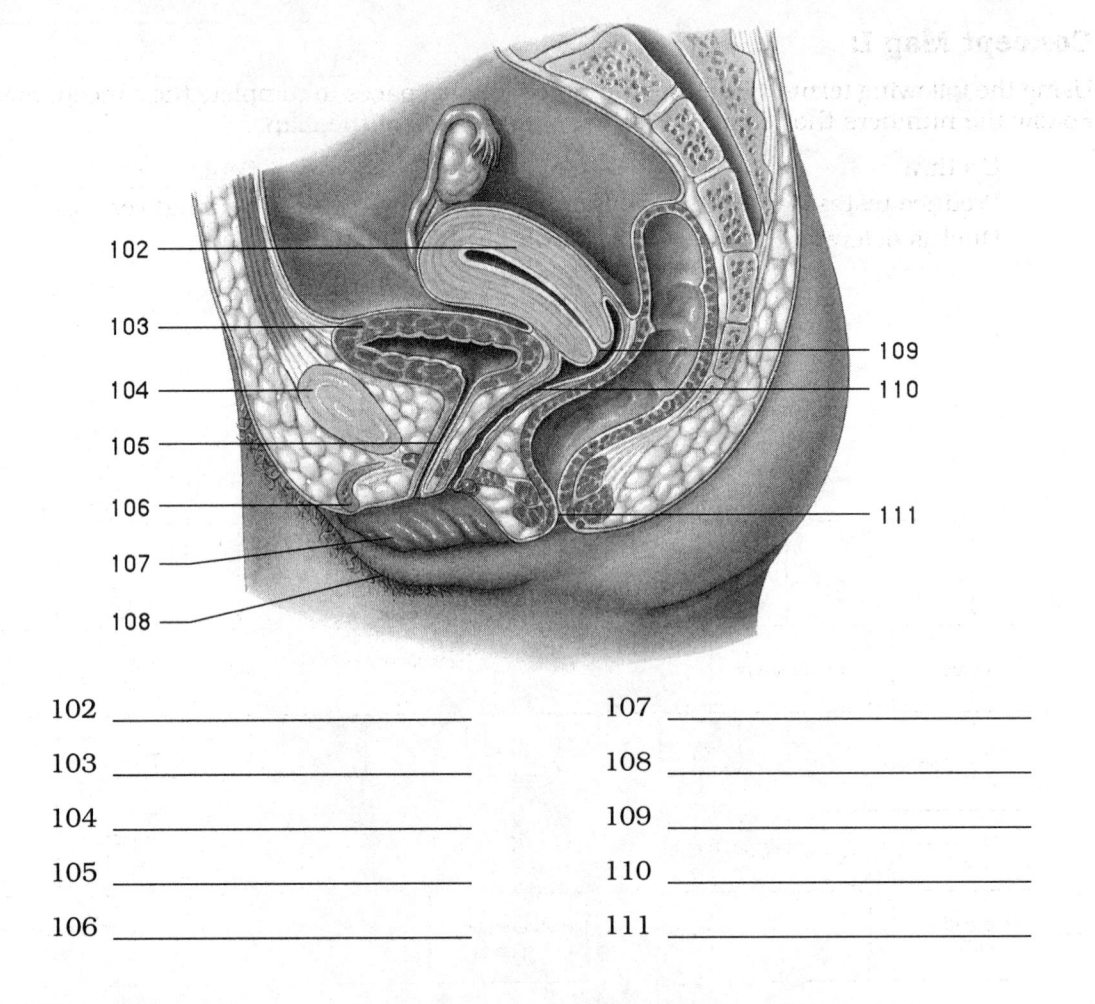

102 _____	107 _____
103 _____	108 _____
104 _____	109 _____
105 _____	110 _____
106 _____	111 _____

OBJ. 6   **FIGURE 20.5** Female Reproductive Organs (frontal section)

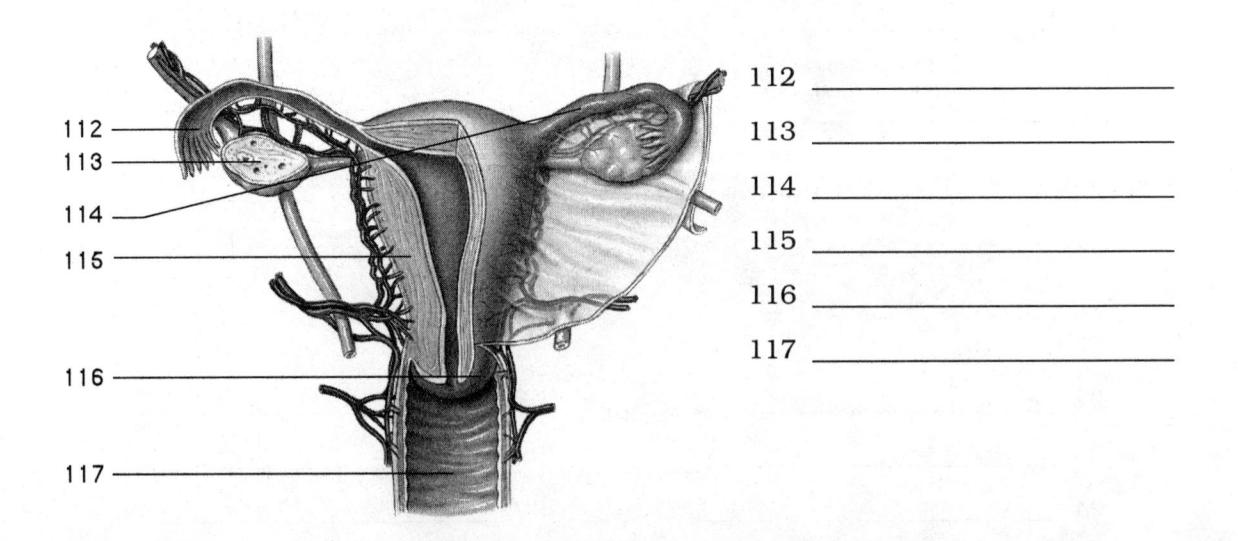

112 _____
113 _____
114 _____
115 _____
116 _____
117 _____

Level -1-   **When you have successfully completed the exercises in L1 proceed to L2.**

LEVEL 2   CONCEPT SYNTHESIS

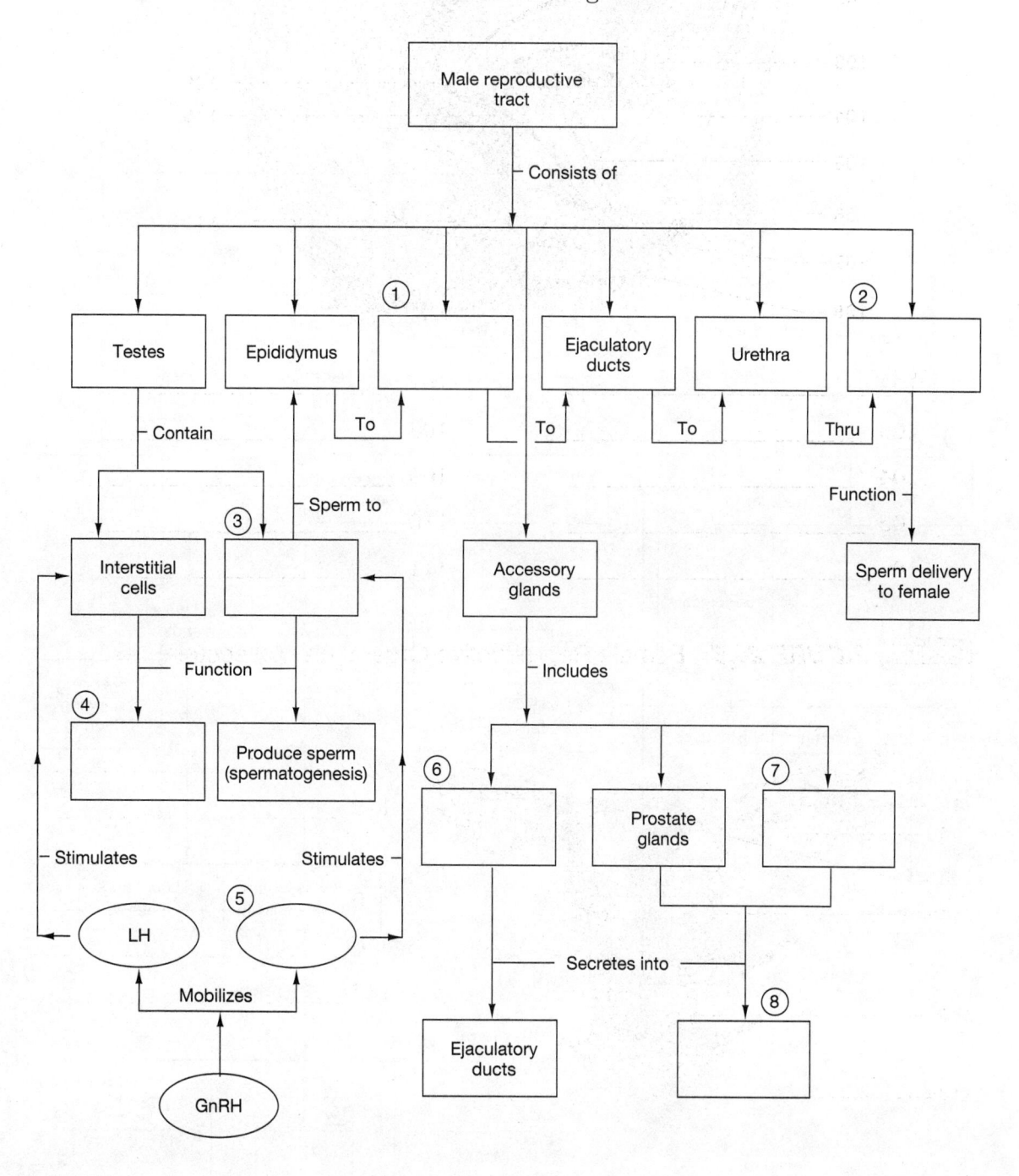

Concept Map I:

Using the following terms, fill in the numbered, blank spaces to complete the concept map. Follow the numbers that comply with the organization of the map.

- Urethra
- Produce testosterone
- Ductus deferens
- Seminiferous tubules
- FSH
- Bulbourethral glands
- Penis
- Seminal vesicles

Chapter 20 The Reproductive System

Concept Map II:

Using the following terms, fill in the blank spaces to complete the concept map. Follow the numbers that comply with the organization of the map.

- nutrients
- vulva
- uterine tubes
- endometrium
- clitoris
- labia majora and minora
- follicle cells
- vagina
- follicles
- supports fetal development

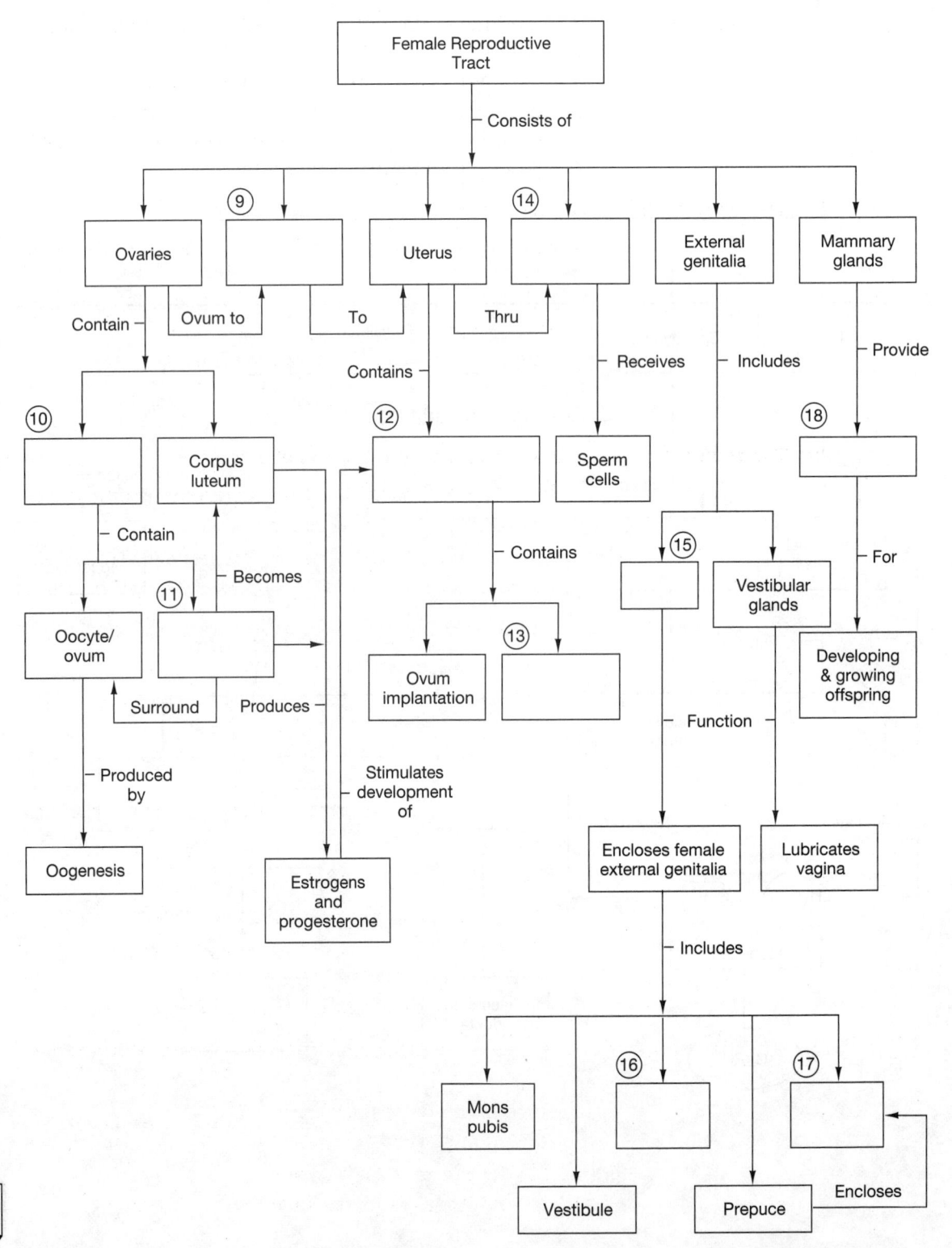

[L2] Multiple Choice:

_____ 19. In a 28-day cycle, estrogen levels peak at:
   a. day 1
   b. day 7
   c. day 14
   d. day 28

_____ 20. The rupture of the follicular wall and ovulation is caused by:
   a. a sudden surge in LH (luteinizing hormone) concentration
   b. a sudden surge in the secretion of estrogen
   c. an increase in the production of progesterone
   d. increased production and release of GnRH (gonadotrophin-releasing hormone)

_____ 21. The body of the spermatic cord is a structure that includes:
   a. epididymis, ductus deferens, blood vessels, and nerves
   b. vas deferens, prostate gland, blood vessels, and urethra
   c. ductus deferens, blood vessels, nerves, and lymphatics
   d. a, b, and c are correct

_____ 22. The tail of the sperm has the unique distinction of being the:
   a. only flagellum in the body that contains chromosomes
   b. only flagellum in the human body
   c. only flagellum in the body that contains mitochondria
   d. only flagellum in the body that contains centrioles

_____ 23. The process of erection involves complex neural processes that include:
   a. increased sympathetic outflow over the pelvic nerves
   b. increased parasympathetic outflow over the pelvic nerves
   c. decreased parasympathetic outflow over the pelvic nerves
   d. somatic motor neurons in the upper sacral segments of the spinal cord

_____ 24. Impotence, a common male sexual dysfunction, is:
   a. the inability to produce sufficient sperm for fertilization
   b. the term used to describe male infertility
   c. the inability of the male to ejaculate
   d. the inability to achieve or maintain an erection

_____ 25. If fertilization is to occur, the ovum must encounter spermatozoa during the first:
   a. 2 - 4 hours of its passage
   b. 6 - 8 hours of its passage
   c. 12 - 24 hours of its passage
   d. 30 - 36 hours of its passage

308 Chapter 20 The Reproductive System

_____ 26. The hormone that acts to reduce the rate of GnRH and FSH production by the anterior pituitary is:

    a. inhibin
    b. LH
    c. ICSH
    d. testosterone

_____ 27. The three sequential stages of the menstrual cycle include:

    a. menses, luteal phase, postovulatory phase
    b. menses, follicular phase, preovulatory phase
    c. menses, proliferative phase, follicular phase
    d. menses, proliferative phase, secretory phase

[L2] Completion:

Using the terms below, complete the following statements.

cervical os	inguinal canals	prepuce	menses
fimbriae	zona pellucida	corona radiata	cremaster
acrosomal cap	corpus luteum		

28. The narrow canals linking the scrotal chambers with the peritoneal cavity are called the _____.
29. The layer of skeletal muscle that contracts and tenses the scrotum, pulling the testes closer to the body, is the _____ muscle.
30. The tip of the sperm containing an enzyme that plays a role in fertilization is the _____.
31. The fold of skin that surrounds the tip of the penis is the _____.
32. Microvilli are present in the space between the developing oocyte and the innermost follicular cells called the _____.
33. Follicular cells surrounding the oocyte prior to ovulation are known as the _____.
34. Degenerated follicular cells proliferate to create an endocrine structure known as the _____.
35. The fingerlike projections on the infundibulum that extend into the pelvic cavity are called the _____.
36. The uterine cavity opens into the vagina at the _____.
37. The period marked by the wholesale destruction of the functional zone of the endometrium is the _____.

[L2] Short Essay:

Briefly answer the following questions in the spaces provided below.

38. (a) What three (3) glands secrete their products into the male reproductive tract?

    (b) What are the primary functions of these glands?

39. What are the primary functions of testosterone in the male?

40. What are the three (3) phases of female sexual function and what occurs in each phase?

41. What are the five (5) steps involved in the ovarian cycle?

42. What are the three (3) stages of the menstrual cycle?

When you have successfully completed the exercises in L2 proceed to L3.

☐ LEVEL 3   CRITICAL THINKING/APPLICATION

Using principles and concepts learned about the reproductive system, answer the following questions. Write your answers on a separate sheet of paper.

1. I. M. Hurt was struck in the abdomen with a baseball bat while playing in a young men's baseball league. As a result, his testes ascend into the abdominopelvic region quite frequently, causing sharp pains. He has been informed by his urologist that he is sterile due to his unfortunate accident.
   a. Why does his condition cause sterility?
   b. What primary factors are necessary for fertility in males?
2. A 19-year-old female visits her gynecologist with the concern that she feels she looks and acts too much like a male. She complains of a low-pitched voice, excess facial hair, and small breasts. Physiologically speaking, what might her problem be related to?
3. A contraceptive pill "tricks the brain" into thinking you are pregnant. What does this mean?
4. Sexually transmitted diseases in males do not result in inflammation of the peritoneum (peritonitis) as they sometimes do in females. Why?

CHAPTER 21

Development and Inheritance

■ Overview

It is difficult to imagine that there is a single cell that in 38 weeks can develop into a complex organism with over 200 million cells organized into tissues, organs, and organ systems. It is the miracle of life!

The previous chapter considered the male and female reproductive systems by which gametes are created and transported and which, in the female, offspring develop and are nourished.

In both males and females, the formation of gametes yields new genetic combinations, similar to, yet different from, their own and those of their parents. The union of gametes therefore results in a unique combination of inherited genes and a unique new individual, who will grow and develop in the mother's womb until birth.

After birth, the offspring will continue to grow and change at a remarkable rate until adulthood. And even throughout adulthood, the body goes through the changes that ultimately result in senescence and death. All of this is the complex process of development.

Chapter 21 highlights the major aspects of development and development processes, as well as the mechanisms and patterns of inheritance, which allows genetic traits to be passed to the next generation.

☐ LEVEL 1   REVIEW OF CHAPTER OBJECTIVES

1. Describe the process of fertilization.
2. List the three prenatal periods and describe the major events associated with each period.
3. Describe the origin of the three primary germ layers and their participation in the formation of the extraembryonic membranes.
4. Describe the interplay between the maternal organ systems and the developing fetus.
5. List and describe the events that occur during labor and delivery.
6. Discuss the major stages of life after delivery.
7. Relate basic principles of genetics to the inheritance of human traits.

[L1] Multiple Choice:

Place the letter corresponding to the correct answer in the space provided.

OBJ. 1 ____ 1. The normal male genotype is ____, and the normal female genotype is ____.
   a. XX; XY
   b. X; Y
   c. XY; XX
   d. Y; X

OBJ. 1 ____ 2. Normal fertilization occurs in the:
   a. lower part of the uterine tube
   b. upper one-third of the uterine tube
   c. upper part of the uterus
   d. antrum of a tertiary follicle

OBJ. 1 ____ 3. Fertilization is completed with the:
   a. formation of a gamete containing 23 chromosomes
   b. formation of the male and female pronuclei
   c. completion of the meiotic process
   d. formation of a zygote containing 46 chromosomes

OBJ. 2 ____ 4. The most dangerous period in prenatal life for congenital malformations to occur is:
   a. the first trimester
   b. the second trimester
   c. the third trimester
   d. during the birth process

OBJ. 2 ____ 5. The four general processes that occur during the first trimester include:
   a. dilation, expulsion, placental, labor
   b. blastocyst, blastomere, morula, trophoblast
   c. cleavage, implantation, placentation, embryogenesis
   d. yolk sac, amnion, allantois, chorion

OBJ. 2 ____ 6. Organs and organ systems complete most of their development during the:
   a. first trimester
   b. second trimester
   c. third trimester
   d. time of placentation

OBJ. 3 ____ 7. Germ-layer formation results from the process of:
   a. embryogenesis
   b. organogenesis
   c. gastrulation
   d. parturition

312 Chapter 21 Development and Inheritance

OBJ. 3 ____ 8. The extraembryonic membranes that develop from the endoderm and mesoderm are:

    a. amnion and chorion
    b. yolk sac and allantois
    c. allantois and chorion
    d. yolk sac and amnion

OBJ. 3 ____ 9. The chorion develops from the:

    a. endoderm and mesoderm
    b. ectoderm and mesoderm
    c. trophoblast and endoderm
    d. mesoderm and trophoblast

OBJ. 4 ____ 10. Blood flows to and from the placenta via:

    a. paired umbilical veins and a single umbilical artery
    b. paired umbilical arteries and a single umbilical vein
    c. a single umbilical artery and a single umbilical vein
    d. two umbilical arteries and two umbilical veins

OBJ. 4 ____ 11. Throughout embryonic and fetal development metabolic wastes generated by the fetus are eliminated by transfer to the:

    a. maternal circulation
    b. amniotic fluid
    c. chorion
    d. allantois

OBJ. 4 ____ 12. Prostaglandins in the endometrium:

    a. stimulate smooth muscle contractions
    b. cause the mammary glands to begin secretory activity
    c. cause an increase in the maternal blood volume
    d. initiate the process of organogenesis

OBJ. 5 ____ 13. During gestation the mother's primary major compensatory adjustment(s) is (are):

    a. increasing respiratory rate and tidal volume
    b. increasing maternal requirements for nutrients
    c. increasing glomerular filtration rate
    d. a, b, and c are correct

OBJ. 6 ____ 14. The sequential stages that identify the features and functions associated with the human experience are:

    a. neonatal, childhood, infancy, maturity
    b. neonatal, postnatal, childbirth, adolescence
    c. infancy, childhood, adolescence, maturity
    d. prenatal, neonatal, postnatal, infancy

OBJ. 6 ____ 15. The systems that were relatively nonfunctional during the fetus's prenatal period that must become functional at birth are the:

    a. circulatory, muscular, skeletal
    b. integumentary, reproductive, nervous
    c. endocrine, nervous, circulatory
    d. respiratory, digestive, excretory

Level 1

Level 1 Review of Chapter Objectives 313

OBJ. 7 ___ 16. The normal chromosome complement of a typical somatic, or body, cell is:

    a. 23
    b. N or haploid
    c. 46
    d. 92

OBJ. 7 ___ 17. Gametes are different from ordinary somatic cells because:

    a. they contain only half the normal number of chromosomes
    b. they contain the full complement of chromosomes
    c. the chromosome number doubles in gametes
    d. gametes are diploid, or 2N

OBJ. 7 ___ 18. Spermatogenesis produces:

    a. four functional spermatids for every primary spermatocyte undergoing meiosis
    b. functional spermatozoa with the diploid number of chromosomes
    c. secondary spermatocytes with the 2N number of chromosomes
    d. a, b, and c are correct

OBJ. 7 ___ 19. Oogenesis produces:

    a. an oogonium with the haploid number of chromosomes
    b. one functional ovum and three nonfunctional polar bodies
    c. a secondary oocyte with the diploid number of chromosomes
    d. a, b, and c are correct

OBJ. 7 ___ 20. If an allele is dominant it will be expressed in the phenotype:

    a. if both alleles agree on the outcome of the phenotype
    b. by the use of lower-case abbreviations
    c. regardless of any conflicting instructions carried by the other allele
    d. by the use of capitalized abbreviations

OBJ. 7 ___ 21. If a single X chromosome of an allelic pair in a female contains the sex-linked gene for color blindness, the individual would be:

    a. normal
    b. color blind
    c. color blind in one eye
    d. a, b, or c could occur

314 Chapter 21 Development and Inheritance

[L1] Completion:

Using the terms below, complete the following statements.

childhood first trimester placenta
capacitation autosomal gametogenesis
dilation heterozygous chorion
infancy homozygous human chorionic
second trimester fertilization hormone

OBJ. 1 22. One chromosome in each pair is contributed by the sperm and the other by the ovum at the time of _____.

OBJ. 1 23. Sperm cannot fertilize an egg until they have undergone an activation in the vagina called _____.

OBJ. 2 24. The time during prenatal development when the fetus begins to look distinctively human is referred to as the _____.

OBJ. 2 25. The period of time during which the rudiments of all the major organ systems appear is referred to as the _____.

OBJ. 3 26. The extraembryonic membrane formed from the mesoderm and trophoblast is the _____.

OBJ. 4 27. The placental hormone present in blood or urine samples that provides reliable indication of pregnancy is _____.

OBJ. 4 28. The vital link between maternal and embryonic systems that support the fetus during development is the _____.

OBJ. 5 29. Rupturing of the amnion or "having the water break" occurs during the late _____ stage.

OBJ. 6 30. The life stage characterized by events that occur prior to puberty is called _____.

OBJ. 6 31. The life stage that follows the neonatal period and continues to 2 years of age is referred to as _____.

OBJ. 7 32. The formation of gametes is called _____.

OBJ. 7 33. Chromosomes with genes that affect only somatic characteristics are referred to as _____ chromosomes.

OBJ. 7 34. If both chromosomes of a homologous pair carry the same allele of a particular gene, the individual is _____ for that trait.

OBJ. 7 35. When an individual has two different alleles carrying different instructions, the individual is _____ for that trait.

Level -1-

Level 1 Review of Chapter Objectives 315

[L1] Matching:

Match the terms in column "B" with the terms in column "A." Use letters for answers in the spaces provided.

COLUMN "A"

OBJ.	#	Term
OBJ. 1	36.	Amphimixis
OBJ. 1	37.	N
OBJ. 2	38.	Gestation
OBJ. 3	39.	Chorion
OBJ. 4	40.	Maternal organ systems
OBJ. 4	41.	Relaxin
OBJ. 5	42.	Parturition
OBJ. 6	43.	Neonate
OBJ. 6	44.	Adolescence
OBJ. 7	45.	2N
OBJ. 7	46.	Meiosis I
OBJ. 7	47.	Meiosis II
OBJ. 7	48.	Phenotype
OBJ. 7	49.	Genotype

COLUMN "B"

A. Softens symphysis pubis
B. Prenatal development
C. Pronuclei fusion
D. Somatic cell
E. Equational Division
F. Newborn infant
G. Visible characteristics
H. Supports developing fetus
I. Reduction division
J. Gamete
K. Chromosomes and component genes
L. Begins at puberty
M. Forcible expulsion of the fetus
N. Mesoderm and trophoblast

316 Chapter 21 Development and Inheritance

[L1] Drawing/Illustration Labeling:

OBJ. 1 **FIGURE 21.1** Spermatogenesis

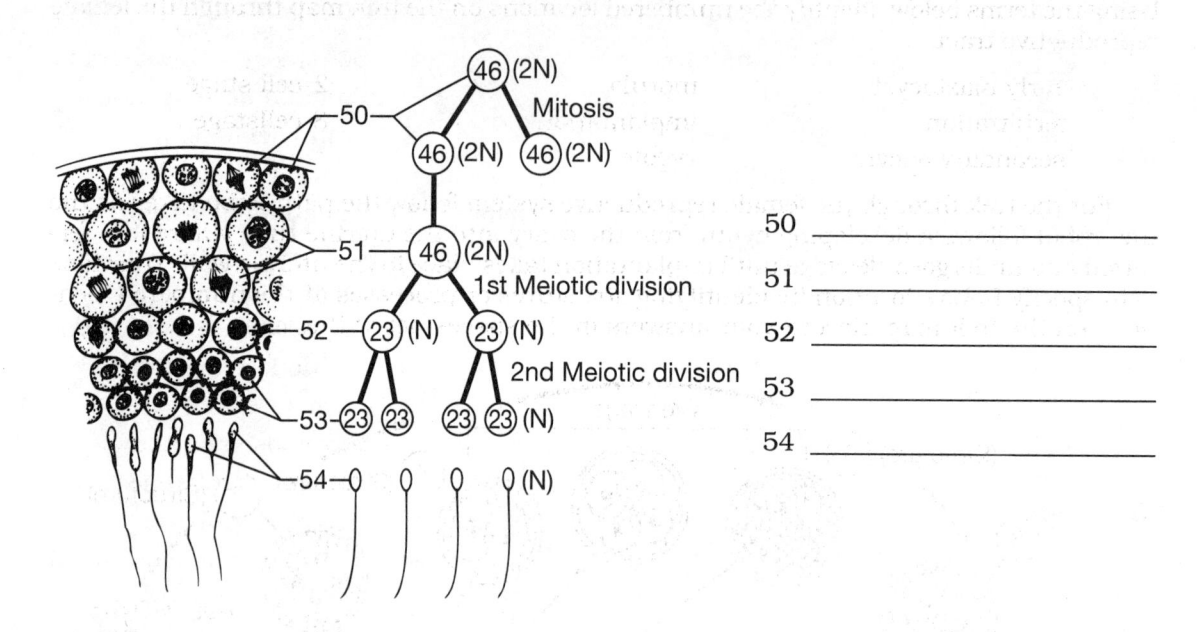

50 _____
51 _____
52 _____
53 _____
54 _____

OBJ. 2 **FIGURE 21.2** Oogenesis

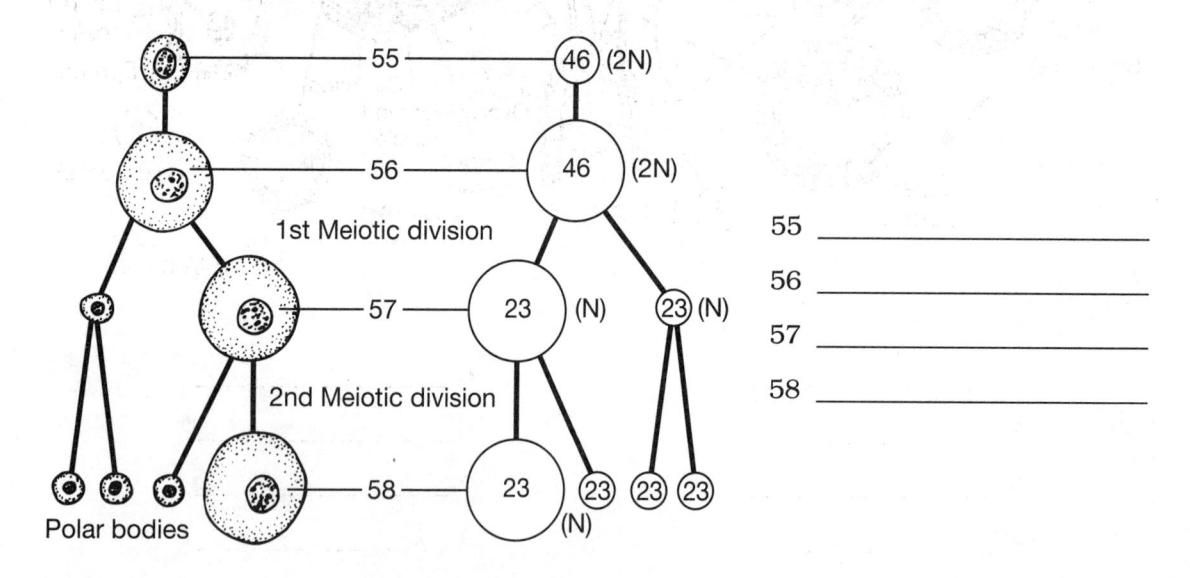

55 _____
56 _____
57 _____
58 _____

Level -1- When you have successfully completed the exercises in L1 proceed to L2.

☐ LEVEL 2   CONCEPT SYNTHESIS

Body Trek:

Using the terms below, identify the numbered locations on the trek map through the female reproductive tract.

early blastocyst   morula   2-cell stage
fertilization   implantation   8-cell stage
secondary oocyte   zygote

For the trek through the female reproductive system follow the path Robo takes as the tiny robot follows a developing ovum from the ovary into the uterine tube where it is fertilized and undergoes cleavage until implantation takes place in the uterine wall. Your task is to specify Robo's location by identifying structures or processes at the numbered locations on the trek map. Record your answers in the spaces below the map.

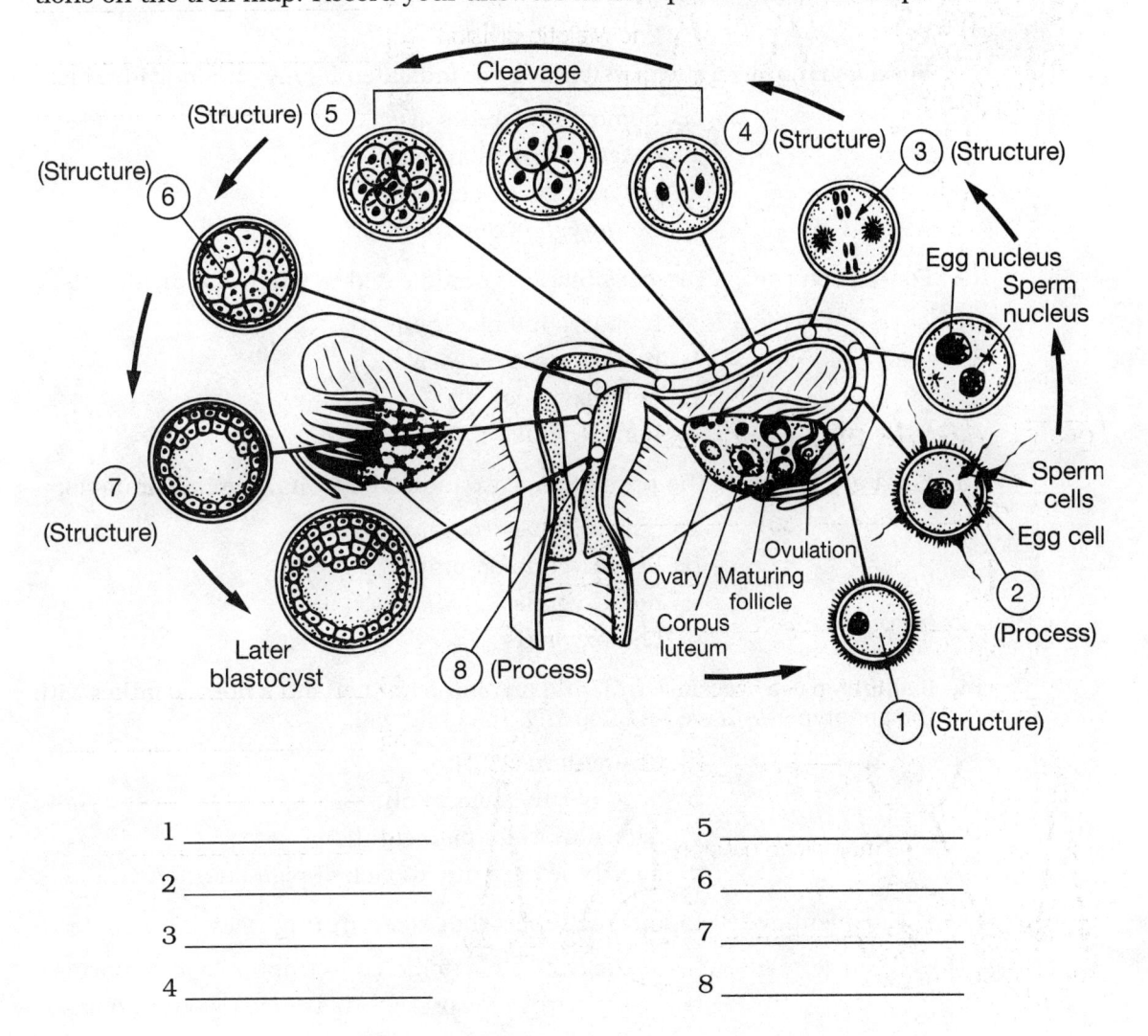

1 _____   5 _____
2 _____   6 _____
3 _____   7 _____
4 _____   8 _____

Chapter 21 Development and Inheritance

[L2] Multiple Choice:

Place the letter corresponding to the correct answer in the space provided.

_____ 9. The completion of metaphase II, anaphase II, and telophase II produces:
   a. four gametes, each containing 46 chromosomes
   b. four gametes, each containing 23 chromosomes
   c. one gamete containing 46 chromosomes
   d. one gamete containing 23 chromosomes

_____ 10. The primary function of the spermatozoa is to:
   a. nourish and program the ovum
   b. support the development of the ovum
   c. carry paternal chromosomes to the site of fertilization
   d. a, b, and c are correct

_____ 11. For a given trait, if the possibilities are indicated by AA, the individual is:
   a. homozygous recessive
   b. heterozygous dominant
   c. heterozygous recessive
   d. homozygous dominant

_____ 12. For a given trait, if the possibilities are indicated by Aa, the individual is:
   a. homozygous dominant
   b. homozygous recessive
   c. heterozygous
   d. homozygous

_____ 13. For a given trait, if the possibilities are indicated by aa, the individual is:
   a. homozygous recessive
   b. homozygous dominant
   c. homozygous
   d. heterozygous

_____ 14. If albinism is a recessive trait and an albino mother and a normal father with the genotype AA have an offspring, the child will:
   a. be an albino
   b. have normal coloration
   c. have abnormal pigmentation
   d. have blue eyes due to lack of pigmentation

_____ 15. The sequential developmental stages that occur during cleavage include:
   a. blastocyst → blastomeres → trophoblast → morula
   b. blastomeres → morula → blastocyst → trophoblast
   c. yolk sac → amnion → allantois → chorion
   d. amnion → allantois → chorion → yolk sac

_____ 16. The zygote arrives in the uterine cavity as a:
   a. morula
   b. blastocyst
   c. trophoblast
   d. chorion

_____ 17. During implantation the inner cell mass of the blastocyst separates from the trophoblast, creating a fluid-filled chamber called the:

        a. blastodisk
        b. blastocoele
        c. allantois
        d. amniotic cavity

_____ 18. In the event of "fraternal" or dizygotic twins:

        a. the blastomeres separate early during cleavage
        b. the inner cell mass splits prior to gastrulation
        c. two separate eggs are ovulated and fertilized
        d. a, b, and c are correct

_____ 19. The important and complex development event(s) that occur during the first trimester is (are):

        a. cleavage
        b. implantation and placentation
        c. embryogenesis
        d. a, b, and c are correct

_____ 20. Exchange between the embryonic and maternal circulations occur by diffusion across the trophoblast layer via:

        a. the umbilicus
        b. the allantois
        c. the chorionic blood vessels
        d. the yolk sac

_____ 21. Embryogenesis is the process that establishes the foundation for:

        a. the formation of the blastocyst
        b. implantation to occur
        c. the formation of the placenta
        d. all the major organ systems

_____ 22. An ectopic pregnancy refers to:

        a. implantation occurring within the endometrium
        b. implantation occurring somewhere other than within the uterus
        c. the formation of a gestational neoplasm
        d. the formation of extraembryonic membranes in the uterus

[L2] Completion:

Using the terms below, complete the following statements.

cleavage	alleles	X-linked
differentiation	inheritance	simple inheritance
genetics	polygenic inheritance	

23. Transfer of genetically determined characteristics from generation to generation refers to _____.
24. The study of the mechanisms responsible for inheritance is called _____.
25. The various forms of any one gene are called _____.
26. Characteristics carried by genes on the X chromosome that affect somatic structures are termed _____.

320 Chapter 21 Development and Inheritance

27. Phenotypic characters determined by interactions between a single pair of alleles are known as _____.
28. Interactions between alleles on several genes involve _____.
29. The sequence of cell division that begins immediately after fertilization and ends at the first contact with the uterine wall is called _____.
30. The creation of different cell types during development is called _____.

[L2]   Short Essay:

Briefly answer the following questions in the spaces provided below.

31. a. What are the four (4) extraembryonic membranes that are formed from the three (3) germ layers?

    b. From which given layer(s) does each membrane originate?

32. What are the major compensatory adjustments necessary in the maternal systems to support the developing fetus?

33. What primary factors interact to produce labor contractions in the uterine wall?

34. What three (3) events interact to promote increased hormone production and sexual maturation at adolescence?

35. What four (4) processes are involved with aging that influence the genetic programming of individual cells?

Level 2

When you have successfully completed the exercises in L2 proceed to L3.

LEVEL 3 CRITICAL THINKING/APPLICATION

Using principles and concepts learned about development and inheritance, answer the following questions. Write your answers on a separate sheet of paper.

1. A common form of color blindness is associated with the presence of a dominant or recessive gene on the X chromosome. Normal color vision is determined by the presence of a dominant gene (C), and color blindness results from the presence of the recessive gene (c). Suppose a heterozygous normal female marries a normal male. Is it possible for any of their children to be color blind? Show the possibilities by using a Punnett square.

2. Albinism (aa) is inherited as a homozygous recessive trait. If a homozygous-recessive mother and a heterozygous father decide to have children, what are the possibilities of their offspring inheriting albinism? Use a Punnett square to show the possibilities.

3. Tongue rolling is inherited as a dominant trait. Even though a mother and father are tongue rollers (T), show how it would be possible to bear children who do not have the ability to roll the tongue. Use a Punnett square to show the possibilities.

ANSWER KEY

Chapter 1

An Introduction to Anatomy & Physiology

[L1] MULTIPLE CHOICE:

1. B	2. C	3. A	4. D	5. B
6. C	7. C	8. D	9. A	10. D
11. C	12. D	13. C	14. A	15. D
16. D	17. C	18. D	19. B	20. B
21. C	22. A			

[L1] COMPLETION:

23. responsivenesss	24. digestion	25. excretion
26. histologist	27. physiology	28. tissues
29. molecules	30. organs	31. urinary
32. digestive	33. integumentary	34. regulation
35. positive feedback	36. endocrine	37. liver
38. medial	39. distal	40. transverse
41. pericardial	42. mediastinum	

[L1] MATCHING:

44. E	45. C	46. H	47. A	48. J
49. I	50. D	51. S	52. F	53. G
54. L	55. K			

[L1] DRAWING/ILLUSTRATION LABELING:

Figure 1.1

56. frontal (coronal)	57. transverse	58. midsagittal

Figure 1.2

59. superior (cephalad)	60. posterior (dorsal)	61. inferior (caudal)
62. anterior (ventral)	63. proximal	64. distal

Figure 1.3

65. occipital
66. deltoid
67. scapular
68. lumbar
69. gluteal
70. popliteal
71. calf
72. axillary
73. brachial
74. abdominal
75. femoral
76. orbital
77. buccal
78. cervical
79. thorax
80. cubital
81. umbilical
82. pubic
83. palmar
84. patellar

Figure 1.4

85. ventral cavity
86. thoracic cavity
87. diaphragm
88. abdominal cavity
89. pelvic cavity
90. cranial cavity
91. spinal cavity
92. dorsal cavity

Figure 1.5

93. left thoracic cavity
94. pericardial cavity
95. right thoracic cavity
96. diaphragm

[L2] CONCEPT MAPS:

I.

1. macroscopic anatomy
2. regional anatomy
3. structure of organ systems
4. surgical anatomy
5. cytology
6. tissues

II.

7. cranial cavity
8. spinal cord
9. two pleural cavities
10. heart
11. abdominopelvic cavity
12. pelvic cavity

III.

13. radiologist
14. high-energy radiation
15. CT scans
16. radio waves
17. echogram

[L2] BODY TREK:

18. atoms
19. molecules
20. organelles
21. cells
22. tissues
23. organs
24. systems
25. organisms

[L2] MULTIPLE CHOICE:

26. A
27. C
28. C
29. B
30. B
31. D
32. D

[L2] COMPLETION:

33. extrinsic regulation
34. nervous
35. knee
36. appendicitis
37. elbow
38. stethoscope
39. sternum

[L2] SHORT ESSAY:

40. Any one of the following might be listed: responsiveness, adaptability, growth, reproduction, movement, absorption, respiration, excretion, digestion, circulation.

41. Subatomic particles - atoms - molecules - organelle - cell(s) - tissue(s) - organ(s) - system(s)

42. In negative feedback a variation outside of normal limits triggers an automatic response that corrects the situation. In positive feedback the initial stimulus produces a response that exaggerates the stimulus.

Chapter 1 An Introduction to Anatomy and Physiology

43. a) They protect delicate organs from accidental shocks and cushion them from the thumps and bumps that occur during walking, jumping and running.

    b) They permit significant changes in the size and shape of visceral organs.

[L3] CRITICAL THINKING/APPLICATION:

1. Since there is a lung in each compartment, if one lung is diseased or infected the other lung may remain functional. Also, if one lung is traumatized due to injury, the other one may be spared and function sufficiently to save the life of the injured person.

2. Stretching of the uterus by the developing embryo stimulates the start of contractions. Contractions push the baby toward the opening of the uterus, causing additional stretching which initiates more contractions. The cycle continues until the baby is delivered and the stretching stimulation is eliminated.

3. pericardial, mediastinal, abdominal, pelvic

4. Barium is very radiodense, and the contours of the gastric and intestinal lining can be seen against the white of the barium solution.

Chapter 2
The Chemical Level of Organization

[L1] MULTIPLE CHOICE:

1. D
2. C
3. B
4. A
5. C
6. C
7. D
8. C
9. A
10. D
11. D
12. B
13. C
14. B
15. A
16. C
17. B
18. D
19. B
20. C

[L1] COMPLETION:

21. Protons
22. atomic weight
23. covalent bonds
24. ionic bonds
25. Na$_2$S$_4$
26. decomposition
27. exergonic, endergonic
28. catalysts
29. organic
30. inorganic
31. solvent, solute
32. acidic
33. buffers
34. salt
35. glucose
36. dehydration synthesis

[L1] MATCHING:

37. I
38. N
39. F
40. L
41. A
42. G
43. D
44. H
45. C
46. B
47. M
48. E
49. K
50. J

[L1] DRAWING/ILLUSTRATION LABELING:

Figure 2.1

51. nonpolar covalent bond
52. polar covalent bond
53. ionic bond

Figure 2.2

54. monosaccharide
55. disaccharide
56. polysaccharide
57. saturated fatty acid
58. polyunsaturated fatty acid
59. amino acid
60. cholesterol
61. DNA

[L2] CONCEPT MAPS:

I. CARBOHYDRATES

1. monosaccharides
2. glucose
3. disaccharide
4. sucrose
5. complex carbohydrates
6. gycogen
7. plants

II. LIPIDS

8. saturated
9. glyceride
10. diglyceride (Di)
11. glycerol + 3 fatty acids
12. phospholipid
13. steroids

III. PROTEINS

14. amino acids
15. amino group
16. -COOH
17. variable group
18. globular proteins
19. enzymes
20. keratin

IV. NUCLEIC ACIDS

21. deoxyribonucleic acid
22. deoxyribose
23. thymine (T)
24. ribonucleic acid
25. ribose
26. N bases
27. uracil (U)

Chapter 2 The Chemical Level of Organization

[L2] BODY TREK:

28. electrons
29. shells
30. nucleus
31. protons
32. neutrons
33. isotope
34. double covalent bond
35. molecule
36. oxygen gas
37. polar covalent
38. negatively

[L2] MULTIPLE CHOICE:

39. B
40. D
41. D
42. C
43. B
44. D
45. D
46. A

[L2] COMPLETION:

47. ionic bond
48. inorganic compounds
49. alkaline
50. hydrolysis
51. dehydration synthesis
52. peptide bond

[L2] SHORT ESSAY:

53.

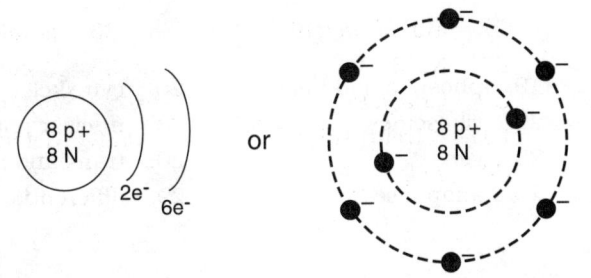

54. The oxygen atom has a much stronger attraction for the shared electrons than do the hydrogen atoms, so the electrons spend most of this time in the vicinity of the oxygen nucleus. Because the oxygen atom has two extra electrons part of the time, it develops a slight negative charge. The hydrogens develop a slight positive charge because their electrons are away part of the time.

55. (1) molecular structure, (2) freezing point 0 degrees C; boiling point 100 degrees C, (3) capacity to absorb and distribute heat, (4) heat absorbed during evaporation, (5) solvent properties, (6) 66 % total body weight.

56. carbohydrates, ex. glucose; lipids, ex. steroids; proteins, ex. enzymes; nucleic acid, ex. DNA

57. (1) adenine nucleotide; (2) thymine nucleotide; (3) cytosine nucleotide; (4) guanine nucleotide

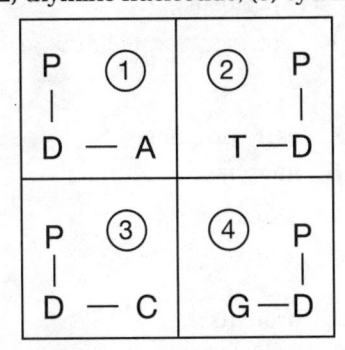

[L3] CRITICAL THINKING/APPLICATION:

1. Baking soda is sodium bicarbonate (NaHCO$_3$). In solution sodium bicarbonate reversibly dissociates into a sodium ion (Na$^+$) and a bicarbonate ion (HCO$_3^-$) [NaHCO $\leftrightarrow$ Na$^+$ + HCO$_3^-$]. The bicarbonate ion will remove an excess hydrogen ion (H$^+$) from the solution and form a weak acid, carbonic acid [H$^+$ + HCO$_3^-$ $\leftrightarrow$ H$_2$CO$_3$].

2. $C_6H_{12}O_6 + C_6H_{12}O_6 \leftrightarrow C_{12}H_{22}O_{11} + H_2O$

3. Carbohydrates are an immediate source of energy and can be metabolized quickly. Those not immediately metabolized may be stored as glycogen or excessses may be stored as fat.

4. The RDA for fat intake per day is 30 % of the total caloric intake. Fats are necessary for good health. They are involved in many body functions and serve as energy reserves, provide insulation, cushion delicate organs, and are essential structural components of all cells.

Chapter 3

The Cellular Level of Organization: Cell Structure

[L1] MULTIPLE CHOICE:

1. D.
2. C
3. D
4. C
5. A
6. A
7. B
8. A
9. D
10. C
11. A
12. B
13. C
14. B
15. A
16. C
17. C

[L1] COMPLETION:

18. cell theory
19. phospholipid bilayer
20. cytoskeleton
21. endocytosis
22. ribosomes
23. nuclear pores
24. nucleus
25. gene
26. translation
27. interphase
28. anaphase
29. differentiation

[L1] MATCHING:

30. M
31. G
32. B
33. K
34. C
35. A
36. L
37. I
38. E
39. D
40. H
41. F
42. J

[L1] DRAWING/ILLUSTRATION LABELING:

Figure 3.1

44. cilia
45. centriole
46. Golgi apparatus
47. smooth endoplasmic reticulum
48. mitochondrion
49. ribosomes
50. rough endoplasmic reticulum
51. nuclear envelope
52. nuclear pores
53. microvilli
54. cytosol
55. nucleolus
56. chromatin

Figure 3.2

57. interphase
58. early prophase
59. late prophase
60. metaphase
61. anaphase
62. telophase

[L2] CONCEPT MAPS:

I.

1. lipid bilayer
2. proteins
3. organelles
4. membranes
5. nucleolus
6. lysosomes
7. centrioles
8. ribosomes
9. fluid component

II.

10. somatic cells
11. DNA replication
12. mitosis
13. metaphase
14. telophase
15. cytokinesis

Chapter 3 The Cellular Level of Organization: Cell Structure

[L2] BODY TREK:

16. extracellular fluid
17. cilia
18. cell membrane
19. membrane proteins
20. channels
21. phospholipid
22. anchor proteins
23. intracellular fluid
24. cytoskeleton
25. organelles
26. protein synthesis
27. cell division
28. mitochondrion
29. cristae
30. matrix
31. energy-producing enzymes
32. ATP
33. nucleus
34. nuclear pores
35. nuclear envelope
36. nucleoli
37. ribosomes
38. nucleoplasm
39. chromosomes
40. endoplasmic reticulum
41. rough endoplasmic reticulum
42. Golgi apparatus

[L2] MULTIPLE CHOICE:

43. C   44. A   45. D   46. A   47. C
48. D   49. D   50. B   51. A   52. A
53. B   54. C

[L2] COMPLETION:

55. channels
56. microvilli
57. cilia
58. rough ER
59. permeability
60. diffusion
61. isotonic

[L2] SHORT ESSAY:

62. (a) Circulatory - RBC; (b) Muscular - muscle cell; (c) Reproductive - sperm cell; (d) Skeletal - bone cell; (e) Nervous - neuron (Other systems and cells could be listed for this answer.)

63. (a) Physical isolation; (b) Regulation of exchange with the environment; (c) Sensitivity; (d) Structural support

64. Cytosol - high concentration of K+; Extra Cellular Fluid (E.C.F.) - high concentration of Na+

    Cytosol - higher concentration of dissolved proteins

    Cytosol - smaller quantities of carbohydrates and lipids

65. Centrioles - move DNA during cell division

    Cilia - move fluids or solids across cell surfaces

    Flagella - move cell through fluids

[L3] CRITICAL THINKING/APPLICATION:

1. In salt water drowning, the body fluid becomes hypertonic to cells. The cells dehydrate and shrink, which causes the victim to go into shock, thus allowing time for resuscitaion to occur. In freshwater drowning, the body fluid is hypotonic to cells causing the cells to swell and burst. The intracellular K+ are released into circulation and when contacting the heart in excessive amounts can cause cardiac arrest, thus allowing little time for the possiblity of resuscitation.

2. MgSO$_4$ —epsom salts—increase the solute concentration in the lumen of the large intestine making the intestine hypertonic to surrounding tissues. The osmosis of water occurs from the surrounding tissues into the intestinal lumen. The fluid helps to soften the stool and the watery environment prepares the intestine for eventual evacuation of the stool from the bowel.

3. Because of the increase of solute concentration in the body fluid, it becomes hypertonic to the RBCs. The red blood cells dehydrate and shrink—crenation. The crenated RBCs lose their oxygen-carrying capacity and body tissues are deprived of the oxygen necessary for cellular metabolism.

4. The vegetables contain a greater solute concentration than does the watery environment surrounding them. The vegetables are hypertonic to the surrounding fluid; therefore, the osmosis of water into the vegetables causes crispness or turgidity.

Chapter 4
The Tissue Level of Organization

[L1] MULTIPLE CHOICE:

1. D	2. C	3. D	4. A	5. D
6. A	7. B	8. C	9. D	10. D
11. B	12. C	13. A	14. D	15. B
16. C	17. B	18. D	19. C	20. B
21. A	22. A	23. C	24. D	25. D
26. B	27. B	28. C	29. A	30. C

[L1] COMPLETION:

31. connective
32. stratified ep.
33. gap junction
34. exocytosis
35. collagen
36. areolar
37. mucous
38. skeletal
39. neuroglia
40. infection
41. osteoporosis

[L1] MATCHING:

42. O	43. H	44. M	45. I	46. A
47. B	48. L	49. F	50. N	51. K
52. C	53. G	54. J	55. D	56. E

[L1] DRAWING/ILLUSTRATION LABELING:

Figure 4.1 Types of Epithelial Tissue

57. simple squamous
58. statified squamous
59. simple columnar
60. simple cuboidal
61. transitional
62. pseudostratified columnar

Figure 4.2 Types of Connective Tissue

63. loose
64. adipose
65. dense
66. hyaline cartilage
67. fibrocartilage
68. elastic cartilage
69. osseous (bone)
70. blood

Figure 4.3 Types of Muscle Tissue

71. smooth
72. cardiac
73. skeletal

Figure 4.4

74. neuron

[L2] CONCEPT MAP:

1. epithelial
2. connective
3. muscle
4. neural

[L2] BODY TREK:

5. stratified squamous ep.
6. trachea mucosa (ciliated)
7. simple squamous ep.
8. simple cuboidal ep.
9. transitional ep.
10. adipose
11. tendons, ligaments
12. hyaline cartilage
13. fibrocartilage
14. elastic cartilage
15. bone or osseous
16. cardiovascular system
17. skeletal muscle
18. cardiac muscle
19. smooth muscle
20. neurons (axons, dendrites, neurogila)

Chapter 4 The Tissue Level of Organization

[L2] MULTIPLE CHOICE:

21. B 22. D 23. A 24. B 25. D
26. C 27. D 28. C 29. B

[L2] COMPLETION:

30. avascular
31. exocrine
32. endocrine
33. desmosomes
34. tight junctions
35. serous
36. mucous
37. exfoliation

[L2] SHORT ESSAY:

38. epithelial, connective, muscle, neural tissue

39. Provides physical protection, controls permeability, provides sensations, and provides specialized secretion.

40. Microvilli are abundant on epithelial surfaces where absorption and secretion take place. A cell with microvilli has at least twenty times the surface area of a cell without them. A typical ciliated cell contains about 250 cilia that beat in coordinated fashion. Materials are moved over the epithelial surface by the synchronized beating of cilia.

41. Merocrine secretion—the product is released through exocytosis. Apocrine secretion — loss of cytoplasm as well as the secretory product.
    Holocrine secretion — product is released, cell is destroyed.
    (Merocrine and apocrine secretions leave the cell intact & are able to continue secreting; holocrine does not.)

42. Specialized cells, extracellular protein fibers, and ground substance.

43. collagen, reticular, elastic

44. Mucous membranes, serous membranes, cutaneous membranes and synovial membranes.

45. skeletal, cardiac, smooth

46. neurons — transmission of nerve impulses from one region to the body to another
    neuroglia — support framework for neural tissue

[L3] CRITICAL THINKING/APPLICATION:

1. Tissues play an important part in diagnosis, which is necessary prior to treatment. As a part of the Allied Health Professional team, the histologist synthesizes anatomical and histological observations to determine the nature and severity of the disease or illness.

2. Integumentary system — sebaceous, sweat, mammary
   Digestive system — salivary, pancreatic

3. *Staphylococcus aureus* secretes the enzyme hyaluronidase which breaks down hyaluronic acid and other proteoglycans (an important part of ground substance). These bacteria are dangerous because they can spread rapidly by liquefying the ground substance of connective tissues and dissolving the intercellular cement that hold epithelial cells together.

4. Because chondrocytes produce a chemical that discourages the formation of blood vessels, cartilage is avascular. All nutrient and waste product exchange must occur by diffusion which is a very slow process) through the matrix. This may cause the healing process to be slow, if it occurs at all.

Chapter 5

The Integumentary System

[L1] MULTIPLE CHOICE:

1. C	2. D	3. D	4. A	5. D
6. C	7. D	8. A	9. B	10. D
11. D	12. B	13. C	14. C	15. D
16. C	17. B	18. A	19. D	20. D
21. D	22. C			

[L1] COMPLETION:

23. skin
24. stratum lucidum
25. stratum corneum
26. dermal blood supply
27. decrease
28. melanin
29. sebum
30. sebaceous glands
31. follicle
32. cyanosis
33. melanocyte
34. glandular

[L1] MATCHING:

35. J	36. H	37. I	38. D	39. A
40. E	41. G	42. C	43. B	44. F

[L1] DRAWING/ILLUSTRATION LABELING:

Figure 5.1 Organization of the Integument

43. dermis
44. subcutaneous layer
45. stratum corneum
46. stratum lucidum
47. stratum granulosum
48. stratum spinosum
49. stratum germinativum
50. epidermis
51. sebaceous gland
52. arrector pili muscle
53. hair follicle
54. sweat gland
55. touch and pressure receptor

[L2] CONCEPT MAPS:

I.

1. dermis
2. vitamin D synthesis
3. sensory reception
4. exocrine glands
5. lubrication
6. produce secretions

II.

7. skin
8. epidermis
9. granulosum
10. papillary layer
11. nerves
12. collagen
13. connective
14. fat

[L2] BODY TREK:

15. lunula
16. cuticle
17. keratin
18. stratum lucidum
19. stratum granulosum
20. desmosomes
21. stratum spinosum
22. stratum germinativum
23. mitosis
24. epidermal ridges
25. papillary
26. dermal papillae
27. sebaceous
28. reticular layer
29. collagen
30. elastic
31. subcutaneous layer

Chapter 5 The Integumentary System

[L2] **MULTIPLE CHOICE:**

32. A 33. D 34. B 35. C 36. D
37. C 38. A

[L2] **COMPLETION:**

39. epidermal ridge 40. lipid-soluble carriers 41. liposomes
42. malignant melanoma 43. melanocytes 44. dandruff

[L2] **SHORT ESSAY:**

45. Palms of hand; soles of feet. These areas are covered with 30 or more layers of cornified cells. The epidermis in these locations may be six times thicker than the epidermis covering the general body surface.

46. Stratum corneum, stratum granulosum, stratum spinosum, stratum germinativum, papillary layer, reticular layer.

47. Long-term damage can result from chronic exposure, and an individual attempting to acquire a deep tan places severe stress on the skin. Alterations in underlying connective tissue lead to premature wrinkling, and skin cancer can result from chromosomal damage or breakage.

48. Hairs are dead, keratinized structures, and no amount of oiling or shampooing with added ingredients will influence either the exposed hair or the follicles buried in the dermis.

[L3] **CRITICAL THINKING/APPLICATION:**

1. The ocean is a hypertonic solution, thus causing water to leave the body by crossing the epidermis from the underlying tissues.

2. Blood with abundant O_2 is bright red, and blood vessels in the dermis normally give the skin a reddish tint. During the frightening experience, the circulatory supply to the skin is temporarily reduced because of the constriction of the blood vessels, thus the skin becomes relatively pale.

3. (a) protects the scalp from ultraviolet light

    (b) cushions a blow to the head

    (c) prevents entry of foreign particles (eyelashes, nostrils, ear canals)

    (d) sensory nerves surrounding the base of each hair provide an early warning sytem that can help prevent injury

4. Perspiration produced by merocrine (eccrine) glands plus a mixture of electrolytes, metabolites and waste products is a clear secretion that is more than 99 % water. When all of the merocrine sweat glands are working at maximum, the rate of perspiration may exceed a gallon per hour, and dangerous fluid and electrolyte losses occur.

5. When the skin is submitted to mechanical stresses, the actively mitotic (stem) cells of the germinabitum layer divide more rapidly, and the depth of the epithelium increases.

6. To reach the underlying connective tissues, a bacterium must: (a) survive the bacteriocidal components of sebum (b) avoid being flushed from the skin's surface by sweat gland secretions (c) penetrate the stratum corneum (d) squeeze between the intercellular spaces of deeper skin layers (e) escape the immune cells of the skin (f) cross the basement membrane of the epidermis

Chapter 6

The Skeletal System

[L1] MULTIPLE CHOICE:

1.	D	2.	B	3.	B	4.	A	5.	C
6.	B	7.	D	8.	B	9.	C	10.	A
11.	B	12.	D	13.	C	14.	A	15.	B
16.	D	17.	A	18.	B	19.	D	20.	B
21.	D	22.	C	23.	A	24.	B	25.	C
26.	A	27.	D	28.	A	29.	D	30.	C
31.	C	32.	A	33.	B	34.	D	35.	B
36.	B	37.	C	38.	B	39.	C	40.	C
41.	B	42.	A	43.	A	44.	B	45.	B
46.	C	47.	C	48.	C	49.	A	50.	C
51.	D	52.	D	53.	B	54.	C	55.	C
56.	B	57.	D	58.	B	59.	D	60.	A
61.	C	62.	D	63.	B	64.	C	65.	B
66.	D								

[L1] COMPLETION:

67.	support	68.	osteon	69.	epiphysis
70.	intramembraneous	71.	endochondral	72.	ossification
73.	calcium	74.	remodeling	75.	minerals
76.	axial	77.	muscles	78.	costal
79.	floating	80.	malleolus	81.	acetabulum
82.	cranium	83.	foramen magnum	84.	paranasal
85.	fontanels	86.	secondary	87.	primary
88.	cervical	89.	clavicle	90.	pectoral girdle
91.	glenoid fossa	92.	coxae	93.	suture
94.	symphysis	95.	bursae	96.	supination
97.	synovial	98.	gliding	99.	scapulohumeral
100.	knee	101.	red bone marrow		

[L1] MATCHING:

102.	G	103.	I	104.	L	105.	A	106.	B
107.	K	108.	E	109.	C	110.	F	111.	J
112.	H	113.	D						

[L1] DRAWING/ILLUSTRATION LABELING:

Figure 6.1 Anterior View of the Skull

114.	coronal suture	115.	parietal bone	116.	frontal bone
117.	nasal bone	118.	lacrimal bone	119.	zygomatic bone
120.	temporal bone	121.	sphenoid bone	122.	ethmoid bone
123.	vomer bone	124.	maxilla bone	125.	mandible bone

Figure 6.2 Lateral View of the Skull

126. coronal suture
127. frontal bone
128. nasal bone
129. zygomatic arch
130. zygomatic bone
131. maxilla bone
132. mandible
133. parietal bone
134. squamosal suture
135. temporal bone
136. lambdoidal suture
137. external auditory canal
138. occipital bone
139. mastoid process
140. styloid process

Figure 6.3 Inferior View of the Skull

141. sphenoid bone
142. vomer bone
143. styloid process
144. foramen magnum
145. occipital bone
146. maxilla bone
147. zygomatic bone
148. occipital condyle

Figure 6.4 The Vertebral Column

149. cervical vertebra
150. thoracic vertebra
151. lumbar vertebra
152. sacrum
153. coccyx
154. intervertebral disks

Figure 6.5 The Ribs

155. sternum
156. manubrium
157. body of sternum
158. xiphoid process
159. floating ribs
160. true ribs
161. false ribs
162. costal cartilage

Figure 6.6 The Scapula

163. coracoid process
164. glenoid fossa
165. lateral border
166. acromium process
167. coracoid process
168. supraspinous fossa
169. spine
170. infraspinous fossa
171. medial border

Figure 6.7 The Humerus

172. greater tubercle
173. lesser tubercle
174. deltoid tuberosity
175. lateral epicondyle
176. capitulum
177. head of humerus
178. coronoid fossa
179. medial epicondyle
180. greater tubercle
181. olecranon fossa
182. lateral epicondyle

Figure 6.8 The Radius and Ulna

183. olecranon process
184. ulna
185. head of the ulna
186. head of the radius
187. radius
188. styloid process of radius
189. trochlear notch
190. coronoid process
191. radial tuberosity
192. ulna
193. styloid process of ulna

Figure 6.9 The Pelvis (anterior & lateral views)

194. pubic symphysis
195. obturator foramen
196. iliac crest
197. sacroiliac joint
198. ilium
199. pubis
200. ischium
201. iliac crest
202. ilium
203. acetabulum
204. pubis
205. ischium

Figure 6.10 The Femur (anterior and posterior views)

206. greater trochanter
207. neck of femur
208. lateral epicondyle
209. lateral condyle
210. head of femur
211. lesser trochanter
212. patellar surface
213. medial epicondyle
214. medial condyle
215. linea aspera
216. lateral condyle
217. lateral epicondyle

Figure 6.11 The Tibia and Fibula

218. lateral condyle
219. fibula
220. lateral malleolus
221. medial condyle
222. tibial tuberosity
223. tibia
224. medial malleolus

Figure 6.12 Movements of the Skeleton

225. elevation
226. depression
227. flexion
228. extension
229. hyperextension
230. rotation
231. abduction
232. adduction
233. opposition
234. pronation
235. abduction
236. adduction
237. adduction
238. abduction
239. circumduction
240. flexion
241. extension
242. inversion
243. eversion
244. retraction
245. protraction
246. dorsiflexion
247. plantar flexion

[L2] CONCEPT MAPS:

I.
1. intramembranous ossification
2. collagen
3. osteocyes
4. hyaline cartilage
5. periosteum

II.
6. skull
7. mandible
8. lacrimal
9. occipital
10. temporal
11. coronal
12. hyoid
13. vertebral column
14. thoracic
15. sacral
16. floating ribs, 2 pair
17. sternum
18. xiphoid process

[L2] BODY TREK:

19. compound
20. yellow marrow
21. endosteum
22. cancellous or spongy
23. trabecula
24. lamella
25. osteocytes
26. canaliculi
27. red blood cells
28. red marrow
29. Volkman's canal
30. periosteum
31. compact bone
32. Haversian canal
33. blood vessels
34. osteon
35. lacunae
36. osteoclasts

[L2] MULTIPLE CHOICE:

37. B
38. D
39. D
40. A
41. B
42. D
43. A
44. A
45. B
46. C
47. C
48. A
49. C
50. B
51. D
52. B
53. B

[L2] COMPLETION:

54. intramembranous
55. endochondral
56. osteopenia
57. depressed
58. kyphosis
59. lordosis
60. scoliosis
61. bursitis
62. arthroscopy
63. arthritis
64. articular cartilage
65. hyperextension

[L2] SHORT ESSAY:

66. Calcification: refers to the deposition of calcium salts within a tissue.
    Ossification: refers specifically to the formation of bone.

67. Intramembranous ossification begins when osteoblasts differentiate within a connective tissue. Endochondral ossification begins with the formation of a cartilaginous model.

68. The bones of the skeleton are attached to the muscular system, extensively connected to the cardiovascular (blood vessels) and lymphatic (lymphatic capillaries) systems, and largely under the physiological control of the endocrine system. The digestive and excretory systems provide the calcium and phosphate minerals needed for bone growth. The skeleton represents a reserve of calcium, phosphate, and other minerals that can compensate for changes in the dietary supply of these ions.

69. (1) create a framework that supports and protects organ systems in the dorsal and ventral body cavities.

    (2) provide a surface area for attachment of muscles that adjust the positions of the head, neck and trunk.

    (3) performs respiratory movements.

    (4) stabilize or position elements of the appendicular system.

70. Provides control over the immediate environmnent; changes your position in space, and makes you an active, mobile person.

71. Muscle contractions can occur only when the extracellular concentration of calcium remains within relatively narrow limits. Most of the body's calcium is tied up in the skeleton.

72. (1) gliding joints - intercarpals

    (2) hinge joints - elbow, knee

    (3) pivot joints - between atlas and axis

    (4) ellipsoidal joints - between metacarpals and phalanges

    (5) saddle joints - base of thumb

    (6) ball-and-socket joints - shoulder, hip

73. Both the elbow and knee are extremely stable joints. Stability for the elbow is provided by the:

    (a) interlocking of the body surfaces of the humerus and ulna

    (b) the thickness of the articular capsule; (c) strong ligaments reinforcing the capsule

    Stability for the hip joint is provided by the:

    (a) almost complete bony socket; (b) strong articular capsule; (c) supporting ligaments

    (d) muscular padding

[L3] CRITICAL THINKING/APPLICATION:

1. In premature or precocious puberty, production of sex hormones escalates early, usually by 8 or earlier. This results in an abbreviated growth spurt, followed by premature closure of the epiphyseal plates. Estrogen and testosterone both cause early uniting of the epiphyses of long bones; thus, the growth of long bones is completed prematurely.

2. Foods or supplements containing vitamins A, C and D are necessary to maintain the integrity of bone. Vitamin D plays an important role in calcium metabolism by stimulating the absorption and transport of calcium and phosphate ions. Vitamins A and C are essential for normal bone growth and remodeling. Any exercise that is weight-bearing or that exerts a pressure on the bones is necessary to retain the minerals in the bones, especially calcium salts. As the mineral content of a bone decreases the bone softens and skeletal support decreases.

3. During whiplash the movement of the head resembles the cracking of a whip. The head is relatively massive, and it sits on top of the cervical vertebra. Small muscles articulate with the bones and can produce significant effects by tipping the balance one way or another. If the body suddenly changes position, the balancing muscles are not strong enough to stabilize the head. As a result, a partial or complete dislocation of the cervical vertebrae can occur, with injury to muscles and ligaments and potential injury to the spinal cord.

4. When the gelatinous interior of the disc leaks through the fibrous outer portion of the disc, the affected disc balloons out from between the bony parts of the vertebrae. If the bulging or herniated area is large enough, it may press on a nerve, causing severe or incapacitating pain. Usually, the sciatic nerve is affected. Sciatica is generally located in the lumbar region and can radiate over the buttock, rear thigh and calf, and can extend into the foot.

5. In the hip joint, the femur articulates with a deep, complete bony socket, the acetabulum. The articular capsule is unusually strong; there are numerous supporting ligaments, and there is an abundance of muscular padding. The joint is extremely stable and mobility is sacrificed for stability.

6. The first patient probably sustained a trochanteric fracture, which usually heals well if the hip joint can stabilize (not always an easy matter because the powerful muscles surrounding the hip joint can prevent proper alignment of the bone fragments). Steel frames, pins and/or screws may be used to preserve alignment and encourage healing. The second patient probably suffered a fracture of the femoral neck; these fractures have a higher complication rate because the blood supply to that area is more delicate. This means that the procedures which succeed in stabilizing trochanteric fractures are often unsuccessful in stabilizing femoral neck fractures. If pinning fails, the entire joint can be surgically replaced in a procedure which removes the damaged portion of the femur. An artificial femoral head and neck are attached by a spike that extends into the marrow cavity of the shaft. Special cement anchors it and provides a new articular surface to the acetabulum.

Chapter 7

The Muscular System

[L1] MULTIPLE CHOICE:

1. D	2. B	3. D	4. C	5. D
6. C	7. A	8. B	9. A	10. D
11. D	12. C	13. D	14. C	15. A
16. D	17. B	18. B	19. D	20. B
21. C	22. A	23. B	24. D	25. B
26. D	27. B	28. C	29. C	30. A
31. A	32. D	33. C	34. B	35. D
36. D	37. C	38. C	39. A	40. B
41. D				

[L1] COMPLETION:

- 42. contraction
- 43. epimyseum
- 44. fascicles
- 45. tendon
- 46. sarcolemma
- 47. T tubules
- 48. sarcomeres
- 49. cross-bridges
- 50. recruitment
- 51. troponin
- 52. twitch
- 53. ATP
- 54. white muscles
- 55. red muscles
- 56. oxygen debt
- 57. endurance
- 58. pacemaker
- 59. origin
- 60. synergist
- 61. diaphragm
- 62. deltoid
- 63. rectus femoris
- 64. atrophy
- 65. hypertrophy
- 66. endocrine

[L1] MATCHING:

67. I	68. D	69. K	70. A	71. J
72. B	73. L	74. F	75. E	76. C
77. I	78. O	79. N	80. R	81. P
82. Q	83. M	84. G		

[L1] DRAWING/ILLUSTRATION LABELING:

Figure 7.1 Organization of Skeletal Muscles

- 85. sarcolemma
- 86. sarcoplasm
- 87. myofibril
- 88. nucleus
- 89. muscle fiber
- 90. muscle fascicle
- 91. muscle fibers
- 92. endomysium
- 93. epimysium
- 94. perimysium
- 95. endomysium
- 96. blood vessels
- 97. muscle fascicle
- 98. body of muscle
- 99. tendon
- 100. bone

Figure 7.2 The Histological Organization of Skeletal Muscles

- 101. myofibril
- 102. mitochondria
- 103. muscle fiber
- 104. nucleus
- 105. sarcoplasmic reticulum
- 106. T tubules
- 107. sarcomere
- 108. thin filament (actin)
- 109. thick filament (myosin)

Figure 7.3 Structure of a Sarcomere

- 110. sarcomere
- 111. Z line
- 112. Z line
- 113. I band
- 114. A band
- 115. myosin (think filament)
- 116. actin (thin filament)

Figure 7.4 Types of Muscle Tissue

117. smooth muscle
118. cardiac muscle
119. skeletal muscle

Figure 7.5 Major Superficial Skeletal Muscles (anterior view)

120. sternocleidomastoid
121. deltoid
122. biceps brachii
123. external oblique
124. brachioradialis
125. rectus femoris
126. vastus lateralis
127. vastus medialis
128. tibialis anterior
129. pectoralis major
130. rectus abdominis
131. gracilis
132. sartorius
133. gastrocnemius
134. soleus

Figure 7.6 Major Superficial Skeletal Muscles (posterior view)

135. sternocleidomastoid
136. teres major
137. latissimus dorsi
138. external oblique
139. semitendinosus
140. biceps femoris
141. tibialis posterior
142. trapezius
143. deltoid
144. triceps brachii
145. gluteus medius
146. gluteus maximus
147. gastrocnemius
148. soleus

Figure 7.7 Superficial View of Facial Muscles (lateral view)

149. occipitalis
150. buccinator
151. temporalis
152. frontalis
153. orbicularis oculi
154. zygomaticus major
155. orbicularis oris
156. platysma
157. sternocleidomastoid

Figure 7.8 Superficial Muscles of the Arm (anterior view)

158. biceps brachii
159. pronator teres
160. brachioradialis
161. flexor carpi radialis
162. palmaris longus
163. flexor carpi ulnaris
164. pronator quadratus

Figure 7.9 Superficial Muscles of Lower Leg (lateral view)

165. gastrocnemius
166. soleus
167. extensor digitorum
168. tibialis anterior
169. peroneus
170. peroneus

Figure 7.10 Superficial Muscles of Thigh (anterior view)

171. sartorius
172. rectus femoris
173. vastus lateralis
174. gracilis
175. vastus medialis

Figure 7.11 Superficial Muscles of Thigh (posterior view)

176. adductor magnus
177. semitendinosus
178. biceps femoris
179. semimembranosus

[L2] CONCEPT MAPS:

I.

1. heart
2. striated
3. smooth
4. involuntary
5. non-striated
6. bones
7. multi-nucleated

II.

8. release of Ca++ from sacs of sarcoplasmic reticulum
9. cross-bridging (heads of myosin attach to turned-on thin filaments)
10. shortening, ie. contraction of myofibrils and muscle fibers they comprise
11. energy + ADP + phosphate

Chapter 7 The Muscular System 341

[L2] BODY TREK:

12. epimysium
13. perimysium
14. fascicles
15. endomysium
16. sarcolemma
17. T tubules
18. nuclei
19. myofibrils
20. myofilaments
21. actin
22. myosin
23. sarcomeres
24. Z line
25. I band
26. A band
27. thick
28. sliding filament
29. contraction

[L2] MULTIPLE CHOICE:

30. A
31. B
32. D
33. C
34. B
35. D
36. C
37. A
38. B
39. C
40. A
41. C
42. C
43. B
44. A
45. D
46. A
47. A
48. B

[L2] COMPLETION:

49. muscle tone
50. fatigue
51. motor unit
52. tetanus
53. isotonic
54. biomechanics
55. innervation
56. sartorius
57. perineum
58. hamstrings
59. quadriceps

[L2] SHORT ESSAY:

60. (a) produce skeletal movement; (b) maintain posture and body position; (c) support soft tissues (d) guard entrances and exits (e) maintain body temperature

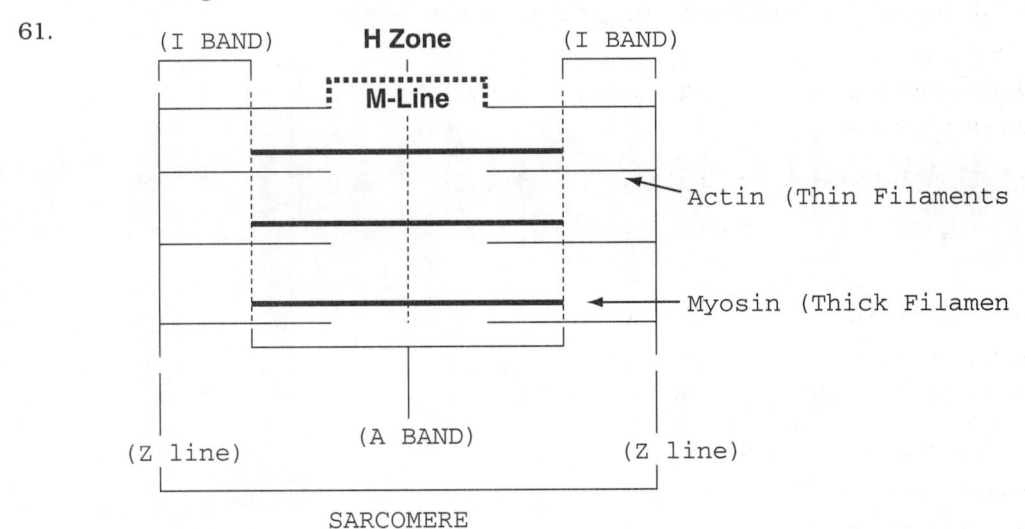

61.

```
        (I BAND)      H Zone      (I BAND)
                    ┊         ┊
                    ┊ M-Line  ┊
                    ┊         ┊
        ━━━━━━━━━━━━━━━━━━━━━━━━
                                    ◀── Actin (Thin Filaments)
        ━━━━━━━━━━━━━━━━━━━━━━━━
                                    ◀── Myosin (Thick Filamen
        
        (Z line)    (A BAND)     (Z line)
                    SARCOMERE
```

62. (a) active site exposure; (b) cross-bridge attachment; (c) pivoting; (d) cross-bridging detachment (e) myosin activation

63. When fatigue occurs and the oxygen supply to muscles is depleted, aerobic respiration ceases owing to the decreased oxygen supply. Anaerobic glycolysis supplies the needed energy for a short period of time. The amount of oxygen needed to restore normal pre-exertion conditions is the oxygen debt.

64. Fast fiber muscles produce powerful contractions, which use ATP in massive amounts. Prolonged activity is primarily supported by anaerobic glycolysis, and fast fibers fatigue rapidly. Slow fibers are specialized to enable them to continue contracting for extended periods. The specializations include an extensive network of capillaries so supplies of O_2 molecules are available, and the presence of myoglobin, which binds O_2 molecules and which results in the buildup of O_2 reserves. These factors improve mitochondrial performance.

65. (a) muscles of the head and neck; (b) muscles of the spine; (c) oblique and rectus muscles; (d) muscles of the pelvic floor

66. (a) muscles of the shoulders and arms; (b) muscles of the pelvic girdle and legs

[L3] CRITICAL THINKING/APPLICATION:

1. Training to improve "aerobic" endurance usually involves sustained low levels of muscular activity. Jogging, distance swimming, biking and other cardiovascular activities that do not require peak tension production are appropriate for developing aerobic endurance. Training to develop "anaerobic" endurance involves frequent, brief, intensive workouts. Activities might include running sprints; fast, short-distance swimming; pole vaulting; or other exercises requiring peak tension production in a short period of time.

2. This diet probably lacks dietary calcium and vitamin D. The resulting condition is hypocalcemia, a lower-than-normal concentration of calcium ions in blood or extracellular fluid. Because of the decreased number of calcium ions, sodium ion channels open and the sodium ions diffuse into the cell, causing depolarization of the cell membranes to threshold and initiates action potentials. Spontaneous reactions of nerves and muscles result in nervousness and muscle spasms.

3. (a) Injecting into tissues rather than circulation allows a large amount of a drug to be introduced at one time because it will enter the circulation gradually. The uptake is usually faster and produces less irritation than when drugs are administered through intradermal or subcutaneous routes; also, multiple injections are possible.

   (b) Bulky muscles containing few large blood vessels or nerves are ideal targets. The muscles that may serve as targets are the posterior, lateral and superior portion of the gluteus maximus; the deltoid of the arm; and the vastus lateralis of the thigh. The vastus lateralis of the thigh is the perferrred site in infants and young children whose gluteal and deltoid muscles are relatively small.

Chapter 8

Neural Tissue and the Central Nervous System

[L1] MULTIPLE CHOICE:

1. A	2. C	3. C	4. A	5. C
6. D	7. D	8. A	9. B	10. C
11. D	12. B	13. D	14. C	15. D
16. B	17. C	18. D	19. A	20. B
21. C	22. B	23. D	24. C	25. A
26. D	27. A	28. C	29. A	30. A
31. D	32. B	33. A	34. A	35. D
36. B	37. A	38. B	39. C	40. C
41. B	42. D			

[L1] COMPLETION:

43. autonomic nervous system
44. microglia
45. collaterals
46. afferent
47. threshold
48. saltatory
49. cholinergic
50. adrenergic
51. divergent
52. neural reflexes
53. receptor
54. nuclei
55. columns
56. cerebral cortex
57. third ventricle
58. choroid plexus
59. shunt
60. postcentral gyrus
61. corpus callosum

[L1] MATCHING:

62. E	63. D	64. F	65. H	66. A
67. J	68. G	69. B	70. C	71. I
72. L	73. O	74. M	75. K	76. N
77. P	78. Q	79. T	80. U	81. S
82. R	83. V			

[L1] DRAWING/ILLUSTRATION LABELING:

Figure 8.1 Structure and Classification of Neurons

84. dendrite
85. soma (cell body)
86. axon hillock
87. nucleus of Schwann cell
88. axon
89. Schwann cell
90. nodes of Ranvier
91. motor neuron (multipolar)
92. sensory neuron (unipolar)

Figure 8.2 Neuron Classification (based on structure)

93. multipolar
94. unipolar
95. bipolar

Figure 8.3 Structure of the Reflex Arc

96. white matter
97. gray matter
98. synapse
99. interneuron
100. sensory neuron (afferent)
101. motor neuron (efferent)
102. effector
103. receptor

344 Answer Key

Figure 8.4 Organization of the Spinal Cord

104. white matter	105. central canal	106. gray matter (anterior horn)
107. spinal nerve	108. posterior gray horn	109. gray commissure

Figure 8.5 Lateral View of the Human Brain

110. central sulcus	111. parietal lobe	112. occipital lobe
113. cerebellum	114. medulla oblongata	115. postcentral gyrus
116. precentral gyrus	117. frontal lobe	118. temporal lobe
119. pons		

Figure 8.6 Sagittal View of the Human Brain

120. cerebral hemisphere	121. corpus callosum	122. pineal body
123. cerebellum	124. thalamus	125. third ventricle
126. optic chiasma	127. pituitary gland	128. pons
129. medulla oblongata		

[L2] CONCEPT MAPS:

I.

1. Schwann cells
2. glial cells
3. transmit nerve impulses
4. central nervous system

II.

5. brain
6. motor system
7. somatic nervous system
8. sympathetic N.S.
9. smooth muscle
10. peripheral N.S.
11. afferent division

III.

12. diencephalon
13. hypothalamus
14. cerebellar hemispheres
15. pons
16. medulla oblongata
17. ascending and descending tracts

[L2] MULTIPLE CHOICE:

18. D	19. A	20. D	21. B	22. B
23. C	24. B	25. A	26. D	27. C
28. A	29. A	30. C	31. D	32. D
33. C	34. D	35. B	36. B	37. D
38. B	39. B	40. B	41. C	

[L2] COMPLETION:

42. ganglia	43. gated	44. nerve impulse
45. preganglionic fibers	46. postganglionic fibers	47. convergence
48. nuclei	49. tracts	50. motor nuclei
51. gray commissures	52. nerve plexus	53. reflexes
54. pituitary gland	55. hippocampus	56. sulci
57. fissures	58. hypothalamus	

[L2] SHORT ESSAY:

59. (a) providing sensation of the internal and external environment; (b) integrating sensory information; (c) coordinating voluntary and involuntary activites; (d) regulating or controlling peripheral structures and systems

60. CNS consists of the brain and spinal cord. PNS consists of the somatic nervous system and the autonomic nervous system.

61. Neurons are responsible for information transfer and processing in the nervous system. Neuroglia are specialized cells that provide support throughout the nervous system.

62. (a) activation of sodium channels and membrane depolarization; (b) sodium channel inactivation; (c) potassium channel activation; (d) return to normal permeability

Chapter 8   Neural Tissue and the Central Nervous System   345

63. (a) sensory neurons - carry nerve impulses to the CNS (b) motor neurons - carry nerve impulses from CNS to PNS (c) association or interneurons - situated between sensory and motor neurons within the brain and spinal cord

64. The white matter contains large numbers of myelinated and unmyelinated axons. The gray matter is dominated by bodies of neurons and glial cells.

65. (a) arrival of a stimulus and activation of a receptor; (b) activation of a sensory neuron; (c) information processing; (d) activation of a motor neuron; (e) response of a peripheral effector

66. (a) The interneurons can control several different muscle groups. (b) The interneurons may produce either excitatory or inhibitory postsynaptic potentials at CNS motor nuclei; thus the response can involve the stimulation of some muscles and the inhibition of others.

67. The brain's versatility results from (a) the tremendous number of neurons and neuronal pools in the brain; and, (b) the complexity of the interconnections between the neurons and neuronal pools.

68. "Higher centers" refers to nuclei, centers and cortical areas of the cerebrum, cerebellum, diencephalon and mesencephalon (midbrain).

69. C.N. I - olfactory; C.N. III - optic; C.N. III - vestibulocochlear

70. Cranial reflexes provide a quick and easy method for checking the condition of cranial nerves and specific nuclei and tracts in the brain.

[L3]   CRITICAL THINKING/APPLICATION:

1. The combination of coffee and cigarette has a strong stimulatory effect, making the person appear to be "nervous" or feeling like he or she is "on edge". The caffeine in the coffee lowers the threshold at the axon hillock, making the neurons more sensitive to depolarizing stimuli. Nicotine stimulates ACh (acetylcholine) recpetors by binding to the ACh receptor sites.

2. Microglia do not develop in neural tissue; they are phagocytic WBCs that have migrated across capillary walls in the neural tissue of the CNS. They engulf cellular debris, waste products, and pathogens. In times of infection or injury their numbers increase dramatically, as other phagocytic cells are attracted to the damaged area.

3. Because the spinal cord extends to the L2 level of the vertebral column and the meninges extend to the end of the vertebral column, a needle can be inserted through the meninges inferior to the medullary cone (the terminus of the spinal cord) into the subarachnoid space with minimal risk to the cauda equina (the collection of spinal nerve roots caudad to the terminus of the spinal cord).

4. (a) eliminates sensation and motor control of the arms and legs; usually results in extensive paralysis quadriplegia
   (b) motor paralysis and major respiratory muscles such as the diaphragm - patient needs mechanical assistance to breath
   (c) the loss of motor control of the legs - paraplegia
   (d) damage to the elements of the cauda equina causes problems with peripheral nerve function

5. Even though cerebrospinal fluid exits in the brain are blocked, CSF continues to be produced. The fluid continues to build inside the brain, causing pressure that compresses the nerve tissue and causes the ventricles to dilate. The compression of the nervous tissue causes irreversible brain damage.

6. The neurotransmitter dopamine is manufactured by neurons in the substantia nigra and carried to synapses in the cerebral nuclei where it has an inhibitory effect. If the dopamine-producing neurons are damaged, inhibition is lost and the excitatory neurons become increasingly active. This increased activity produces the motor symptoms of spasticity and/or tremor associated with Parkinson's disease.

7. The objects serve as stimuli initiating tactile sensations that travel via sensory neurons to the spinal cord. From the ascending tracts in the spinal cord the impulses are transmitted to the peripheral sensory association cortex of the left cerebral hemisphere where the objects are "recognized". The impulses are then transmitted to the speech comprehension area (Wernicke's area) where the objects are given names. From there the impulses travel to Broca's area for formulation of the spoken words, and finally the impulses arrive at the premotor and motor cortex for programming and for producing movements to form and say the words that identify the objects.

Chapter 9

The Peripheral Nervous System and Integrated Neural Function

[L1] MULTIPLE CHOICE:

1. C	2. B	3. D	4. A	5. C
6. C	7. B	8. C	9. A	10. C
11. A	12. B	13. D	14. B	15. C
16. D	17. C	18. D	19. B	20. D
21. D	22. C	23. B	24. C	25. B
26. C	27. D	28. B	29. C	30. A
31. D	32. C	33. C	34. D	

[L1] COMPLETION:

35. hypoglossal
36. spinal accessory
37. epineurim
38. cranial reflexes
39. somatic reflexes
40. flexor reflex
41. Babinski reflex
42. sensation
43. pyramidal system
44. cerebral nuclei
45. cerebellum
46. synapses
47. involuntary
48. "fight or flight"
49. "rest and respose"
50. acetylcholine
51. opposing
52. autonomic tone
53. visceral reflexes
54. limbic
55. Parkinson's disease
56. Alzheimer's disease

[L1] MATCHING:

57. K	58. I	59. L	60. A	61. E
62. C	63. J	64. B	65. H	66. P
67. Q	68. F	69. G	70. O	71. N
72. D	73. M			

[L1] DRAWING/ILLUSTRATION LABELING:

Figure 9.1 Preganglionic and Postganglionic Cell Bodies of Sympathetic Neurons

74. T1
75. L2
76. preganglionic cell body in gray matter of spinal cord
77. preganglionic axon
78. sympathetic chain ganglia
79. postganglionic neuron
80. celiac ganglion
81. superior mesenteric ganglion
82. inferior mesenteric ganglion
83. collateral ganglion

[L2] CONCEPT MAP:

1. sympathetic
2. motor neurons
3. smooth muscle
4. ganglia outside CNS
5. postganglionic

[L2] BODY TREK:

6. receptor
7. dorsal root ganglion
8. posterior horn
9. medulla oblongata
10. pons
11. midbrain
12. diencephalon
13. thalamus
14. synapse
15. cerebral cortex
16. pyramidal

Chapter 9 The Peripheral Nervous System and Integrated Neural Function

[L2] MULTIPLE CHOICE:

17. C   18. B   19. A   20. B   21. D
22. C   23. A   24. D   25. A   26. D
27. A   28. A   29. C   30. B   31. D
32. D

[L2] COMPLETION:

33. postganglionic
34. norepinephrine
35. splanchnic
36. hypothalamus
37. cerebral nuclei
38. electroencephalogram
39. dyslexia
40. arousal
41. dopamine

[L2] SHORT ESSAY:

42. (a) overseeing the postural muscles of the body, and
    (b) adjusting voluntary and involuntary motor patterns.

43. (a) a reduction in brain size and weight; (b) a decrease in blood flow to the brain;
    (c) changes in synaptic organization of the brain;
    (d) intracellular and extracellular changes in CNS neurons.

44. (a) the sympathetic division stimulates tissue metabolism, increases alertness, and generally prepares the body to deal with emergencies;
    (b) the parasympathetic division conserves energy and promotes sedentary activities, such as digestion.

45. (a) preganglionic neurons located between segments T1 and L2 of the spinal cord;
    (b) ganglionic neurons located in ganglia near the vertebral column (sympathetic chain ganglia, collateral ganglia).

46. (a) preganglionic neurons in the brain stem and in sacral segments of the spinal cord;
    (b) ganglionic neurons in peripheral ganglia located within or adjacent to the target organs.

47. When dual innervation exists, the two divisions of the ANS often but not always have opposite effects. Sympathetic-parasympathetic opposition can be seen along the digestive tract, at the heart, in the lungs and elsewhere throughout the body.

[L3] CRITICAL THINKING/APPLICATION:

1. The organized distribution of sensory information on the sensory cortex enables us to determine what specific portion of the body's "surface" has been affected by a stimulus. The surface pattern of distribution of individual spinal sensory nerve innervation is termed a "dermatome," and the resulting dermatome pattern follows a basic series of bands around the trunk, proceeding from the neck region (the cervical spinal nerves), through the thoracic, lumber, and sacral nerves, and terminating with the coccygeal spinal nerve in the region of the perineum. In the case of the arm pains during a heart attack, the pain is "referred" to the left shoulder and arm surface areas due to the embryological origin of the arms which arise as arm buds from the thoracic wall, and which "drag" along their original innervation from those dermatomes lying on the surface of the chest, which coincidently lie on the surface ventral to the heart.

2. Injuries to the motor corex eliminate the ability to exert fine control over motor units, but gross movements may still be produced by the cerebral nuclei using alternate spinal tracts than those used prior to the damage.

3. Initial symptoms might include moodiness, irritability, depression and general lack of energy. There may be difficulty in making decisions, and with the gradual deterioration of mental organization the individual loses memories, verbal and reading skills, and emotional control. She may experience difficulty in performing even the simplest motor tasks.

4. Sympathetic postganglionic fibers that enter the thoracic cavity in autonomic nerves cause the heart rate to accelerate (thus increasing the force of cardiac contractions) and dilate the respiratory passageways. Because of these functions the heart works harder, moving blood faster. The muscles receive more blood, and their utilization of stored and absorbed nutrients accelerates. Lipids, a potential energy source, are released. The lungs deliver more oxygen and prepare to eliminate the carbon dioxide produced by contracting muscles. Sweat glands become active and the eyes look for approaching dangers.

5. Even though most sympathetic postganglionic fibers are adrenergic, releasing norepinephrine, a few are cholinergic, releasing acetylcholine. The distribution of the cholinergic fibers via the sympathetic division provides a method of regulating sweat gland secretion and selectively controlling blood flow to skeletal muscles while reducing the flow to certain other tissues in the body.

Chapter 10

Sensory Function

[L1] MULTIPLE CHOICE:

1. C	2. A	3. B	4. D	5. B
6. C	7. C	8. B	9. A	10. C
11. A	12. A	13. B	14. C	15. C
16. D	17. C	18. C	19. A	20. D
21. B	22. B	23. C	24. B	25. C
26. B	27. C	28. B	29. D	

[L1] COMPLETION:

30. somatosensory	31. cerebral cortex	32. sensitivity	33. thermoreceptors
34. mechanoreceptors	35. bipolar	36. taste buds	37. sclera
38. pupil	39. rods	40. cones	41. occipital
42. saccule, utricle	43. otoliths	44. endolymph	45. round window

[L1] MATCHING:

46. K	47. N	48. E	49. I	50. B
51. M	52. F	53. H	54. J	55. G
56. A	57. C	58. D	59. L	

[L1] DRAWING/ILUSTRATION LABELING:

Figure 10.1 Sectional Anatomy of the Eye

60. posterior chamber	61. choroid	62. fovea	63. optic nerve
64. optic disk	65. retina	66. sclera	67. ciliary body
68. iris	69. lens	70. cornea	71. suspensory ligaments

Figure 10.2 Anatomy of the Ear: External, Middle and Inner Ears

72. pinna	73. external auditory canal	74. external auditory meatus
75. tympanic membrane	76. auditory ossicles	77. middle ear
78. cranial nerve VIII	79. inner ear	80. eustachian tube

Figure 10.3 Anatomy of the Ear (Bony Labyrinth)

81. semicircular canals	82. utricle	83. oval window	84. saccule
85. round window	86. vestibule	87. cochlea	

Figure 10.4 Gross Anatomy of the Cochlea: Details Visible in Section

88. scala vestibuli	89. scala media	90. tectorial membrane
91. organ of Corti	92. basilar membrane	93. scala tympani
94. spiral ganglion	95. cochlear nerve	

Chapter 10 Sensory Function **349**

[L2] CONCEPT MAP:

1. olfaction
2. smell
3. tongue
4. taste buds
5. ears
6. balance and hearing
7. hearing
8. retina
9. rods and cones

[L2] BODY TREK:

10. pinna
11. exteral auditory meatus
12. ceruminous
13. tympanic membrane
14. external ear
15. middle ear
16. auditory ossicles
17. malleus
18. incus
19. stapes
20. pharyngotympanic
21. masopharynx
22. oval window
23. endolymph
24. scala vestibuli
25. scala tympani
26. basilar membrane
27. round window
28. organ or Corti
29. tectorial
30. hairs atop hair cell
31. cochlear

[L2] MULTIPLE CHOICE:

32. B
33. A
34. B
35. A
36. C
37. D
38. C
39. A
40. B
41. D
42. B
43. D
44. C
45. B
46. A
47. C

[L2] COMPLETION:

48. sensory receptor
49. adaptation
50. referred pain
51. ampulla
52. pupil
53. aqueous humor
54. retina
55. cataract
56. accommodation
57. myopia
58. hyperopia

[L2] SHORT ESSAY:

59. sensations of temperature, pain, touch, pressure, vibration and proprioception
60. smell (olfaction), taste (gustation), balance (equilibrium), hearing (audition), vision (sight)
61. (a) nociceptors - variety of stimuli usually associated with tissue damage
    (b) thermoreceptors - changes in temperature
    (c) mechanoreceptors - stimulated or inhibited by physical distortion, contact or pressure on their cell membranes
    (d) chemoreceptors - respond to presence of specific molecules
62. Baroreceptors monitor changes in pressure. Proprioceptors monitor the position of joints, the tension in tendons and ligaments, and the state of muscular contraction.
63. Receptors in the saccule and utricle provide sensations of gravity and linear acceleration.
64. During accommodation the lens becomes rounder to focus the image of a nearby object on the retina.

[L3] CRITICAL THINKING/APPLICATION:

1. The total number of olfactory receptors declines with age, and elderly individuals have difficulty detecting odors unless excesssive quantities are used. Younger individuals can detect the odor in lower concentrations because the olfactory receptor population is constantly producing new receptor cells by division and differentiation of basal cells in the epithelium.

2. The middle ear contains the auditory ossicles including the *malleus*, or "hammer," the *incus*, or "anvil," and the *stapes*, or "stirrup."

3. When light falls on the eye, it passes through the cornea and strikes photoreceptor cells in the retina, bleaching many molecules of the pigment rhodopsin that lie within them. Vitamin A, a part of the rhodopsin molecule, is broken off when bleaching occurs. After an intense exposure to light, a photoreceptor cannot respond to further stimulation until its rhodopsin molecules have been regenerated.

Chapter 11

The Endocrine System

[L1] MULTIPLE CHOICE:

1. A	2. C	3. D	4. B	5. B
6. D	7. B	8. B	9. D	10. C
11. C	12. A	13. C	14. B	15. B
16. C	17. D	18. D	19. D	20. D
21. B	22. D	23. B		

[L1] COMPLETION:

24. neurotransmitters
25. adrenal gland
26. amino acid derivative
27. testosterone
28. reflex
29. hypothalamus
30. parathyroids
31. thymus
32. cytoplasm
33. gigantism
34. exhaustive
35. general adaptation syndrome
36. diabetes mellitus
37. sex hormones

[L1] MATCHING:

38. D	39. G	40. K	41. M	42. J
43. A	44. E	45. O	46. C	47. I
48. B	49. R	50. P	51. S	52. H
53. Q	54. N	55. F	56. L	

[L1] DRAWING/ILLUSTRATION LABELING:

Figure 11.1 Structural Classification of Hormones

57. amino acid derivative
58. steroid
59. peptide

Figure 11.2 The Endocrine System

60. parathyroid glands
61. adrenal
62. hypothalamus
63. pituitary
64. thyroid
65. thymus
66. pancreas
67. gonads (female - ovary; male - testes)

[L2] CONCEPT MAPS:

I.

1. hormones
2. epinephrine
3. peptide hormones
4. testosteone
5. pituitary
6. parathyroids
7. heart
8. male/female gonads
9. pineal
10. blood stream

II.

11. cellular communication
12. homeostasis
13. target cells
14. formation of second messenger
15. hormones

[L2] BODY TREK:

16. pineal
17. melatonin
18. infundibulum
19. pituitary
20. sella turcica
21. thyroid
22. parathyroid
23. thymus
24. heart
25. pancreas
26. insulin
27. adrenal
28. kidneys
29. erythropoietin
30. RBCs
31. ovaries
32. estrogen
33. progesterone
34. testes
35. testosterone

[L2] MULTIPLE CHOICE:

36. D	37. B	38. C	39. A	40. C
41. A	42. D	43. B	44. D	45. A
46. A	47. B	48. C	49. B	

[L2] COMPLETION:

50. hypothalamus   51. target cells   52. nucleus   53. cyclic-AMP
54. portal   55. aldosterone   56. epinephrine   57. glucocorticods

[L2] SHORT ESSAY:

58. The hypothalamus: (a) contains autonomic centers that exert direct neural control over the endocrine cells of the adrenal medulla. Sympathetic activation causes the adrenal medulla to release hormones into the bloodstream; (b) acts as an endocrine organ to release hormones into the circulation at the posterior pituitary; (c) secretes regulatory hormones that control activities of endocrine cells in the pituitary gland.

59. (a) control by releasing hormones; (b) control by inhibiting hormones; (c) regulation by releasing and inhibiting hormones.

60. Thyroid hormones elevate oxygen consumption and rate of energy consumption in peripheral tissues, causing an increase in the metabolic rate. As a result, more heat is generated, replacing the heat lost to the environment.

61. Erythropoietin stimulates the production of red blood cells by the bone marrow. The increase in the number of RBCs elevates the blood volume, causing an increase in blood pressure.

62. (a) The two hormones may have opposing, or antagonistic, effects; (b) the two hormones may have an additive, or synergistic, effect; (c) one can have a permissive effect on another. In such cases the first hormone is needed for the second to produce its effect; (d) the hormones may have integrative effect, i.e., the hormones may produce different but complementary results in specific tissues and organs.

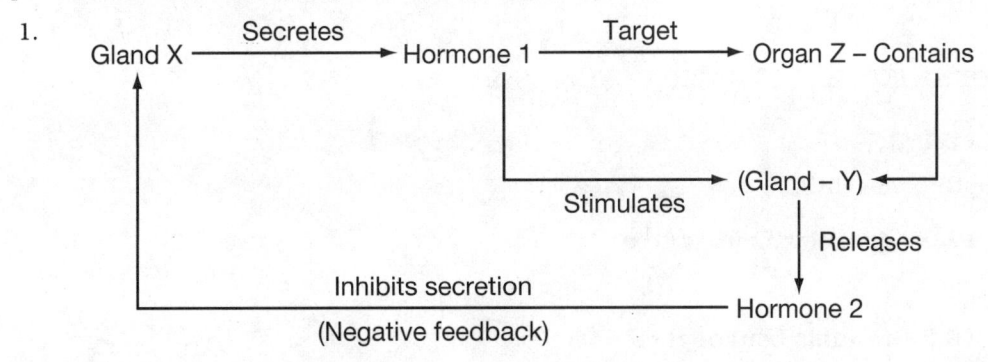

[L3] CRITICAL THINKING/APPLICATION:

1.

```
              Secretes              Target
Gland X ─────────────► Hormone 1 ─────────► Organ Z – Contains
   ▲                                             │
   │                                             ▼
   │                                        (Gland – Y) ◄────
   │                        Stimulates          │
   │                                            │ Releases
   │                                            ▼
   │     Inhibits secretion                  Hormone 2
   └──────────────────────────────────────────┘
          (Negative feedback)
```

2. (a) Patient A: underproduction of ADH; diabetes insipidus
       Patient B: underproduction of thyroid hormone; myxedema
       Patient C: overproduction of glucocorticoids; Cushing's disease
   (b) Patient A: pituitary disorder
       Patient B: thyroid disorder
       Patient C: adrenal disorder

3. Structurally, the hypothalamus is a part of the diencephalon; however, this portion of the brain secretes ADH and oxytocin that target peripheral effectors; the hypothalamus controls secretory output of the adrenal medulla, and it releases hormones that control the pituitary gland.

4. The anti-inflammatory activites of these steroids result from their effects on white blood cells and other components of the immune system. The glucocorticoids (steroid hormones) slow the migration of phagocytic cells into an injury site, and phagocytic cells already in the area become less active. In addition, most cells exposed to these steroids are less likely to release the chemicals that promote inflammation, thereby slowing the wound healing process. Because the region of the open wound's defenses are weakened, the area becomes an easy target for infecting organisms.

5. Anxiety, anticipation, and excitement may stimulate the sympathetic division of the ANS or release of epinephrine from the adrenal medulla. The peripheral effect of epinephrine results from interactions with particular receptors on cell membranes. The result is increased cellular energy utilization and mobilization of energy reserves. Hormone secretion triggers a mobilization of glycogen reserves in skeletal muscles and accelerates the breakdown of glucose to provide ATP. This combination increases muscular power and endurance.

Chapter 12

Blood

[L1] MULTIPLE CHOICE:

1. B
2. A
3. D
4. C
5. C
6. B
7. C
8. B
9. B
10. C
11. D
12. A
13. C
14. B
15. A
16. A
17. D
18. C
19. A
20. A
21. C
22. D
23. A
24. B
25. D
26. C
27. B

[L1] COMPLETION:

28. plasma
29. formed elements
30. venepuncture
31. viscosity
32. serum
33. hemopoiesis
34. vitamin B12
35. hematocrit
36. agglutinins
37. lymphocytes
38. fixed macrophages
39. lymphopoiesis
40. platelets
41. vascular

[L1] MATCHING:

42. H
43. C
44. G
45. F
46. A
47. K
48. D
49. E
50. B
51. J

[L1] DRAWING/ILLUSTRATION LABELING:

Figure 12.1

52. erythrocytes - RBCs

Figure 12.2 Agranular Leukocytes

53. lymphocyte
54. monocyte

Figure 12.3 Granular Leukocytes

55. basophil
56. neutrophil
57. eosinophil

[L2] CONCEPT MAP:

1. plasma
2. solutes
3. albumins
4. gamma
5. leukocytes
6. neutrophils
7. monocytes

[L2] BODY TREK:

8. endothelium
9. vascular spasm
10. thrombocytes
11. platelet plug
12. vascular
13. platelet
14. coagulation
15. fibrinogen
16. fibrin
17. RBCs
18. clot
19. clot retraction
20. fibrinolysis
21. plasminogen
22. plasmin

[L2] MULTIPLE CHOICE:

23. A
24. B
25. C
26. C
27. A
28. B
29. B
30. C
31. B
32. A
33. C
34. B
35. A

[L2] COMPLETION:

36. fractionated
37. fibrin
38. lipoproteins
39. hemolysis
40. leukopenia
41. leukocytosis
42. differential

Chapter 12   Blood   353

[L2]   SHORT ESSAY:

43. Blood: (a) "transports" dissolved gases; (b) "distributes" nutrients; (c) "transports" metabolic wastes; (d) "delivers" enzymes and hormones; (e) "regulates" the pH and electrolyte composition of intersititial fluid; (f) "restricts" fluid losses through damaged vessels; (g) "defends" the body against toxins and pathogens; (h) helps "regulate" body temperature by absorbing and redistributing heat.

44. (a) water; (b) electrolytes; (c) nutrients; (d) organic wastes; (e) proteins.

45. Granular leukocytes: neutrophils, eosinophils, basophils
    Agranular leukocytes: monocytes, lymphocytes

46. (a) transport of chemicals important to the clotting process
    (b) formation of a plug in the walls of damaged blood vessels
    (c) active contraction after clot formation has occurred.

47. (a) vascular phase: spasm in damaged smooth muscle
    (b) platelet phase: platelet aggregation and adhesion
    (c) coagulation phase: activation of clotting system and clot formation
    (d) clot retraction: contraction of blood clot
    (e) clot destruction: enzymatic destruction of clot

48. embolus: a drifting blood clot
    thrombosis: a blood clot that sticks to the wall of an intact blood vessel

[L3]   CRITICAL THINKING/APPLICATION:

1. (a) 154 lb ÷ 2.2 kg/lb = 70 kg,
       and 1 kg blood = approximately 1 liter
       therefore, 70 kg × 0.07 = 4.9 kg or 4.9 l
       4.9 l × 1 l = 4.9 l
   (b) Hematocrit: 45%
       therefore, total cell vol = 0.45 × 4.9 l = 2.2
   (c) plasma volume = 4.9 l – 2.2 l = 2.7 l
   (d) plasma volume in % = 2.7 l ÷ 4.9 l = 55%
   (e) % formed elements = 2.2 l ÷ 4.9 l = 45%

2. (a) increasing hematocrit; (b) increasing hematocrit; (c) decreasing hematocrit; (d) decreasing hematocrit

3. The patient with type B blood has type B antigens and type A antibodies. The donor's blood (type A) has type A antigens and type B antibodies. When the patient receives the type A blood, the B antibodies in the donor's blood will bind to the B antigen of the patient's blood and a transfusion reaction will occur. Also, the patient's type A antibodies can bind to the type A antigens of the donor's blood.

4. (a) Vitamin K deficiencies are rare because vitamin K is produced by bacterial synthesis in the digestive tract; (b) dietary sources include liver, green leafy vegetables, cabbage-type vegetables, and milk; (c) adequate amounts of vitamin K must be present for the liver to be able to synthesize four of the clotting factors, including prothrombin. A deficiency of vitamin K leads to the breakdown of the common pathway, inactivating the clotting system.

Chapter 13

The Cardiovascular System: The Heart

[L1] MULTIPLE CHOICE:

1. D	2. B	3. A	4. D	5. C
6. A	7. A	8. B	9. D	10. B
11. C	12. C	13. D	14. A	15. B
16. D	17. B	18. C	19. C	20. B
21. A	22. C	23. D	24. C	

[L1] COMPLETION:

25. atria
26. fibrous skeleton
27. pericardium
28. carbon dioxide
29. pulmonary veins
30. pulmonary
31. myocardium
32. repolarization
33. automaticity
34. electrocardiogram
35. chemoreceptors
36. autonomic nervous system

[L1] MATCHING:

37. F	38. A	39. I	40. J	41. E
42. G	43. H	44. C	45. D	46. B

[L1] DRAWING/ILLUSTRATION LABELING:

Figure 13.1 Anatomy of the Heart (ventral view)

47. pulmonary semilunar valve
48. superior vena cava
49. right pulmonary arteries
50. right atrium
51. right pulmonary veins
52. coronary sinus
53. tricuspid valve
54. chordae tendinae
55. right ventricle
56. inferior vena cava
57. aortic arch
58. pulmonary trunk
59. left atrium
60. left pulmonary arteries
61. left pulmonary veins
62. bicuspid valve
63. aortic semilunar valve
64. interventricular septum
65. left ventricle
66. myocardium

[L2] BODY TREK:

1. superior vena cava
2. right atrium
3. tricuspid valve
4. right ventricle
5. pulmonary similunar valve
6. pulmonary arteries
7. pulmonary veins
8. left atrium
9. bicuspid valve
10. left ventricle
11. aortic semilunar valve
12. L. common carotid artery
13. aorta
14. systemic arteries
15. systemic veins
16. inferior vena cava

[L2] MULTIPLE CHOICE:

17. A	18. B	19. B	20. A	21. B
22. D	23. B	24. D	25. C	26. C
27. D	28. B			

[L2] COMPLETION:

29. systemic
30. endocardium
31. nodal
32. cardiac reserve
33. diuretics
34. angina pectoris

[L2] SHORT ANSWER:

35. SV = EDV − ESV

Chapter 13 The Cardiovascular System: The Heart

SV = 140 ml − 60 ml = 80 ml

36. CO = SV × HR

Therefore, $\dfrac{CO}{HR} = \dfrac{SV \times HR}{HR}$;

Therefore, SV = $\dfrac{CO}{HR}$;

SV = $\dfrac{5 \; l/min.}{100 \; B/min.}$ = 0.05 l/beat

37. (a) epicardium; (b) myocardium; (c) endocardium

38. SA node → AV node → bundle of His → bundle branches → Purkinje cells → cardiac fibers

[L3] CRITICAL THINKING/APPLICATION:

1. In cardiac muscle tissue there are no antagonistic muscle groups to extend the cardiac muscle fibers after each contraction. The necessary stretching force is provided by the blood pouring into the heart, aided by the elasticity of the fibrous skeleton. As a result, the amount of blood entering the heart is equal to the amount ejected during the next contraction.

2. If a coronary artery is obstructed by a clot, the myocardial cells that the artery supplies do not receive sufficient amounts of blood (ischemia). Chest pains (angina pectoris) are usually a symptom of ischemia. When the heart tissue is deprived of oxygen due to ischemia, the affected portion of the heart dies. This is called a myocardial infarction (heart attack).

3. Cardiac muscle cells have an abundance of mitochondria, which provide enough ATP energy to sustain normal myocardial energy requirements. Most of the ATP is provided from the metabolism of fatty acids when the heart is resting. During periods of strenuous exercise muscle cells use lactic acid as an additional energy source.

4. Anastomeses are the interconnections between arteries in coronary circulation. Because of the interconnected arteries, the blood supply to the cardiac muscle remains relatively constant, regardless of pressure fluctuations within the left and right coronary arteries.

Chapter 14

Blood Vessels and Circulation

[L1] MULTIPLE CHOICE:

1. A	2. D	3. B	4. C	5. D
6. B	7. D	8. A	9. B	10. C
11. B	12. D	13. B	14. A	15. D
16. C	17. C	18. D	19. B	20. C
21. C	22. A	23. B	24. D	

[L1] COMPLETION:

25. arterioles
26. venules
27. precapillary sphincter
28. vasomotion
29. hydrostatic pressure
30. osmotic pressure
31. pulse pressure
32. sphygmomanometer
33. total peripheral pressure
34. autoregulation
35. vasoconstriction
36. shock
37. hepatic portal system
38. aortic arch
39. arteriosclerosis

[L1] MATCHING:

40. G	41. I	42. L	43. J	44. M
45. A	46. E	47. C	48. B	49. H
50. F	51. K	52. D		

[L1] DRAWING/ILLUSTRATION LABELING:

Figure 14.1 The Arterial System

53. brachiocephalic
54. aortic arch
55. ascending aorta
56. abdominal aorta
57. common iliac
58. internal iliac
59. external iliac
60. common carotid
61. descending aorta
62. subclavian
63. axillary
64. brachial
65. thoracic aorta
66. celiac
67. renal
68. superior mesenteric
69. gonadal
70. inferior mesenteric
71. femoral
72. popliteal

Figure 14.2 The Venous System

73. subclavian
74. axillary
75. brachial
76. inferior vena cava
77. internal jugular
78. external jugular
79. brachiocephalic
80. superior vena cava
81. renal
82. gonadal
83. lumbar
84. common iliac
85. internal iliac
86. eternal iliac
87. femoral
88. great saphenous
89. popliteal
90. posterior tibial
91. small saphenous
92. plantar venous network

Figure 14.3 Major Arteries of the Head and Neck

93. superficial temporal
94. circle of Willis
95. posterior cerebral
96. basilar
97. internal carotid
98. vertebral artery
99. subclavian
100. internal thoracic
101. anterior cerebral
102. maxillary
103. facial
104. external carotid
105. common carotid
106. brachiocephalic

Figure 14.4 Major Veins Draining the Head and Neck

107. superior sagittal sinus
108. vertebral vein
109. external jugular vein
110. temporal vein
111. maxillary vein
112. facial vein
113. internal jugular vein
114. brachiocephalic vein
115. internal thoracic vein

Chapter 14 Blood Vessels and Circulation

[L2] CONCEPT MAPS:

I.
1. pulmonary veins
2. arteries and arterioles
3. veins and venules
4. pulmonary arteries
5. systemic circuit

II.
6. ascending aorta
7. brachiocephalic artery
8. L. subclavian artery
9. thoracic aorta
10. celiac trunk
11. superior mesenteric artery
12. R. gonadal artery
13. L. common iliac artery

[L2] BODY TREK:
14. aortic semilunar valve
15. aortic arch
16. descending aorta
17. brachiocephalic
18. L. common carotid
19. L. subclavian
20. phrenic
21. celiac
22. renal
23. superior mesenteric
24. gonadal
25. inferior mesenteric
26. lumbar
27. common iliacs

[L2] MULTIPLE CHOICE:
28. B
29. D
30. B
31. C
32. A
33. D
34. C
35. D
36. B
37. D
38. B
39. A
40. D
41. C
42. B
43. A
44. B

[L2] COMPLETION:
45. circle of Willis
46. edema
47. precapillary sphincters
48. endothelium
49. veins
50. venous return
51. brachial
52. radial
53. great saphenous

[L2] SHORT ESSAY:
54. heart —> arteries —> arterioles —> capillaries —> venules —> veins —> heart
55. (a) In the pulmonary circuit, oxygen stores are replenished, carbon dioxide is excreted, and the "reoxygenated" blood is returned to the heart for distribution in the sytemic circuit.
    (b) The sytemic circuit supplies the capillary beds in all parts of the body with oxygenated blood, and returns deoxygenated blood to the heart of the pulmonary circuit for removal of carbon dioxide.
56. (a) vascular resistance, viscosity, turbulence
    (b) only vascular resistance can be adjusted by the nervous and endocrine systems
57. (a) distributes nutrients, hormones, and dissolved gases throughout tissues
    (b) transports insoluble lipids and tissue proteins that cannot enter circulation by crossing capillary linings
    (c) speeds removal of hormones and carries bacterial toxins and other chemical stimuli to cells of the immune system
58. cardiac output, blood volume, peripheral resistance
59. aortic baroreceptors, carotid sinus baroreceptors, atrial baroreceptors
60. epinephrine and norepinephrine, ADH, angiotensin II, erythropoietin, and atrial natriuretic peptide
61. Arteries lose their elasticity, the amount of smooth muscle they contain decreases, and they become stiff and relatively inflexible.

[L3] CRITICAL THINKING/APPLICATION:

1. L. ventricle → aortic arch → L. subclavian artery → axillary artery → brachial artery → radial and ulnar arteries → palmar arterial system → digital arteries → digital veins → palmar venous system → radius and ulnar veins → brachial vein → axillary vein → L. subclavian vein → brachiocephalic vein → superior vena cava → R. atrium

2. When a person rises rapidly from a lying position, a drop in blood pressure in the neck and thoracic regions occurs because of the pull of gravity on the blood. Owing to the sudden decrease in blood pressure, the blood flow to the brain is reduced enough to cause dizziness or loss of consciousness.

3. By applying pressure on the carotid artery at frequent intervals during exercise, the pressure to the region of the carotid sinus may be sufficient to stimulate the baroreceptors. The increased action potentials from the baroreceptors initiate reflexes in parasympathetic impulses to the heart, causing a decrease in the heart rate.

Chapter 15

The Lymphatic System and Immunity

[L1] MULTIPLE CHOICE:

1. D	2. C	3. D	4. B	5. A
6. A	7. C	8. B	9. D	10. A
11. C	12. A	13. A	14. D	15. B
16. A	17. C	18. A	19. C	20. B
21. D	22. B	23. D	24. D	

[L1] COMPLETION:

- 25. lacteals
- 26. lymph capillaries
- 27. cytotoxic T cells
- 28. phagocytes
- 29. diapedesis
- 30. passive
- 31. cell-mediated
- 32. active
- 33. suppressor T
- 34. helper T
- 35. plasma cells
- 36. immunological competence
- 37. lymphokines
- 38. IgG
- 39. immunodeficiency disease
- 40. vaccinated

[L1] MATCHING:

41. G	42. F	43. L	44. D	45. I
46. C	47. K	48. B	49. M	50. N
51. H	52. E	53. J	54. A	

[L1] DRAWING/ILLUSTRATION LABELING:

Figure 15.1 Nonspecific Defenses

- 55. physical barriers
- 56. phagocytes
- 57. immunological surveillance
- 58. complement system
- 59. inflammatory response

[L2] CONCEPT MAP:

- 1. nonspecific immunity
- 2. phagocytic cells
- 3. inflammation
- 4. specific immunity
- 5. innate
- 6. acquired
- 7. active
- 8. active immunization
- 9. transfer of antibodies via placenta
- 10. passive immunization

[L2] BODY TREK:

- 11. viruses
- 12. macrophages
- 13. natural killer cells
- 14. helper T cells
- 15. B cells
- 16. antibodies
- 17. killer T cells
- 18. suppressor T cells
- 19. memory T and B cells

[L2] MULTIPLE CHOICE:

20. B	21. C	22. B	23. A	24. C
25. D	26. D	27. C	28. B	29. C
30. C	31. B	32. D		

[L2] COMPLETION:

- 33. Langerhans cells
- 34. cytokines
- 35. mast
- 36. tumor necrosis factor
- 37. NK cells
- 38. interferon
- 39. IgG
- 40. IgM
- 41. helper T

[L2] SHORT ESSAY:

42. (a) production, maintenance, and distribution of lymphocytes
    (b) maintenance of normal blood volume
    (c) elimination of local variations in the composition of the interstitial fluid

43. Stimulated B cells differentiate into plasma cells that are responsible for production and secretion of antibodies. B cells are said to be responsible for humoral immunity.

44. (a) physical barriers; (b) phagocytes; (c) immunological surveillance; (d) complement system; (e) inflammatory response; (f) fever

45. NK (natural killer) cells are sensitive to the presence of abnormal cell membranes and respond immediately. When the NK cell makes contact with an abnormal cell it releases secretory vesicles that contain proteins called perforins. The perforins create a network of pores in the target cell membrane. These pores result in the loss of intracellular materials from the target cell necesary for homeostasis, thus causing the target cell to die and disintegrate.

46. (a) specificity; (b) versatility; (c) memory; (d) tolerance

47. Active immunity appears following exposure to an antigen, as a consequence of the immune response. Passive immunity is produced by transfer of antibodies from another individual.

48. (a) IgG (b) IgE (c) IgD (d) IgM (e) IgA

[L3] CRITICAL THINKING/APPLICATION:

1. Tissue transplants normally contain protein molecules called human lymphocyte antigen (HLA) genes that are foreign to the recipient. These antigens trigger the recipient's immune responses, activating the cellular and humoral mediated responses that may act to destroy the donated tissue.

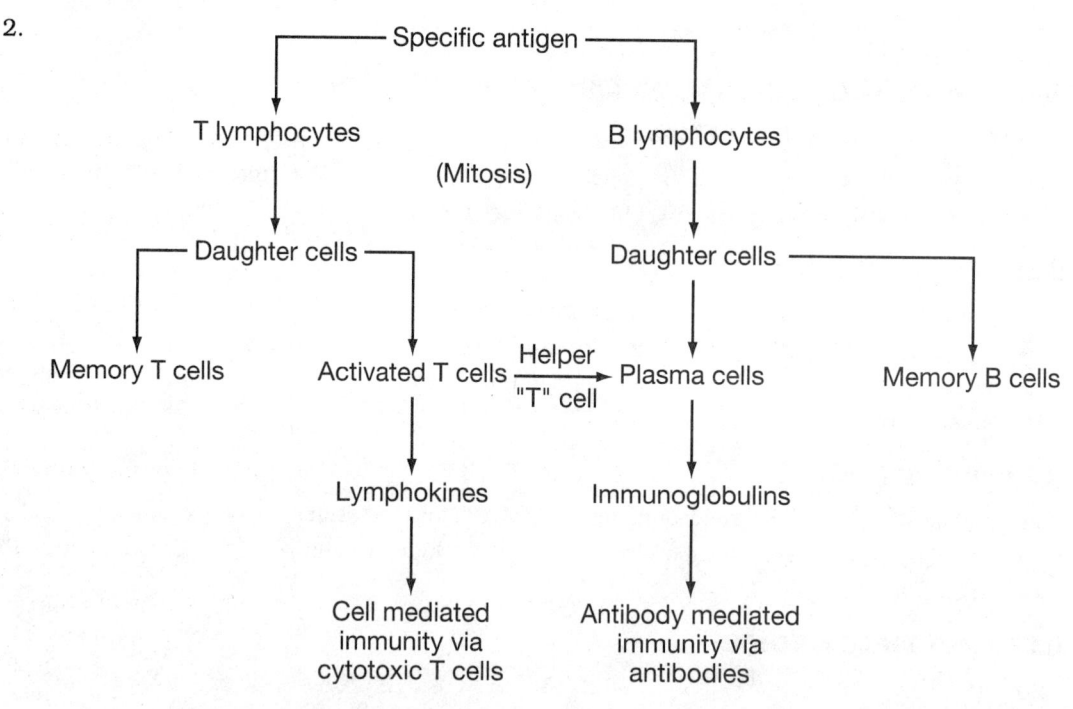

2.

```
                    ── Specific antigen ──
                   ↓                      ↓
            T lymphocytes            B lymphocytes
                   │     (Mitosis)         │
                   ↓                       ↓
         ── Daughter cells ──     ── Daughter cells ──
        ↓                    ↓     ↓                   ↓
  Memory T cells    Activated T cells ──Helper──→ Plasma cells    Memory B cells
                          │          "T" cell         │
                          ↓                           ↓
                    Lymphokines                 Immunoglobulins
                          ↓                           ↓
                   Cell mediated              Antibody mediated
                   immunity via                 immunity via
                   cytotoxic T cells             antibodies
```

3. Viruses reproduce inside living cells, beyond the reach of lymphocytes. Infected cells incorporate viral antigens into their cell membranes. NK cells recognize these infected cells as abnormal. By destroying virally-infected cells, NK cells slow or prevent the spread of viral infection.

4. High body temperatures may inhibit some viruses and bacteria, or may speed up their reproductive rates to that the disease runs its course more rapidly. The body's metabolic processes are accelerated, which may help mobilize tissue defenses and speed the repair process.

Chapter 16

The Respiratory System

[L1]   MULTIPLE CHOICE:

1. D	2. B	3. C	4. D	5. C
6. B	7. B	8. A	9. B	10. A
11. C	12. A	13. A	14. A	15. C
16. B	17. B	18. C	19. C	20. D
21. C	22. D	23. D	24. C	25. C
26. B	27. B	28. D		

[L1]   COMPLETION:

29. expiration
30. inspiration
31. surfactant
32. glottis
33. larynx
34. bronchioles
35. external respiration
36. internal respiration
37. vital capacity
38. alveolar ventilation
39. carbamino-hemoglobin
40. apnea
41. mechanoreceptor
42. chemoreceptor
43. exercise performance

[L1]   MATCHING:

44. D	45. E	46. J	47. F	48. L
49. H	50. G	51. M	52. A	53. B
54. I	55. K	56. C		

[L1]   DRAWING/ILLUSTRATION LABELING:

Figure 16.1 Upper Respiratory Tract

57. internal nares
58. nasopharynx
59. eustachian tube opening
60. hard palate
61. soft palate
62. palatine tonsil
63. oropharynx
64. epiglottis
65. glottis
66. vocal fold (cord)
67. laryngopharynx
68. trachea
69. nasal concha
70. nasal vestibule
71. oral cavity
72. tongue
73. thyroid cartilage
74. cricoid cartilage

Figure 16.2 Lower Respiratory Tract

75. epiglottis
76. "Adam's" apple
77. thyroid cartilage
78. cricoid cartilage
79. terminal bronchioles
80. alveoli
81. larynx
82. trachea
83. L. primary bronchus
84. secondary bronchi
85. tertiary bronchi

[L2]   CONCEPT MAP:

1. upper respiratory tract
2. pharynx and larynx
3. paranasal sinuses
4. speech production
5. lungs
6. ciliated mucous membrane
7. alveoli
8. blood
9. O_2 from alveoli into blood

[L2]   BODY TREK:

10. external nares
11. nasal cavity
12. nasal conchae
13. hard palate
14. soft palate
15. nasopharynx
16. pharynx
17. epiglottis
18. larynx
19. vocal folds (cords)
20. phonation
21. trachea
22. cilia
23. oral cavity
24. primary bronchus
25. smooth muscle
26. bronchioles
27. alveolus
28. oxygen
29. carbon dioxide
30. pulmonary capillaries

362 Answer Key

[L2] MULTIPLE CHOICE:

31. C	32. B	33. D	34. B	35. D
36. A	37. C	38. C	39. B	40. B
41. C	42. A			

[L2] COMPLETION:

43. laryngopharynx
44. epiglottis
45. thyroid cartilage
46. cribriform plate
47. hypoxia
48. pneumothorax
49. intrapleural
50. anatomic dead space
51. alveolar ventilation

[L2] SHORT ESSAY:

52. (a) provides an area for gas exchange between air and blood; (b) to move air to and from exchange surfaces; (c) protects respiratory surfaces from abnormal changes or variations; (d) defends the respiratory system and other tissues from pathogenic invasion: (e) permits communication via production of sound; (f) participates in the regulation of blood volume, pressure and body fluid pH.

53. The air is warmed to within 1 degree of body temperature before it enters the pharynx. This results from the warmth of rapidly flowing blood in an extensive vasculature of the nasal mucosa. For humidifying the air, the nasal mucosa is supplied with small mucus glands that secrete a mucoid fluid inside the nose. The warm and humid air prevents drying of the pharynx, trachea and lungs, and facilitates the flow of air through the respiratory passageways without affecting environment changes.

54. Hairs, cilia and mucus traps in the nasal cavity; mucus escalator in the larynx, trachea and bronchi moves trapped "junk" downward to be passed by swallowing into the esophagus. These areas have a mucus lining and contain cilia that beat toward the pharynx; phagocytes by alveolar macrophages.

55. Increasing volume; decreasing pressure and decreasing volume; increasing pressure.

56. A rise in arterial P_{CO2} immediately elevates cerebrospinal fluid CO_2 levels and stimulates the chemoreceptor neurons of the medulla. These receptors then stimulate the respiratory center causing an increase in the rate and depth of respiration, or hyperventilation.

[L3] CRITICAL THINKING/APPLICATION:

1. Running usually requires breathing rapidly through the mouth, which eliminates much of the preliminary filtration, heating and humidifying of inspired air. When these conditions are eliminated by breathing through the mouth, the delicate respiratory surfaces are subject to chilling, drying out and possible damage.

2. The esophagus lies immediately posterior to the cartilage-free posterior wall of the trachea. Distention of the esophagus due to the passage of the bolus of food exerts pressure on surrounding structures. If the tracheal cartilages were complete rings, the tracheal region of the neck and upper thorax would not accommodate the necessary compression to allow the food bolus to pass freely through the esophagus.

3. In emphysema, respiratory bronchi and alveoli are functionally eliminated. The alveoli expand and their walls become infiltrated with fibrous tissue. The capillaries deteriorate and gas exchange ceases. During the later stages of development bronchitis may develop, especially in the bronchioles. Emphysema and bronchitis produce a particularly dangerous combination known as chronic obstructive pulmonary disease (COPD). These conditions have been linked to the inhalation of air containing fine particulate matter or toxic vapors, such as those found in cigarette smoke.

Chapter 17

The Digestive System

[L1] MULTIPLE CHOICE:

1. C	2. C	3. D	4. D	5. B
6. B	7. B	8. D	9. B	10. A
11. B	12. C	13. C	14. B	15. D
16. D	17. A	18. B	19. A	20. A
21. B	22. A			

[L1] COMPLETION:

23. esophagus
24. digestion
25. lamina propria
26. peristalsis
27. gastrin
28. cuspids
29. carbohydrates
30. chyme
31. duodenum
32. cholecystokinin
33. pyloric sphincter
34. acini
35. haustrae
36. lipase
37. pepsin
38. diarrhea and constipation

[L1] MATCHING:

39. R	40. S	41. D	42. T	43. L
44. M	45. O	46. N	47. G	48. B
49. F	50. E	51. H	52. I	53. A
54. P	55. J	56. C	57. U	58. K

[L1] DRAWING/ILLUSTRATION LABELING:

Figure 17.1 The Digestive Tract

59. sublingual gland
60. submandibular gland
61. liver
62. hepatic duct
63. gall bladder
64. cystic duct
65. common bile duct
66. pancreatic duct
67. duodenum
68. transverse colon
69. ascending colon
70. ileocecal valve
71. cecum
72. appendix
73. ileum
74. parotid gland
75. oropharynx
76. esophagus
77. lower esophageal sphincter
78. fundus of stomach
79. body of stomach
80. pyloric sponcter
81. pylorus
82. pancreas
83. jejunum
84. descending colon
85. sigmoid colon
86. rectum
87. anus

[L2] CONCEPT MAPS:

I.

1. amylase
2. pancreas
3. bile
4. hormones
5. digestive tract movements
6. stomach
7. large intestine
8. hydrochloric acid
9. intestinal mucosa

II.

10. esophagus
11. small intestine
12. polypeptides
13. amino acids
14. complex sugars and starches
15. disaccharides, trisaccharides
16. simple sugars
17. monoglycerides, fatty acids in micelles
18. triglycerides
19. lacteal

364 Answer Key

[L2] BODY TREK:

20.	oral cavity	21.	lubrication	22.	mechanical processing		
23.	gingivae (gums)	24.	teeth	25.	mastication	26.	palates
27.	tongue	28.	saliva	29.	salivary amylase	30.	carbohydrates
31.	pharynx	32.	uvula	33.	swallowing	34.	esophagus
35.	peristalsis	36.	stomach	37.	gastric juices	38.	chyme
39.	rugae	40.	mucus	41.	hydrochloric	42.	pepsin
43.	protein	44.	pylorus	45.	duodenum	46.	lipase
47.	pancreas	48.	large intestine	49.	feces		

[L2] MULTIPLE CHOICE:

50.	D	51.	B	52.	C	53.	A	54.	D
55.	D	56.	D	57.	A	58.	B		

[L2] COMPLETION:

59.	visceral peritoneum	60.	mesenteries	61.	adventitia	62.	segmentation
63.	lacteals	64.	enamel	65.	intestinal	66.	cephalic

[L2] SHORT ESSAY:

67. (a) ingestion; (b) mechanical processing; (c) digestion; (d) secretion; (e) absorption; (f) compaction; (g) excretion (defecation)

68. (a) incisors - clipping or cutting; (b) cuspids (canines) - tearing or slashing; (c) bicuspids (premolars) - crushing, mashing, grinding; (d) molars - crushing, mashing, grinding

69. (a) cephalic, gastric, intestinal; (b) CNS regulation; release of gastrin into circulation; enterogastric reflexes, secretion of cholecystokinin (CCK) and secretin.

70. (a) metabolic regulation; (b) hematological regulation; (c) bile production.

71. (a) endocrine function - pancreatic islets secret insulin and glucagon into the bloodstream; (b) exocrine function - secrete a mixture of water, ions and digestive enzymes into the small intestine.

[L3] CRITICAL THINKING/APPLICATION:

1. Swelling in front of and below the ear is an obvious symptom of the mumps, a contagious viral disease. It is a painful enlargement of the parotid salivary glands and is far more severe in adulthood and can occasionally cause infertility in males. Today there is a safe mumps vaccine, MMR (measles, mumps, and rubella), which can be administered after the age of 15 months.

2. Heartburn, or acid indigestion, is not related to the heart, but is caused by a backflow, or reflux, of stomach acids into the esophagus, a condition called gastroesophygeal reflux. Caffeine and alcohol stimulate the secretion of HCl in the stomach. When the HCl is refluxed into the esophagus, it causes the burning sensation.

3. I. M. Nervous probably experienced a great deal of stress and anxiety while studying anatomy and physiology. If a person is excessively stressed, an increase in sympathetic nervous activity may inhibit duodenal gland secretion, increasing susceptibility to a duodenal ulcer. Decreased duodenal gland secretion reduces the duodenal wall's coating of mucus, which protects it against gastric enzymes and acid.

Chapter 18
Nutrition and Metabolism

[L1] MULTIPLE CHOICE:

1. A   2. B   3. C   4. A   5. B
6. A   7. C   8. B   9. D   10. B
11. B   12. B   13. C   14. B   15. D
16. C   17. A   18. A

[L1] COMPLETION:

19. anabolism
20. oxidative phosphorylation
21. liver
22. insulin
23. glucagon
24. triglycerides
25. beta oxidation
26. essential
27. TCA cycle
28. nutrition
29. minerals
30. avitaminosis
31. hypervitaminosis
32. sodium ions
33. iron
34. niacin
35. cobalamin
36. vitamin C
37. vitamin D
38. Vitamin K
39. Vitamin B1
40. calorie
41. basal metabolic rate
42. thermoregulation

[L1] MATCHING:

43. O   44. P   45. Q   46. E   47. I
48. D   49. K   50. G   51. M   52. A
53. L   54. J   55. N   56. B   57. F
58. R   59. S   60. H   61. C

[L2] CONCEPT MAP:

1. lipolysis   2. lipogenesis   3. glycolysis   4. beta oxidation
5. gluconeogenesis   6. amino acids

[L2] MULTIPLE CHOICE:

7. C   8. B   9. D   10. C   11. B
12. A   13. C   14. D   15. C

[L2] COMPLETION:

16. nutrient pool
17. lipoproteins
18. chylomicrons
19. LDLs
20. HDLs
21. deamination
22. uric acid
23. metabolic rate
24. acclimatization

[L2] SHORT ESSAY:

25. (a) proteins are difficult to break apart; (b) their energy yield is less than that of lipids; (c) the byproduct, ammonia, is a toxin that can damage cells; (d) proteins form the most important structural and functional components of any cell; extensive protein catabolism threatens homeostasis at the cellular and system levels.

26. When nucleic acids are broken down, only the sugar and pyrimidine bases (cytosine, thymine, uracil) provide energy. Purine bases (adenine, guanine) cannot be catabolized; instead, they are deaminated (the amine is removed) and excreted as uric acid, a nitrogenous waste.

27. (a) liver; (b) adipose tissue; (c) skeletal muscle; (d) neural tissue; (e) other peripheral tissue

28. (a) milk group; (b) meat group; (c) vegetable and fruit group; (d) bread and cereal group

29. minerals (i.e., inorganic ions) are important because they: (a) determine the osmolarities of fluids; (b) play major roles in important physiological processes; (c) are essential cofactors in a variety of enzymes.

30. (a) fat soluble: ADEK; (b) water-soluble: B complex and C (ascorbic acid)

[L3] CRITICAL THINKING/APPLICATION:

1. Because of a normal total cholesterol and triglyceride level, Greg's low HDL level implies that excess cholesterol delivered to the tissues cannot be easily returned to the liver for excretion. The amount of cholesterol in peripheral tissues, and especially in arterial walls, is likely to increase.

2. Diets too low in calories, especially carbohydrates, will bring about physiological responses that are similar to fasting. During brief periods of fasting or low calorie intake, the increased production of ketone bodies resulting from lipid catabolism results in ketosis, a high concentration of ketone bodies in body fluids. When keto-acids dissociate in solution, they release a hydrogen ion. The appearance of ketone bodies in the circulation presents a threat to the plasma pH. During prolonged starvation or low calorie dieting, a dangerous drop in pH occurs. This acidification of the blood is called ketoacidosis. Charlene's symptoms represent warning signals to what could develop into more disruptive normal tissue activities, ultimately causing coma, cardiac arrhythmias and death, if left unchecked.

3. A temperature rise accompanying a fever increases the body's metabolic energy requirements and accelerates water losses stemming from evaporation and perspiration. For each degree the temperature rises above normal, the daily water loss increases by 200 ml. Drinking fluids helps to replace the water loss.

Chapter 19

The Urinary System

[L1] MULTIPLE CHOICE:

1. A	2. C	3. C	4. B	5. D
6. C	7. D	8. C	9. A	10. A
11. D	12. B	13. A	14. B	15. B
16. A	17. B	18. B	19. B	20. C
21. D	22. B	23. D	24. A	25. B
26. A	27. D	28. B	29. C	30. D
31. C	32. B	33. A	34. C	35. D
36. A				

[L1] COMPLETION:

37. kidneys	38. glomerulus	39. filtrate
40. interlobar veins	41. glomerular hydrostatic	42. antidiuretic hormone
43. composition	44. concentration	45. urethra
46. internal sphincter	47. micturition reflex	48. cerebral cortex
49. integumentary	50. fluid	51. electrolyte
52. osmoreceptors	53. aldosterone	54. acidosis
55. alkalosis	56. incontinence	

[L1] MATCHING:

57. I	58. O	59. E	60. P	61. N
62. F	63. K	64. A	65. B	66. D
67. C	68. H	69. M	70. J	71. L
72. G				

[L1] DRAWING/ILLUSTRATION LABELING:

Figure 19.1 Components of the Urinary System

73. kidney   74. ureter   75. urinary bladder

Figure 19.2 Sectional Anatomy of the Kidney

76. minor calyx	77. renal pelvis	78. ureter	79. renal column
80. renal pyramid	81. renal vein	82. major calyx	83. renal capsule
84. cortex			

Figure 19.3 Structure of a Typical Nephron (including circulation)

85. efferent arteriole	86. glomerulus	87. afferent arteriole
88. proximal convoluted tubule	89. peritubular capillaries	90. distal convoluted tubule
91. collecting duct	92. loop of Henle	93. proximal convoluted tubule
94. peritubular capillaries	95. Bowman's capsule	96. glomerulus
97. distal convoluted tubule	98. loop of Henle	

368 Answer Key

[L2] CONCEPT MAP:

I.
1. decreasing volume of body H₂O
2. increasing H₂O retention at kidneys
3. aldosterone secretion by adrenal cortex

[L2] BODY TREK:

4. proximal	5. glomerulus	6. protein-free	7. descending limb
8. filtrate	9. ascending limb	10. active transport	11. ions
12. distal	13. aldosterone	14. ADH	15. collecting
16. urine	17. ureters	18. urinary bladder	19. urethra

[L2] MULTIPLE CHOICE:

20. D	21. B	22. D	23. D	24. B
25. D	26. C	27. C	28. C	29. B
30. C	31. B	32. A	33. B	34. C
35. B	36. C			

[L2] SHORT ESSAY:

37. (a) regulates plasma concentrations of ions; (b) regulates blood volume and blood pressure; (c) contributes to stabilization of blood pH; (d) conserves valuable nutrients; (e) eliminates organic wastes; (f) assists liver in detoxification and deamination.

38. (a) produces a powerful vasoconstriction of the afferent arteriole, thereby decreasing the glomerular filtration rate and slowing the production of filtrate; (b) stimulation of renin release; (c) direct stimulation of water and sodium ion reabsorption.

39. (a) autoregulation; (b) hormonal regulation; (c) autonomic regulation.

40. (a) ADH - decreased urine volume; (b) renin - causes angiotensin II production; stimulates aldosterone production; (c) aldosterone - increased sodium ion reabsorption; decreased urine concentration and volume; (d) atrial natriuretic peptide (ANP) - inhibits ADH production; results in increased urine production.

41. (a) stimulates water conservation at the kidney, reducing urinary water losses; (b) stimulates the thirst center to promote the drinking of fluids; the combination of decreased water loss and increased water intake gradually restores normal plasma osmolarity.

42. (a) secrete and/or absorb hydrogen ions; (b) control excretion of acids and bases; (c) generate additional buffers when necessary

[L3] CRITICAL THINKING/APPLICATION:

1. The alcohol acts as a diuretic. It inhibits ADH secretion from the posterior pituitary causing the distal convoluted tubule and the collecting duct to be relatively impermeable to water. Inhibiting the osmosis of water from the tubule along with the increased fluid intake results in an increase in urine production, and increased urination becomes necessary.

2. (a) filtration; (b) primary site of nutrient reabsorption; (c) primary site for secretion of subtances into the filtrate; (d) loop of Henle and collecting system interact to regulate the amount of water and the number of sodium and potassium ions lost in the urine.

3. (a) metabolic acidosis; (b) respiratory alkalosis; (c) respiratory acidosis; (d) metabolic alkalosis

Chapter 20

The Reproductive System

[L1] MULTIPLE CHOICE:

1. D	2. B	3. D	4. B	5. C
6. D	7. D	8. A	9. A	10. D
11. B	12. C	13. A	14. C	15. D
16. B	17. C	18. D	19. B	20. C
21. A	22. C	23. A	24. C	25. A

[L1] COMPLETION:

26. fertilization
27. seminiferous tubules
28. testes
29. spermiogenesis
30. ductus deferens
31. fructose
32. ICSH
33. ovaries
34. areola
35. progesterone
36. placenta
37. Graafian
38. ovulation
39. infundibulum
40. implantation
41. cardiovascular
42. menopause
43. climacteric
44. testosterone

[L1] MATCHING:

45. G	46. C	47. F	48. A	49. J
50. O	51. R	52. L	53. P	54. Q
55. M	56. H	57. I	58. N	59. D
60. K	61. E	62. S	63. B	

[L1] DRAWING/ILLUSTRATION LABELING:

Figure 20.1 Male Reproductive Organs

64. prostatic urethra
65. pubic symphysis
66. ductus deferens
67. corpora cavernosa
68. corpus spongiosum
69. penile urethra
70. glans penis
71. prepuce
72. testis
73. epididymis
74. urinary bladder
75. rectum
76. seminal vesicle
77. seminal vesicle
78. ejaculatory duct
79. prostate gland
80. anus
81. anal sphincters
82. bulbourethral gland
83. membranous urethra
84. bulb of penis
85. scrotum

Figure 20.2 The Testis

86. septum (internal wall)
87. epididymis (head)
88. ductus deferens
89. rete testis
90. seminiferous tubule
91. tunica albuginea

Figure 20.3 Female External Genitalia

92. mons pubis
93. clitoris
94. labia minora
95. vaginal orifice
96. vestibule
97. perineum
98. prepuce
99. urethral orifice
100. labia majora
101. hymen

Figure 20.4 Female Reproductive Organs (sagittal section)

102. uterus
103. urinary bladder
104. pubic symphysis
105. urethra
106. clitoris
107. labium minora
108. labium majora
109. cervix
110. vagina
111. anus

Figure 20.5 Female Reproductive Organs (frontal section)

112. infundibulum
113. ovary
114. uterine tube
115. myometrium
116. cervix
117. vagina

[L2] CONCEPT MAPS:

I.

1. ductus deferens
2. penis
3. seminiferous tubules
4. produce testosterone
5. FSH
6. seminal vesicles
7. bulbourethral glands
8. urethra

II.

9. uterine tubes
10. follicles
11. follicle cells
12. endometrium
13. supports fetal development
14. vagina
15. vulva
16. labia majora and minora
17. clitoris
18. nutrients

[L2] MULTIPLE CHOICE:

19. C
20. A
21. C
22. B
23. B
24. D
25. C
26. A
27. D

[L2] COMPLETION:

28. inguinal canals
29. cremaster
30. acrosomal cap
31. prepuce
32. zona pellucida
33. corona radiata
34. corpus luteum
35. fimbriae
36. cervical os
37. menses

[L2] SHORT ESSAY:

38. (a) seminal vesicles, prostate gland, bulbourethral glands; (b) activates the sperm, provides nutrients for sperm motility, provides sperm motility, produces buffers to counteract acid conditions.

39. (a) promotes the functional maturation of spermatozoa; (b) maintains accessory organs of male reproductive tract; (c) responsible for male secondary sexual characteristics; (d) stimulates bone and muscle growth; (e) stimulates sexual behaviors and sexual drive.

40. (a) arousal - parasympathetic activation leads to an engorgement of the erectile tissues of the clitoris and increased secretion of the greater vestibular glands; (b) coitus - rhythmic contact with the clitoris and vaginal walls provides stimulation that eventually leads to orgasm; (c) orgasm - accompanied by peristaltic contractions of vaginal muscles giving rise to pleasurable sensations.

41. Step 1: formation of primary follicles; Step 2: formation of secondary follicle; Step 3: formation of a tertiary follicle; Step 4: ovulation; Step 5: formation and degeneration of the corpus luteum.

42. (a) menses; (b) proliferative phase; (c) secretory phase.

[L3] CRITICAL THINKING/APPLICATION:

1. (a) The normal temperature of the testes in the scrotum is 1 to 2 degrees lower than the internal body temperature—the ideal temperature for developing sperm. Mr. Hurt's infertility is caused by the inability of sperm to tolerate the higher temperature in the abdominopelvic cavity. (b) Three major factors are necessary for fertility in the male: (1) adequate motility of sperm: 30 to 35 % motility necessary; (2) adequate numbers of sperm: 20,000,000/ml minimum; (3) sperm must be morphologically perfect: sperm cannot be malformed.

2. The 19-year-old female has a problem with hormonal imbalance in the body. Females, like males, secrete estrogens and androgens; however, in females, estrogen secretion usually "masks" the amount of androgen secreted in the body. In females an excess of testosterone secretion may cause a number of conditions such as sterility, fat distrubution like a male, beard, low-pitched voice, skeletal muscle enlargement, male skeletal configuration, clitoral enlargement and a diminished breast size.

3. Progesterone inhibits FSH secretion by the pituitary and without FSH, no follicles mature to be ovulated. If a woman becomes pregnant, the corpus luteum, which secretes progesterone, is maintained; otherwise the corpus luteum disintegrates, progesterone levels fall off, and the cycle begins again. This artificially high progesterone level thus "tricks" the brain into believing a pregnancy has occurred. Most contraceptive pills contain large quantities of progesterone and a small quantity of estrogen. Birth control pills are usually taken for 20 days beginning day 5 of a 28-day cycle. The increased level of progesterone and decreased levels of estrogen prepare the uterus for ovum implantation. (And remember, FSH causes follicles to produce estrogen and without FSH there will be less estrogen in circulation.) On day 26 the progesterone level decreases. If taken as directed, the Pill will allow for a normal menstrual cycle.

4. In males the disease-causing organism can move up the urethra to the bladder or into the ejaculatory duct to the ductus deferens. There is no direct connection into the pelvic cavity in the male. In females the pathogen travels from the vagina to the uterus, to the uterine tubes, and into the pelvic cavity where it can infect the peritoneal lining, resulting in peritonitis.

Chapter 21

Development and Inheritance

[L1] MULTIPLE CHOICE:

1. C	2. B	3. D	4. A	5. C
6. B	7. C	8. B	9. D	10. B
11. A	12. A	13. D	14. C	15. D
16. C	17. A	18. A	19. B	20. C
21. A				

[L1] COMPLETION:

22. fertilization
23. capacitation
24. second trimester
25. first trimester
26. chorion
27. human chorionic gonadotropin
28. placenta
29. dilation
30. childhood
31. infancy
32. gametogenesis
33. autosomal
34. homozygous
35. heterozygous

[L1] MATCHING:

36. C	37. J	38. B	39. N	40. H
41. A	42. M	43. F	44. L	45. D
46. I	47. E	48. G	49. K	

[L1] DRAWING/ILLUSTRATION LABELING:

Figure 21.1 Spermatogenesis

50. spermatogonia
51. primary spermatocyte
52. secondary spermatocyte
53. spermatids
54. spermatozoa

Figure 21.2 Oogenesis

55. oogonium
56. primary oocyte
57. secondary oocyte
58. mature ovum

[L2] BODY TREK:

1. secondary oocyte
2. fertilization
3. zygote
4. 2-cell stage
5. 8-cell stage
6. morula
7. early blastocyst
8. implantation

[L2] MULTIPLE CHOICE:

9. B	10. C	11. D	12. C	13. A
14. B	15. B	16. A	17. D	18. C
19. D	20. C	21. D	22. B	

[L2] COMPLETION:

23. inheritance
24. genetics
25. alleles
26. X-linked
27. simple inheritance
28. polygenic inheritance
29. cleavage
30. differentiation

[L2] SHORT ESSAY:

31.
    (a)   (b)
    - yolk sac — endoderm and mesoderm
    - amnion — ectoderm and mesoderm
    - allantois — endoderm and mesoderm
    - chorion — mesoderm and trophoblast

32. (a) the respiratory rate goes up and the tidal volume increases; (b) the maternal blood volume increases; (c) the maternal requirements for nutrients increase; (d) the glomerular filtration rate increases; (e) the uterus increases in size.

33. (a) secretion of relaxin by the placenta - softens symphysis pubis; (b) weight of the fetus - deforms cervical orifice; (c) rising estrogen levels; (d) both b anc c promote release of oxytocin.

34. (a) hypothalamus - increasing production of GnRH; (b) increasing circulatory levels of FSH and LH (ICSH) by the anterior pituitary; (c) FSH and LH initiate gametogenesis and the production of male or female sex hormones that stimulate the appearance of secondary sexual characteristics and behaviors.

35. (a) some cell populations grow smaller throughout life; (b) the ability to replace other cell populations decreases; (c) genetic activity changes over time; (d) mutations occur and accummulate.

[L3] CRITICAL THINKING/APPLICATION:

1. Color blindness is an X-linked trait. The Punnett square shows that sons produced by a normal father and a heterozygous mother will have a 50 % chance of being color blind, while the daughters will all have normal color vision. (X^C = normal allele; X^c = color-blind allele.)

	Maternal alleles	
	X^C	X^c
X^C	$X^C X^C$	$X^C X^c$
Y	$X^C Y$	$X^c Y$ (color blind)

Paternal alleles

2. The Punnett square reveals that 50 % of their offspring have the possiblity of inheriting albinism.

	Maternal alleles	
	a	a
A	Aa	Aa
a	aa (albino)	aa (albino)

Paternal alleles

3. Both the mother and father are heterozygous-dominant.

T = tongue roller; t = non-tongue roller.

The Punnett square reveals that there is a 25 % chance of having children who are not tongue rollers and a 75 % chance of having children with the ability to roll the tongue.

	Maternal alleles	
	T	t
T	TT (yes)	Tt (yes)
t	Tt (yes)	tt (no)

Paternal alleles